Jack,

Thanks so much for your help with the Campaign for Women + Infants!

Cordially,

Bob

Neonatal Intensive Care

CLINICS IN CRITICAL CARE MEDICINE

General Series Editors: *Iain McA Ledingham MD FRCS,* Professor, Department of Surgery, Western Infirmary, Glasgow, UK
Ake Grenvik MD, Professor of Anesthesiology and Surgery, Presbyterian-University Hospital, Pittsburgh, Pennsylvania, USA

Volumes Already Published

Chapman: Acute Renal Failure
Grenvik & Safar: Brain Failure and Resuscitation
Gregory: Respiratory Failure in the Child
Spence: Respiratory Monitoring in Intensive Care
Geelhoed & Chernow: Endocrine Aspects of Acute Illness
Meakins: Surgical Infections
Sprung & Grenvik: Invasive Procedures in Critical Care
Cousins & Phillips: Acute Pain Management
Williams: Liver Failure
Swedlow & Raphaely: Cardiovascular Problems in Pediatric Critical Care
Imre & Moossa: Gastrointestinal Emergencies
Farber: Infection Control in Intensive Care

Forthcoming Volumes in the Series

Fallat & Luce: Cardiopulmonary Critical Care
Shires: Fluids, Electrolytes, and Acid Bases
Henning & Grenvik: Critical Care Cardiology
Kaye & Bircher: Cardiopulmonary Resuscitation: Scientific Basis, Current Standards, and Future Trends

Neonatal Intensive Care

EDITED BY

Robert D. Guthrie, M.D.

Associate Professor
Departments of Pediatrics and
Obstetrics/Gynecology
University of Pittsburgh
School of Medicine
Chief, Department of Pediatrics
Director, Division of Neonatology
Magee-Womens Hospital
Pittsburgh, Pennsylvania

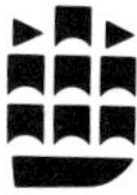

CHURCHILL LIVINGSTONE
NEW YORK, EDINBURGH, LONDON, MELBOURNE 1988

Library of Congress Cataloging in Publication Data

Neonatal intensive care.

(Clinics in critical care medicine ; 13)
Includes bibliographies and index.
1. Neonatal intensive care. I. Guthrie, Robert D., date. II. Series. [DNLM: 1. Critical Care— in infancy & childhood. 2. Infant, Newborn, Diseases. 3. Infant, Premature, Diseases. W1 CL831AI v.13 / WS 420 N4379]
RJ253.5.N46 1987 618.92'01 87-23833
ISBN 0-443-08528-5

Distributed in the United Kingdom by Churchill Livingstone, Robert Stevenson House, 1–3 Baxter's Place, Leith Walk, Edinburgh EH1 3AF, and by associated companies, branches, and representatives throughout the world.

Accurate indications, adverse reactions, and dosage schedules for drugs are provided in this book, but it is possible that they may change. The reader is urged to review the package information data of the manufacturers of the medications mentioned.

Acquisitions Editor: *Linda Panzarella*
Copy Editor: *Ann Ruzycka*
Production Designer: *Jill Little*
Production Supervisor: *Jocelyn Eckstein*

Printed in the United States of America

First published in 1988

Preface

Research advances in the care of high-risk neonates continue at a rapid pace. As the results from these basic and clinical research studies are applied in the clinical arena, neonatal mortality rates in Europe and the United States have shown a progressive decline over the last decade and are now approaching a plateau.

Concomitant with these improvements in survival of high-risk neonates has evolved an increasing emphasis on prevention or amelioration of the short- and long-term complications associated with neonatal intensive care. As many as 20 to 25 percent of high-risk neonates will suffer long-term developmental sequelae, including visual or hearing loss, cerebral palsy, or mild-to-profound developmental retardation. Of infants weighing less than 1500 grams at birth, as many as 50 percent might require special education when they reach school age because of delays in speech and language development, global and specific intellectual deficits, or behavior problems. Clearly, amelioration of the long-term outcome of these high-risk infants must be a clinical and research priority for the next decade.

The purpose of this volume is twofold. First, we hope to provide the reader a concise review of the recent surge in clinical advances in neonatology. It is the intent of this review to move new knowledge from clinical and basic research laboratories into the clinical arena as rapidly as possible. Second, by reviewing our basic scientific understanding of the pathophysiology of many important clinical problems, we propose to shine a light on areas in which there are gaps in our knowledge. A more lucid understanding of the unknown areas in pathophysiologic processes will stimulate future research focused on these problems and will stimulate continued improvements in the outcome of high-risk infants.

To accomplish this purpose, outstanding researchers and clinicians have contributed chapters in their areas of expertise and have reviewed the latest information on pathogenesis, diagnosis, and management of major clinical problems in the high-risk infant.

I wish to acknowledge the tolerance of the chapter authors in agreeing to suggested revisions and clarifications in the interest of making this volume as lucid as possible. I also acknowledge the dedicated support and talent of my administrative assistant, Marge Guzik, in making this volume organized and readable.

Robert D. Guthrie, M.D.

Contributors

Forrest C. Bennett, M.D.

Associate Professor, Department of Pediatrics, and Director, High Risk Infant Follow-Up Program, Child Development and Mental Retardation Center, University of Washington School of Medicine, Seattle, Washington

Beverly S. Brozanski, M.D.

Assistant Professor, Departments of Pediatrics and Obstetrics/Gynecology, University of Pittsburgh School of Medicine; Attending Neonatologist, Department of Pediatrics, Division of Neonatology, Magee-Womens Hospital, Pittsburgh, Pennsylvania

Britton Chance, Ph.D.

Professor Emeritus, Department of Biochemistry and Biophysics, University of Pennsylvania School of Medicine, Philadelphia, Pennsylvania

Robert D. Christensen, M.D.

Associate Professor, Department of Pediatrics, and Co-Director, Division of Developmental Biology and Aging, University of Utah School of Medicine, Salt Lake City, Utah

Ronald David, M.D.

Assistant Professor, Departments of Pediatrics and Obstetrics/Gynecology, University of Pittsburgh School of Medicine; Attending Neonatologist, Department of Pediatrics, Division of Neonatology, Magee-Womens Hospital, Pittsburgh, Pennsylvania

Maria Delivoria-Papadopoulos, M.D.

Professor, Departments of Pediatrics and Physiology, University of Pennsylvania School of Medicine, Philadelphia, Pennsylvania

William W. Fox, M.D.

Professor, Department of Pediatrics, University of Pennsylvania School of Medicine; Department of Pediatrics, Division of Neonatology, The Children's Hospital of Philadelphia, Philadelphia, Pennsylvania

Robert D. Guthrie, M.D.

Associate Professor, Departments of Pediatrics and Obstetrics/Gynecology, University of Pittsburgh School of Medicine; Chief, Department of Pediatrics, and Director, Division of Neonatology, Magee-Womens Hospital, Pittsburgh, Pennsylvania

Harry R. Hill, M.D.

Professor, Departments of Pediatrics and Pathology, and Head, Division of Clinical Immunology and Allergy, University of Utah School of Medicine, Salt Lake City, Utah

M. Douglas Jones, Jr., M.D.

Associate Professor, Departments of Pediatrics and Anesthesiology and Critical Care Medicine, and Assistant Professor, Department of Obstetrics-Gynecology, The Johns Hopkins Medical Institutions, Baltimore, Maryland

Kenneth W. Klesh, M.D.

Assistant Professor, Departments of Pediatrics and Obstetrics/Gynecology, University of Pittsburgh School of Medicine; Attending Neonatologist, Department of Pediatrics, Division of Neonatology, Magee-Womens Hospital, Pittsburgh, Pennsylvania

Raymond C. Koehler, Ph.D.

Associate Professor, Department of Anesthesiology and Critical Care Medicine, and Assistant Professor, Department of Environmental Health Sciences, The Johns Hopkins Medical Institutions, Baltimore, Maryland

Walker A. Long, M.D.

Research Assistant Professor, Department of Pediatrics, Division of Cardiology, University of North Carolina at Chapel Hill, Chapel Hill, North Carolina; Senior Clinical Research Scientist, Clinical Research Division, Wellcome Research Laboratories, Burroughs Wellcome Co., Research Triangle Park, North Carolina

Trevor A. Macpherson, M.B., Ch.B., M.R.C.O.G.

Associate Professor, Department of Pathology, University of Pittsburgh School of Medicine; Director of Laboratories, Department of Pathology, Magee-Womens Hospital, Pittsburgh, Pennsylvania

Michael J. Painter, M.D.

Associate Professor, Departments of Pediatrics and Neurology, University of Pittsburgh School of Medicine; Chief of Child Neurology, Children's Hospital of Pittsburgh, Pittsburgh, Pennsylvania

Robert H. Perelman, M.D.

Associate Professor, Department of Pediatrics, University of Wisconsin School of Medicine; South Central Wisconsin Perinatal Center, Madison General Hospital, Madison, Wisconsin

Henry J. Rozycki, M.D.

Instructor, Department of Pediatrics, University of Pennsylvania School of Medicine; Division of Neonatology, The Children's Hospital of Philadelphia, Philadelphia, Pennsylvania

Ronald L. Sanders, Ph.D.

Adjunct Assistant Professor, Department of Radiology, Duke University, Durham, North Carolina; Clinical Research Scientist, Clinical Research Division, Wellcome Research Laboratories, Burroughs Wellcome Co., Research Triangle Park, North Carolina

Mark S. Scher, M.D.

Assistant Professor, Departments of Pediatrics, Neurology, and Psychiatry, University of Pittsburgh School of Medicine; Director, Neonatal EEG and Clinical Neurophysiology Laboratories, Department of Pediatrics, Division of Neonatology, Magee-Womens Hospital, Pittsburgh, Pennsylvania

Susan Shen-Schwarz, M.B., B.S.

Associate Professor, Department of Pathology, University of Pittsburgh School of Medicine; Director of Perinatal Pathology, Magee-Womens Hospital, Pittsburgh, Pennsylvania

Alan R. Spitzer, M.D.

Associate Professor, Departments of Pediatrics and Obstetrics and Gynecology, University of Pennsylvania School of Medicine; Division of Neonatology, The Children's Hospital of Philadelphia, Philadelphia, Pennsylvania

Richard J. Traystman, Ph.D.

Professor, Departments of Anesthesiology and Critical Care Medicine and Environmental Health Sciences, The Johns Hopkins Medical Institutions, Baltimore, Maryland

Marie Valdes-Dapena, M.D.

Professor and Director of Education, Department of Pathology, and Professor, Department of Pediatrics, University of Miami School of Medicine, Miami, Florida

Contents

1
Neonatal Resuscitation: Historical Perspective and Current Practice

Ronald David

HISTORICAL PERSPECTIVE

The earliest texts on midwifery and obstetrics and gynecology are graphic and poetic in their descriptions of the clinical presentations and management of the asphyxiated newborn. These treatises are replete with anecdotes that leave little doubt in the reader's mind that the authors were indeed writing about the condition asphyxia neonatorum as we know it today. In retrospect, there is equally little doubt that the prescriptions for revivification were as irrational as they were odious.

We've come a long way since the resuscitation kits equipped with "an elaborate fumigator with a bowl which held one and one-half ounces of tobacco and the necessary tubes and bellows for inflating the rectum."[1] Still, delivery-room management of the compromised newborn is more an art than a science. A few practices have withstood the test of time and scientific validation in the twentieth century. Other fads have fortunately faded with time. In this chapter, the historic and scientific foundations of current practices will be reviewed, persisting myths will be debunked, and unresolved controversies will be highlighted. With this approach, I hope to stimulate the reader and potential rescuer to think prospectively about resuscitation strategies currently used or evolving. It is hoped that a future backward glance at modern day resuscitation will not be with consternation.

PATHOPHYSIOLOGY

Early views of the pathophysiology of asphyxia were simplistic. The asphyxiated newborn was either likened to a nearly drowned adult,[1] or its condition held to be the consequence of anemia (asphyxia pallida) or congestion (asphyxia livida).[2] The respective remedies for these conditions were vigorous afferent stimulation, delay in umbilical cord clamping, and blood letting via the cut cord or placing leeches behind the ears. In 1928, Yandell Henderson[3] decried these practices as reprehensible and unphysiologic. He was equally emphatic in his declaration that respiratory depression occurred for want of carbon dioxide as the essential chemical stimulus to drive the respiratory center. He aggressively championed the use of gas mixtures containing 5 percent or more carbon dioxide as "not only the phys-

Table 1.1. Potential Systemic Effects of Hypoxia-Ischemia

Cardiopulmonary
Myocardial necrosis
Systemic and/or pulmonary hypertension
Pulmonary edema
Increased surfactant catabolism
Gastrointestinal
Small and large bowel ischemia
Hematologic
Thrombocytopenia w/wo coagulopathy
Hepatic
Centrolobular necrosis
Metabolic
Lactic acidemia
Hypercapnea
Hypoglycemia
Renal
Tubular and medullary necrosis

iologic and therefore best method; in its essential features it is really the only possible method that nature and science have to offer."

Twenty years later, Little and Tovel[4] wrote a comprehensive and up-to-date review of the definition, etiology, pathophysiology, and rationale for therapies in asphyxia neonatorum. They were considerably less declarative in their understanding of the pathophysiology of this condition. Despite their admitted ignorance, their summary recommendations still pertain today (vide infra).

Asphyxia literally means without pulse. However, asphyxia neonatorum has come generically to mean hypoxemia with or without hypercapnia in the fetus or newly born infant. It occurs as a consequence of failed gas exchange across the placenta or lungs, for any of a variety of reasons. Data from animals thus far studied reveal a characteristic redistribution of fetal blood flow—the diving reflex—in response to hypoxemia. Specifically, blood flow to the brain, myocardium, adrenals, and placenta increases with a concomitant reduction of flow to the carcass. These flow changes are most pronounced when acidemia complicates the hypoxic state.[5]

Depending on the severity and duration of the hypoxemia and blood flow changes that may cause ischemia, asphyxia neonatorum may lead to multi-organ-system failure.[6] Potential systemic effects of hypoxia-ischemia are outlined in Table 1-1. The best studied hypoxic-ischemic insult is that sustained by the brain. The spectrum of insults suffered in asphyxia may include dysregulation of cerebral blood flow,[7] intraperiventricular hemorrhage, neuronal necrosis, cerebral infarction, encephalomalacia, and encephalopathy.[8] Disturbances in cerebral blood flow during perinatal asphyxia have been especially well studied in primates. Specifically, there may initially be as much as a threefold increase in cerebral blood flow in the first five minutes of severe asphyxia. With prolongation of the insult there occurs a loss of vascular autoregulation and blood flow falls.[8] Despite this, it is evident that newborn animals tolerate asphyxia better than do adults.[9] This resilience is related, in part, to the newborn's ability to maintain cardiac output and systemic blood pressure for longer periods of hypoxemia. This, in turn, is related to the rich glycogen stores in the developing myocardium.[10]

There remain significant gaps in our knowledge of the pathophysiology of perinatal asphyxia. Clearly, as our understanding improves, so too can recommendations for the support of cardiocirculatory, respiratory, and neurologic integrity during and subsequent to hypoxic-ischemic insults.

MANAGEMENT

"The establishment and maintenance of an airway is the first requirement in resuscitating the asphyxiated newborn. This may be followed by extremely gentle stimulation. Oxygen must then be administered, by a form of artificial respiration, if necessary. . . . Warmth should be maintained throughout the resuscitative period and thereafter. Stimulatory drugs may do more harm than good, and should not be used."[4] With some modification, these 1948 recommendations by Little and Tovel seem most apropos in 1987. In approaching management of the compromised neonate, the priority concerns are (1) assessment, (2) maintenance of warmth and temperature stability, (3) gentle stimulation, (4) establishment of an airway and provision of oxygen therapy, with artificial ventilation if necessary, (5) support of the circulation, and (6) to a limited extent, administration of supportive drugs.

Assessment

Virginia Apgar has provided us the most practical means of assessing the newly born infant. Among other things, her scoring system, developed in 1953, was designed to define the incidence, causes, and outcome of neonatal depression.[11] The score included items of established value in the assessment of anesthetized patients. They were the physiologic functions or variables most obviously affected by anesthetic agents—heart rate, respiratory effort, muscle tone, reflex irritability, and color. This assessment tool is perhaps most useful when interpreted in the context of the perinatal history. For example, if it is known with currently available techniques of fetal monitoring that the fetus has been stable without compromise, and the mother has received a narcotic analgesic just prior to delivery, limited support of a subsequently depressed newborn is likely to be effective. Contrariwise, the infant with a history of prolonged fetal distress is likely to require more aggressive and sustained resuscitation efforts for successful transition to extrauterine life. In other words, the Apgar score provides clinical confirmation of problems anticipated from the perinatal history. In this way the score helps to guide management in the immediate postpartum period. It is important to note that scores on some items in the Apgar assessment, such as tone and reflex irritability, are partially determined by the physiologic maturity of the infant. Therefore, premature infants may receive a low score because of their immaturity, with no evidence of perinatal compromise.

The practical utility of the Apgar scoring system is in the speed and ease of assessment it permits. The infant can be assessed simultaneously with efforts to stimulate it and provide warmth or a neutral thermal environment, or both. Gentle toweling of the infant to dry it should prove adequate as a means to assess reflex irritability. If the infant is unresponsive, and has a history of perinatal compromise and a low (global) Apgar score, then more vigorous attempts at stimulation are ill advised, will probably be ineffective, and serve only to delay initiating appropriate resuscitation measures. Moreover, premature infants are easily bruised with excessive cutaneous stimulation. Such bruising is likely to contribute to an exaggerated hyperbilirubinemia at 48 to 72 hours of age.

Maintenance of Temperature

> They enter the world naked,
> Cold, uncertain of all
> Save that they enter. All about them
> The cold, unfamiliar wind. . .
>
> William Carlos Williams
> "Spring and All," 1951

The need for warmth cannot be overemphasized. In 1792, Hosack noted that for the support of life are necessary "1st heat; 2nd respiration; 3rd a regular circulation of the blood; and 4th a due excitement of the brain and nervous system."[1] An oft-quoted biblical text, describing the resuscitation of a boy by the prophet Elisha, is cited as the first written historical record of mouth-to-mouth resuscitation.[12] However, Talmudic interpretation has it that this was an example of revivification by rewarming from hypothermia.[13] Midwives of the eighteenth and nineteenth century frequently extolled the virtues of swaddling and warmth for "feeble" (premature) infants when no other supports were available. Curiously, in some midwifery texts the recommendations were made to alternately bathe the moribund infant in hot and cold water.[2] This was done to provide vigorous afferent stimulation. As late as 1962, Miller and co-workers[14] investigated the role of hypothermia in the management of asphyxia experimentally induced in a number of infant animal models. They extended their observations in a limited clinical trial with human newborns, and concluded inappropriately that hypothermia could mitigate the effects of asphyxia.

Budin[15] was the first to document the difference in mortality for warm- versus cold-stressed low-birthweight infants. Ample confirmation of this phenomenon has been provided more recently.[16,17] Incubators were developed when this survival advantage was first recognized. Although the same advantage does not accrue to the full-term infant, there can be a significant reduction in morbidity for this group. Most notably, hypoglycemia and slow resolution of hypoxic lactic acidosis are less likely to occur in the warm, asphyxiated, full-term infant.[18]

Establishing an Airway

> We should in this case, first,
> carefully remove any mucous
> that may be in the mouth, fauces,
> or trachea, by wiping them
> carefully as far as we can reach
> with the little finger armed
> with a piece of fine dry rags. . .
>
> W. DeWees
> "Of the Diseases of
> Children," 1826

Freeing the neonatal airway of mucus and liquor amnii has long been a concern in neonatal resuscitation. This led to the practice of hanging infants from their feet and the design of resuscitation cots with the head of the bed inclined downward at a 30- to 45-degree angle to promote gravity drainage. The most complex instrument designed for this purpose was the Bloxsom positive-pressure airlock[19]—a chamber into which an infant was placed and subjected to alternating atmospheric pressure to simulate uterine contractions and "squeeze out" fetal lung fluid.

The roots of this concern are not entirely clear, but are presumably related to the once prevalent view that newborns, emerging from a fluid-filled environment, are at risk for drowning in their own secretions.[1] There are data to suggest that amniotic fluid may increase the catabolism of pulmonary surfactant in vitro.[20] However, there is no evidence that, in vivo, significant quantities of amniotic fluid move beyond the conducting airways to catabolize surfactant. Moreover, resorption of fetal lung fluid occurs primarily across the pulmonary lymphatic and capillary vessels.[21] The volume of fetal lung fluid appearing in the proximal airway is relatively insignificant. In essence, there are no data to support the current practice of vigorous pulmonary toilet for the removal of amniotic or fetal lung fluid from the proximal airway, even in compromised newborns. Indeed, there is evidence to suggest that such efforts may trigger a vagally mediated bradycardia, and that this reflex response is amplified in the already depressed or hypoxic newborn.[22] At best, overzealous efforts to cleanse the neonatal trachea may delay initiation of more meaningful resuscitation efforts.

The removal of potentially obstructing, particulate meconium from the airway is another issue altogether. Here there is a consensus that suctioning the airway with an endotracheal tube prior to artificial ventilation is advisable and probably reduces the morbidity associated with obstructive airway disease, such as pneumothorax and pneumomediastinum. Despite a series of earlier studies advocating aggressive airway cleansing,[23–25] a more recent spate of clinical case reports raises questions about the efficacy of airway suctioning in reducing mortality in the so-called meconium aspiration syndrome.[26,27]

Several lines of evidence converge to raise doubts about the presumed primary role of meconium aspiration, per se, in neonatal mortality. Null et al.[28] were the first to suggest that meconium aspiration syndrome might be a misnomer. They reviewed evidence for the primary role of intrapartum asphyxia in death and morbidity previously attributed to the aspiration of meconium. In a yet unpublished review of cases from our own institution, we were able to reach this same conclusion. Specifically, in an effort to determine the relationship between meconium aspiration and the development of chemical pneumonitis, we reviewed autopsy data for 18 newborn infants with an antemortem diagnosis of meconium aspiration syndrome (MAS). One of us, a perinatal pathologist blind to the purpose of the study, reviewed lung histopathology sections from these infants and a control group of 18 infants matched for gestational age and time of death. The latter infants did not have a history of antepartum or peripartum meconium release. The histopathology sections were graded for the presence and severity of hemorrhage, emphysema, hyaline membranes, inflammatory infiltrates, and aspiration of fetal squames, meconium, or both. Meconium aspiration was not associated with the development of an inflammatory infiltrate or other evidence of chemical pneumonitis up to 55 hours of age. This finding is consistent with data from most animal models of MAS.[29–31] The exception to this finding is reported in a study that did not include a control group of animals and in which the inflammatory

Table 1.2. Mortality Associated with Meconium Aspiration: Perinatal History, Clinical Course

Mean birth weight = 3.1 kg		
Mean gestational age = 38.8 wks		
Mean age at death = 54.9 hrs		
Perinatal history:	Abnormal fetal heart tone (FHT)	10/12
	1 min Apgar ≤5	13/20
	5 min Apgar ≤7	13/20
	Direct laryngoscopy	8/20
Clinical course:	Postmature/intrauterine growth retardation (IUGR)	7/20
	"Clinical" persistent fetal circulation (PFC)	6/20
	Abnormal chest x-ray (CXR)	13/20

response noted might well have been due to mechanical ventilator support or oxygen therapy.[32]

Murphy et al.[33] have documented abnormal muscularization of the pulmonary arterioles in infants dying with MAS. They concluded that this pathologic change was the cause of the syndrome of persistent pulmonary hypertension frequently noted in infants with MAS. Further, the pathology developed in response to chronic hypoxia and was unlikely to be related to acute peripartum events in general or meconium aspiration in particular. A review of the clinical course and gross and histopathology of the infants in our own study is summarized in Tables 1-2, 1-3, and 1-4. On the basis of these data, we would concur with Murphy and coworkers that hypoxia, acute or chronic, accounts for the major clinical pathology seen in infants dying from MAS. The pathophysiologic events often seen in association with the release and aspiration of meconium are related as diagrammed in Figure 1-1.

In summary, pulmonary toilet during neonatal resuscitation should be limited to the removal of potentially obstructing particulate meconium with an endotracheal tube. All other efforts serve no definable purpose, and may delay the start

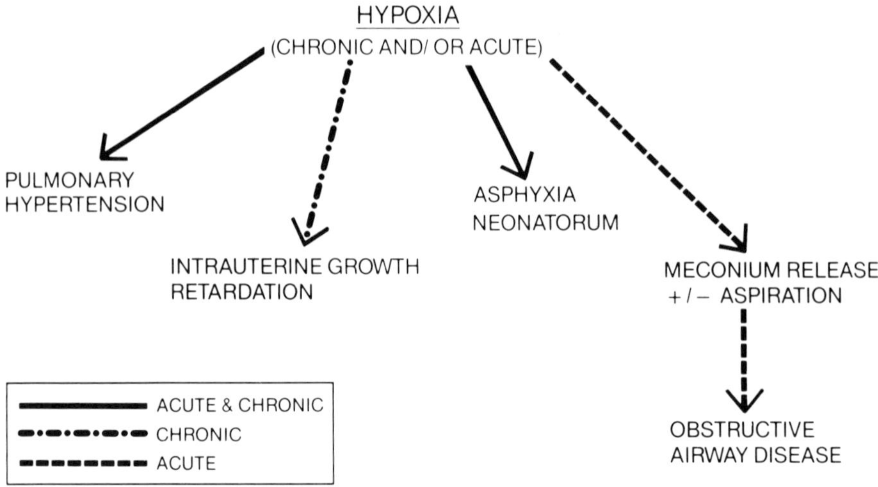

Fig. 1-1. Meconium aspiration syndrome: Suggested scheme of pathophysiologic events.

Table 1.3. Mortality Associated with Meconium Aspiration: Pathology

Hypoxic-ischemic encephalopathy	7/18
Myocardial ischemia	4
Acute tubular necrosis	1
Necrotizing enterocolitis	1
"Pneumonia" (inflammation)	6[a]
Meconium and/or amniotic fluid aspiration	12/18

[a] One each of *Toxoplasma*, *Escherichia coli*, *Klebsiella*, β-Strep; two pneumonia *without* histopathologic evidence of meconium.

of effective support measures. Attention must, then, promptly turn to the management of asphyxia and its sequelae.

Oxygen Therapy and Artificial Ventilation

> It remains a most necessary accomplishment that the obstetrician should be dexterous with laryngoscope and 'Tracheal Pipe'.
>
> E.A. Williams
> Resuscitation of the newborn.
> Guy's Hospital Gazette
> 80:536, 1966

What is purported to be the first written description of mouth-to-mouth resuscitation must now be questioned.[13] Still, this method of artificial respiration has long been noted. Lozes, quoting from the work of the French physician Chaussier, described the resuscitation of a child delivered of a woman reportedly dead for two hours prior to delivery.[34] In this 1743 clinical case report, midwives provided mouth-to-mouth breathing for three and a quarter hours, after which the infant "cried lustily." The use of mouth-to-mouth resuscitation in stillborn infants was supported by the Royal Humane Society in its publications circa 1776. Although known to be efficacious, the practice was discouraged by some authorities.[1]

Table 1.4. Mortality Associated with Meconium Aspiration Syndrome: Histopathology

Meconium aspiration syndrome vs. controls	P Value
Aspiration	
Fetal squames	<.005
Meconium	<.01
Inflammation	
PMN	NS
Mono	NS
Macrophage/giant cells	NS
Emphysema	
Interstitial	NS
Alveolar	NS
Hemorrhage	
Interstitial	NS
Alveolar	NS
Edema	NS

Recommendations for the regular use of "tracheal pipes" for the support of respiration in the newborn began to appear early in the nineteenth century. Here again Chaussier figures prominently in the annals of newborn resuscitation, as he described his experiences with the intubation of apparently asphyxiated infants.[34] In 1816, Haighton further supported the use of the tracheal pipe, but advised the rescuer to consider first mouth-to-mouth breathing or pressing the sternum and ribs toward the spine.[34] Gairal's "Pulmonaire Aerophore" is thought to be the first device designed specifically for the resuscitation and short-term ventilation of the compromised newborn.[35] Pharyngoscopes to facilitate the insertion of these instruments were developed early in the twentieth century.[36]

The best efforts to study the physiology of pulmonary inflation and ventilation in the spontaneously breathing newborn appear in the literature in the late 1950s. Studies of the mechanics of ventilation during the resuscitation of newborn infants followed.[37] Vyas et al. reported a series of clinical studies that serve as the background for current recommendations in providing positive-pressure breathing in infants who have not breathed spontaneously from birth.[38,39] To achieve the best tidal volume and functional residual capacity, with the least opening pressure, a prolonged or slow-rise inflation pressure is applied (Fig. 1-2). Further, Vyas et al. note that artificial ventilation with a bag and mask is less efficient than with endotracheal intubation.[40] However, most compromised newborns will respond to the simplest measure, bag-and-mask ventilation, with a characteristic "rejection" response (Head's paradoxic reflex) followed by inspiratory gasps. These spontaneous respiratory efforts are associated with greater and more rapidly developed lung volumes. The slow rise or prolonged inflation technique should apply whether one is using mouth-to-mouth, bag-and-mask, or bag-and-endotracheal tube ventilation.

Two disadvantages accrue to the use of mouth-to-mouth breathing. First, the airway pressures delivered are more difficult to gauge, thereby increasing the risk of barotrauma, such as pneumothorax and pneumomediastinum. Second, there is the small but real risk to the rescuer of contracting communicable diseases such as hepatitis, cytomegalovirus infection, and other viral illnesses. However, it is worth noting that resuscitation equipment occasionally fails. In these circumstances, it is perfectly appropriate to use mouth-to-mouth or mouth-to-tube ventilation with supplemental oxygen flowing directly into the rescuer's mouth. On more than one occasion I have witnessed utter chaos in the resuscitation of a child when the ventilation bag has failed. Would-be rescuers continue to provide closed-chest cardiac massage with no ventilatory support while someone runs off in search of functional equipment!

Support of the Circulation

> The heart is the ultimum moriens, and I do not believe efforts to restore its pulsations, when once completely extinguished, have ever been found with success.
>
> P. Cazeaux
> "A Theoretical and Practical Treatise on Midwifery," 1866

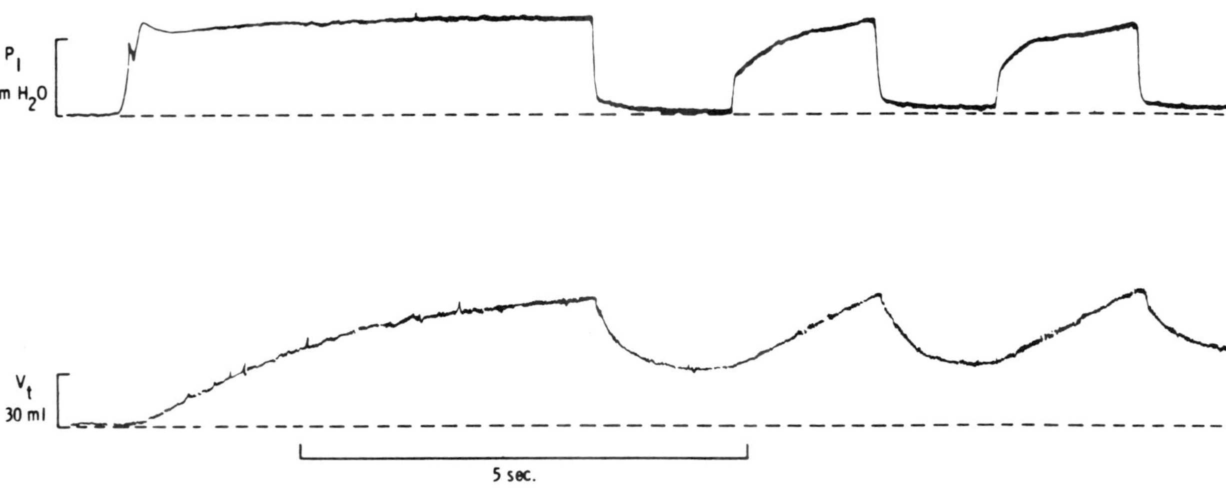

Fig. 1-2. Longitudinal trace of pressure and volume showing prolonged square-wave inflation with formation of a functional residual capacity. (Vyas H, Milner AD, Hopkin IE, Boon AW: Physiologic responses to prolonged and slow rise inflation in the resuscitation of the asphyxiated newborn infant. J Pediatr 99:635, 1981.)

The earliest efforts at external chest compression were directed toward providing artificial ventilation.[34] Closed-chest massage to achieve cardiac output is a relatively new therapy. Serendipitously, while engaged in studies on resuscitating the fibrillating heart, Kouwenhoven and co-workers[41] noted that a rise in blood pressure could be effected when defibrillator paddles were pressed to the chest walls of their experimental animals. Additional studies were undertaken to assess the effect of rhythmic pressure on the lower third of the sternum on blood circulation. The technique was first applied to a human patient by Dr. Henry Bahnson of the University of Pittsburgh School of Medicine when he resuscitated a child whose heart was in ventricular fibrillation. Although Bahnson used the heel of his hand to apply sternal pressure in that seminal effort, his Chief-of-Service, Dr. Alfred Blalock, advised the use of the middle and index fingers in smaller children. The technique was not tested for efficacy in achieving adequate cardiac output (personal communication, H. Bahnson, M.D., 6 June 1986). A series of clinical case reports then appeared in the literature describing the utility of closed-chest massage in apparently stillborn infants.[42,43]

Thaler and Stobie[44] were the first to question the safety and efficacy of sternal depression with two fingers in the resuscitation of newborn infants. As a result of their studies on infant cadavers, they recommended that rescuers encircle the infant's chest with both hands while the thumbs were apposed at mid-sternum. Todres and Rogers[45] again demonstrated the superiority of this technique in producing sustained elevations in blood pressure. David[46] described two additional case reports documenting the superiority of the Thaler-Stobie maneuver in improving aortic blood flow as assessed by mean arterial pressure and the area under the arterial pressure trace curve. Encircling the chest and depressing the sternum by approximately one-half to one inch at a rate of 80 to 100 times per minute with a compression ratio of about 50 percent achieves apparently adequate cardiac output. This approach is more effective than the traditional two-finger technique (Fig. 1-3).

Echoing the admonition of Moya et al.,[43] it cannot be overemphasized that "Maintaining the circulation without adequate oxygenation is futile; however, ventilation of the lungs alone in many infants with no audible heartbeat has resulted in recovery."

Supportive Drugs

Drug therapy in neonatal resuscitation may be fraught with hazard. Few drugs have actually been tested for safety and efficacy. Most have been tried empirically. Medicaments employed for the "due excitement of the central nervous system" have included tobacco-smoke insufflation via the rectum, brandy douches spat from the mouth of the rescuer upon the infant's chest, and spirits of sal ammoniac wafted into the nostrils of the (already) moribund infant. What follows is a review of the potential uses, hazards, and routes of administration of the drugs most commonly used in neonatal resuscitation today.

Atropine

The bradycardia noted in asphyxia neonatorum is largely vagally mediated. Reportedly, atropine can reverse vagal cardiac slowing.[47] However, it is not clear that

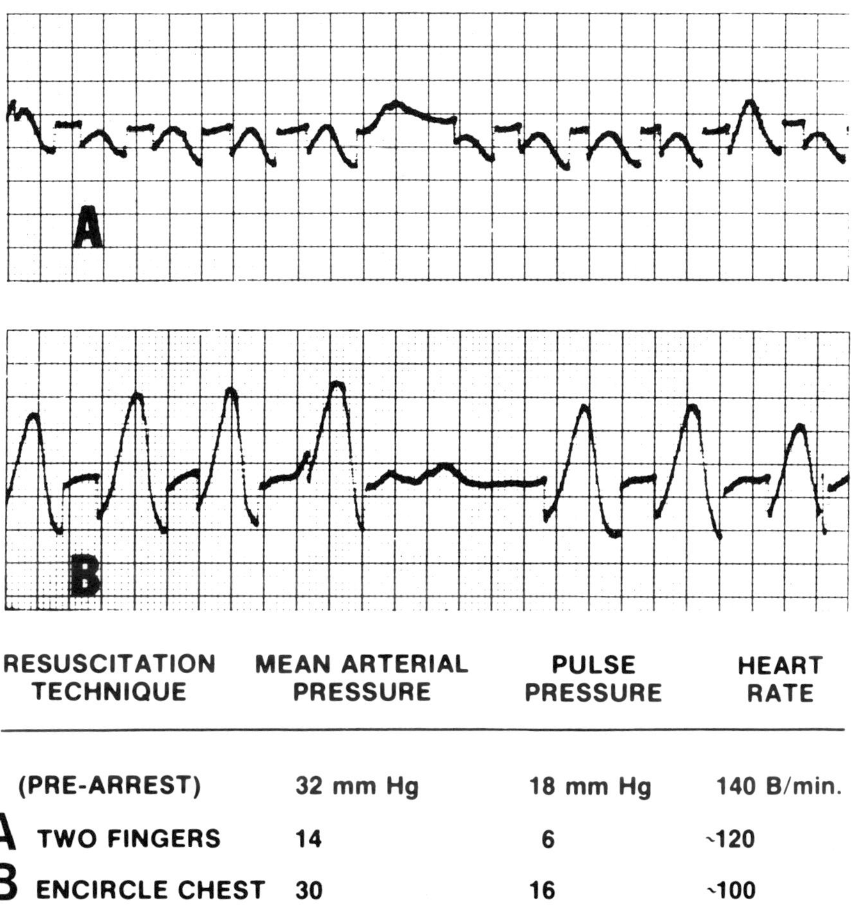

RESUSCITATION TECHNIQUE	MEAN ARTERIAL PRESSURE	PULSE PRESSURE	HEART RATE
(PRE-ARREST)	32 mm Hg	18 mm Hg	140 B/min.
A TWO FINGERS	14	6	~120
B ENCIRCLE CHEST	30	16	~100

Fig. 1-3. Hemodynamic changes associated with different CPR techniques, Case 1: (**A**) Two-finger sternal depression. (**B**) Encircling the chest.

this reversal has been demonstrated when hypoxia is the trigger event for the bradycardia. Moreover, atropine can cause dysrhythmias and, in vitro, block the constricting effect of oxygen on the ductus arteriosus.[48] It is also noteworthy that the return of a normal heart rate is often the only clinical tool available to assess the effectiveness of cardiopulmonary resuscitation. When resuscitation efforts are suboptimal, bradycardia recurs. If atropine is effective in abolishing this response, it is possible that the use of this drug may mask an immediately available clinical sign of inadequate cardiorespiratory support. The use of atropine in neonatal resuscitation requires further study.

Calcium

Newborn infants suffering asphyxial insults characteristically develop a greater degree of hypocalcemia than do their gestational-age-matched, uncompromised cohorts.[49] Calcium, administered as calcium gluconate or calcium chloride, is a cardiotonic drug that increases blood pressure and improves cardiac contractility in healthy preterm infants.[50,51] These observations provide the rationale for recommendations to administer calcium intravenously during and subsequent to cardiorespiratory failure in the newborn. However, the movement of calcium from the extra- to the intracellular compartment during hypoxic-ischemic or other metabolic insults may be the final common pathway for cell death.[52] Clinical support for this experimental finding is suggested in a study by Changaris et al.[53] These investigators reported morphologic evidence of calcium salts within the brains of stressed neonates given parenteral calcium therapy. Further, there have been recent efforts to determine the role of calcium-channel blockers in ameliorating the adverse effects of hypoxia and ischemia on the brain and myocardium.[54] It would seem prudent, therefore, to limit use of calcium in the stressed newborn and consider other cardiotonic agents for the support of blood pressure and cardiac output. Such drugs might include epinephrine and low-dose dopamine.[55] In any event, contrary to recommendations made in a recent textbook on neonatology,[56] this drug should never be administered via the intracardiac route. It has the potential for stimulating an arrhythmia, and can cause tissue necrosis if accidentally injected into the myocardium.

Epinephrine

During hypoxic stress, blood flow is rerouted to vital organs and away from the carcass. This response is amplified in the face of acidemia and is mediated by endogenous catecholamines. In a newborn experimental animal model, epinephrine was shown to significantly improve myocardial and cerebral perfusion during cardiopulmonary resuscitation (CPR).[57] The drug may be administered directly into the heart but, like calcium, can be arrhythmogenic and cause tissue necrosis if injected into the myocardium. The intratracheal route of administration is strongly recommended, since it is safe and effective.[58] The onset of action of epinephrine given in this way is rapid, and may be significantly prolonged as compared to the intravenous route.[47] The recommended dose is 0.1 to 0.2 ml/kg of a 1:10,000 solution. The available evidence suggests that the therapeutic advantages of epinephrine exceed the risks of using this drug in neonatal CPR.

Glucose

A rich supply of intracardiac glycogen stores contributes to the ability of the neonatal myocardium to withstand hypoxic injury. Asphyxiated newborns who have developed myocardial ischemia are typically those who are growth-retarded (postmature with depleted glycogen stores) and prone to postpartum hypoglycemia.[59] Support of myocardial function reduces the risk of central nervous system injury. Further, hypoxia-induced metabolic derangements of the brain are amplified in the presence of hypoglycemia.[60] Therefore, glucose administration may help to protect myocardial function and ameliorate metabolic dysfunction of the central nervous system (CNS). This therapy is not without its potential hazards. Blomstrand et al.[61] present data, from studies on fetal lambs, showing that hyperglycemia reduces the tolerance of the fetal brain to asphyxia. Specifically, during hyperglycemia, asphyxia was associated with the rapid development of acidosis, reduced cerebral oxygen consumption, and deterioration in the neurophysiologic characteristics of the brain. This same concern had been previously raised in adult animal model and human clinical studies.[62] If administered, glucose can be provided as the 10 percent dextrose solution, 5 cc/kg via the intravenous route. Glucose homeostasis should then be carefully monitored for evidence of hyperglycemia or rebound hypoglycemia.

Naloxone

Newborn infants may be depressed by narcotics administered to the mother in the peripartum period. While the use of a narcotic antagonist such as naloxone hydrochloride seems justified or reasonable in this circumstance, there are limited data to document the efficacy of this therapy in reversing profound central nervous system and respiratory depression in newborns. Moreover, there are data to indicate that naloxone may adversely affect the fetus' and newborn's response to the stress of hypoxemia. LaGamma and co-workers[63] noted an exaggerated bradycardia and reduction in biventricular cardiac output and placental blood flow in fetal sheep exposed to naloxone in the face of hypoxemia. Young and co-workers[64] found that naloxone exacerbates the hypoxic-ischemic brain injury in neonatal rat pups. It appears that endogenous opioids may be important in regulating circulation during hypoxia. Recommendations made by the Committee on Drugs of the American Academy of Pediatrics are worth reiterating. Because CNS and respiratory depression may be caused by factors other than the administration of narcotics to the mother, "it is imperative that customary resuscitation efforts be immediately initiated when signs of neonatal depression are present, to insure adequate oxygenation."[65]

Sodium bicarbonate

Acidemia may reduce cardiac output and ventricular contractility.[66] However, the role of bicarbonate therapy in correcting acidemia, particularly hypoxic lactic acidemia, is controversial.[67] In one study of the use of liberal versus restricted use of sodium bicarbonate in the treatment of acidemia in high-risk premature infants, the investigators concluded that the correction of acidemia was not more rapid and that mortality was not decreased in the aggressively treated group.[68] Indeed, there was a somewhat increased risk of death in the treated group of infants. In addition, there are data to indicate a detrimental effect of bicarbonate therapy in lactic acidosis.[69] Specifically, Graf and co-workers noted exacerbations in blood lactate concentrations and decreases in cardiac output and blood pressure in a canine animal model of hypoxic lactic acidosis. The potential relationship between bicarbonate administration and neonatal intraventricular hemorrhage remains unresolved.

Volume repletion

In describing the congestive form of apoplexy (asphyxia livida) in the newborn, Cazeaux[2] recommended cutting the umbilical cord and allowing a few spoonfuls of blood to escape as treatment. He notes "however, in practice, which sometimes finds the circulation so infeebled or benumbed, as it were, that the blood will not run from the umbilical arteries; its effusion may then be encouraged by plunging the child into a warm bath, or by squeezing the cord several times from the insertion toward the cut extremity; and when this does not prove successful in obtaining blood, some advise the application of a leech behind each ear." The use of blood-

Table 1.5. Neonatal Conditions Associated with Inadequate Circulating Blood Volume

Type of Shock	Mechanism of Cardiocirculatory Failure	Examples
Hemorrhagic		
RBCs and plasma	Loss of oxygen carrying capacity and plasma volume	Vasa previa, abruption, twin-twin transfusion
RBCs alone	Loss of oxygen carrying capacity	Rh-isoimmunization
Plasma alone	Decreased plasma volume	Meconium peritonitis, omphalocele, or ruptured gastroschisis
Cardiogenic		
Cardiomyopathy	Mechanical pump failure	Myocardial ischemia
Pulmonary	Decreased venous return to right heart	Tension pneumothorax
Septic	Loss of peripheral vasomotor tone and/or pump failure	β-hemolytic streptococcal septicemia

letting was undoubtedly tied to the observation that loss of blood resulted in tachycardia.[1] In contrast, for asphyxia pallida, Grandin[70] recommended the "injection into the rectum of a pint of hot (115°F) saline (2 percent) solution."

Designing rational fluid therapy for the compromised newborn infant can be complicated, and requires some appreciation of the potential cause(s) of volume depletion, the infant's physiologic responses and capacities for coping with such losses, and the hazards and advantages of the available fluid therapies.

Some of the conditions that may be associated with inadequacy of the circulating blood volume are outlined in Table 1-5. Of the conditions listed, only hemorrhagic shock has been systematically studied in the newborn animal model.[71–74] In these studies, experimentally induced hemorrhage caused a relative or absolute decrease in mean arterial and central venous blood pressures. The heart rate may increase or decrease from the resting, pre-hemorrhage level. It appears that some of the homeostatic mechanisms for restoring an adequate blood volume are functional in the newborn. Further, plasma volume restoration may occur faster than it does in the mature animal.[74]

Peripartum blood loss may be the most common cause of shock in the newborn infant. Still, volume repletion with type-specific or O-negative packed red blood cells must be carried out aggressively but cautiously. The neonate's cardiovascular response to volume overloading is limited and characterized by decreased left ventricular compliance and a paradoxical increase in peripheral vascular resistance.[75] This combination of decreased inotropy and increased afterload reduces the myocardium's ability to increase stroke volume and stroke work. In addition, hypoxic-ischemic myocardial dysfunction may be more common in the human newborn than is clinically recognized.[76,77] If there is clinical, electro-, or echocardiographic evidence of pump failure, pharmacologic support of the cardiac output should be considered.

Recommendations for repletion of plasma volume are not clear-cut. The controversy surrounding the merits of crystalloids versus colloids remains unresolved.[78–81] There appears to be no advantage of albumin-containing solutions over balanced-salt solutions such as Ringer's lactate or normal saline. In particular, there is no justification for the use of fresh-frozen plasma as a volume expander.[82] Infusing albumin in infants with respiratory distress due to surfactant deficiency may lead to impaired oxygen exchange.[83] Albumin containing blood products may increase the risk of contracting infectious illnesses such as hepatitis, infection cytomegalovirus, and acquired immunodeficiency syndrome (AIDS). With these disadvantages, and no clear advantages, I recommend the use of Ringer's lactate as a plasma volume expander in newborn infants. If the infant's liver is healthy, and adequate oxygen made available, the lactate should be metabolized, mole for mole, to bicarbonate. Restoration of plasma proteins may occur spontaneously and within 24 hours of the onset of clinical shock.[71]

Laptook and co-workers[84] studied the effects of different rates of plasmanate infusions on brain blood flow after asphyxia and hypotension in newborn piglets. They observed that both rapid and slow infusion of plasmanate (15 ml/kg over 3 or 30 minutes, respectively) was associated with adequate improvement in brain blood flow. In addition, there were no significant differences in hematocrit, arterial blood gases, and pH between the fast and slow infusion groups. Again, it seems appropriate to recommend that fluid therapy in resuscitation be carried out aggressively but prudently.

OUTCOME

> The softness and flaccidity of the tissues, and coldness of the body and face, are no reason for abandoning the child, provided that the heart still beats, however feebly, slowly or irregularly.
>
> P. Cazeaux
> "A Theoretical and Practical Treatise on Midwifery," 1866

Mortality rates following cardiopulmonary resuscitation in the general pediatric population are significant—fewer than 20 percent of children requiring CPR survive.[85] Judging from limited data, it appears that survival rates for newborns requiring CPR while in neonatal intensive care (exclusive of those resuscitated in the delivery suite) are equally discouraging.[86] However, recovery from perinatal cardiac arrest is significantly greater. Steiner and Neligan[87] and Scott[88] reported on the quality of survival for infants requiring CPR in the peripartum period. The data from these two studies are outlined in Table 1-6. In summary, newborn infants requiring positive-pressure ventilation and closed-chest cardiac massage immediately postpartum have a survival rate of 52 percent. Seventy-eight percent of the

Table 1.6. Quality of Survival for Infants Needing Peripartum CPR

Author	No. Severely Asphyxiated[a]	No. Died	No. Abnormal	No. Normal
Scott	48	25	6	17
Steiner	39	17	4	18
Total	87	42	10[b]	35

[a] Required positive-pressure breathing and closed-chest massage.
[b] Failure to establish spontaneous respiration before 30 minutes a useful predictor in 40 percent of this group.

survivors in the two studies were neurologically intact at 3 to 7 years of follow-up. In these studies, failure to establish spontaneous respirations before 30 minutes of age was a useful predictor of poor outcome for 40 percent of the handicapped survivors. In a case control study, Thomson and co-workers[89] reported on an additional 31 children surviving severe perinatal asphyxia. At 5 to 10 years of follow-up, 93 percent of asphyxiated infants were free of serious neurologic or mental handicap. External cardiac massage was used on only 2 of the 31 infants reported in the study. All infants had a 5-minute Apgar score of less than 4, and required positive-pressure breathing.

It is equally important to note that of infants who may initially be resuscitated but ultimately succumb, 65 percent to 95 percent die within the first week of life. Fewer than 5 percent of infants in whom death appears inevitable are alive at 2 years of age.

The prognosis for intact survival in infants requiring aggressive CPR in the perinatal period is good. It does not appear that such management is necessarily associated with prolonged stays in the neonatal intensive care unit (NICU) that end only with the death of the child, the wasteful spending of health-care dollars, or both.

FUTURE DIRECTIONS

Normal or near-normal neurologic recovery following resuscitation is the outcome toward which we ultimately strive. Indeed, we have entered an era of intense study of what is referred to as neuroresuscitation.[90,91] Advances in this arena have been possible because of increasing knowledge of the pathophysiology of hypoxic-ischemic injury to the mature and developing CNS.[92] The focus of research efforts in suitable animal models has been to safely reduce cerebral metabolism, eliminate potentially hazardous metabolic waste products, maintain brain blood flow following ischemia, and prevent cerebral edema formation. Drug therapy trials with high-dose barbiturates[93] and calcium channel blockers[94] have received the greatest attention in this regard. Goldberg and co-workers,[95] in a randomized controlled trial with a small number of subjects, have determined that there is no apparent benefit from barbiturate therapy in severe perinatal asphyxia. Trials involving calcium channel blockers seem to offer the greatest potential. Such therapy would potentially ameliorate the irreversible toxic injury to cells resulting from the intracellular movement of calcium, improve postischemic brain blood flow, and enhance myocardial contractility.[54]

SUMMARY

Cardiopulmonary resuscitation of the newborn is more an art than a science. Further developments in this area will depend on the elucidation of major pathophysiologic events occurring in asphyxia neonatorum. The simplest techniques have been associated with good outcomes, measured both in terms of survival and neurodevelopmental function. Obtaining a history of fetal well-being, assessing the infant at the time of delivery, attending to maintenance of normothermia, establishing and maintaining an airway, providing oxygen with or without positive-pressure ventilation, and effecting adequate cardiac output with minimal use of drugs are all that seem warranted with currently available data.

The history of neonatal resuscitation is replete with therapeutic misadventures. The rationale for the genesis of some therapies has been lost to time. Fortunately, so too has the implementation of those therapies. The efficacy of the management outlined in this review is such that the addition of new therapies can and should await thorough testing in the appropriate animal models. If suggested approaches to managing the compromised newborn have some theoretical basis, however tenuous, then continuing or modifying the approach becomes easier. Years hence, the backward glance at modern-day resuscitation need not be with consternation.

REFERENCES

1. Lee RV: Cardiopulmonary resuscitation in the eighteenth century: A historical perspective on present practice. J Hist Med 27:418, 1972
2. Cazeaux P: A Theoretical and Practical Treatise on Midwifery. p. 513. Linsday and Blakiston, Philadelphia, 1866
3. Henderson Y: The prevention and treatment of asphyxia in the new-born. JAMA 90:583, 1928
4. Little DM, Tovell RM: The physiological basis for the resuscitation of the newborn. Int Abstr Surg 86:417, 1948
5. Cohn HE, Sacks EJ, Heymann MA, et al: Cardiovascular responses to hypoxemia and acidemia in fetal lambs. Am J Obstet Gynecol 120:817, 1974
6. Cassady G: The pathophysiologic picture of the postasphyxiated infant. p. 66. In Peckham GJ, Heymann MA (eds): Cardiovascular Sequelae of Asphyxia in the Newborn. Ross Lab Publishers, Columbus, 1982
7. Lou HC, Lassen NA, Friis-Hansen B: Impaired autoregulation of cerebral blood flow in the distressed newborn infant. J Pediatr 94:118, 1979
8. Volpe JJ: Hypoxic-ischemic encephalopathy: Neuropathology and clinical aspects. p. 180. In Neurology of the Newborn. WB Saunders, Philadelphia, 1981
9. Himwich HE, Alexander FAD, Fazekas JF: Tolerance of the newborn to hypoxia and anoxia. Am J Physiol 133:327, 1941
10. Dawes GS, Mott JC, Shelley HJ: The importance of cardiac glycogen for the maintenance of life in foetal lambs and new-born animals during anoxia. J Physiol 146:516, 1959
11. Apgar V: A proposal for a new method of evaluation of the newborn infant. Curr Res Anesth Analg 32:260, 1953
12. Schechter DC: Role of the humane societies in the history of resuscitation. Surg Gynecol Obstet 129:811, 1969
13. Wislicki L: A biblical case of hypothermia-resuscitation by rewarming (Elisha's method). Clio Med 9:213, 1974
14. Miller JA Jr, Miller FS, Westin B: Hypothermia in the treatment of asphyxia neonatorum. Biol Neonat 6:148, 1964
15. Budin P: "Le Nourrisson." Alimentation et Hygiene des Enfants Debiles—Enfants nes a Terme. Octave Doin, Paris, 1900
16. Silverman WA, Fertig JW, Berger AP: The influence of the thermal environment upon the survival of newly born premature infants. Pediatrics 22:876, 1958
17. Jolly H, Molyneux P, Newell DJ: A controlled study of the effect of temperature on premature babies. J Pediatr 60:889, 1962
18. Perlstein PH: The thermal environment: Temperature and survival. p. 259. In Fanaroff AA, Martin RJ (eds): Neonatal-Perinatal Medicine. CV Mosby Company, St. Louis, 1983
19. Bloxsom A: Resuscitation of the newborn infant: Use of the positive pressure oxygen-air lock. J Pediatr 37:311, 1950
20. Sheldon G, Brazy J, Tuggle B, et al: Fetal lamb lung lavage and its effect on lung phosphatidylcholine. Pediatr Res 13:599, 1979
21. Strang LB: Neonatal Respiration: Physiological and Clinical Studies. Blackwell Scientific Publications, Oxford, 1977
22. Cordero L Jr, Hon EH: Neonatal bradycardia following nasopharyngeal stimulation. J Pediatr 78:441, 1971

23. Gregory GA, Gooding CA, Phibbs RH, Tooley WH: Meconium aspiration in infants—A prospective study. J Pediatr 85:848, 1974
24. Ting P, Brady JP: Tracheal suction in meconium aspiration. Am J Obstet Gynecol 122:767, 1975
25. Carson BS, Losey RW, Bowes WA Jr, Simmons MA: Combined obstetric and pediatric approach to prevent meconium aspiration syndrome. Am J Obstet Gynecol 126:712, 1976
26. Davis RO, Philips JB III, Harris BA Jr, et al: Fatal meconium aspiration syndrome occurring despite airway management considered appropriate. Am J Obstet Gynecol 151:731, 1985
27. Dooley SL, Pesavento DJ, Depp R, et al: Meconium below the vocal cords at delivery: Correlation with intrapartum events. Am J Obstet Gynecol 153:767, 1985
28. Null DM, deLemos RA: Meconium aspiration syndrome; A misnomer. Pediatr Res 14:607, Abstract No. 1090, 1980
29. Goodlin RC: Meconium aspiration. Obstet Gynecol 32:94, 1968
30. Lauweryns J, Bernat R, Lerut A, Detournay G: Intrauterine pneumonia: An experimental study. Biol Neonate 22:301, 1973
31. Frantz ID, Wang NS, Thach BT: Experimental meconium aspiration: Effects of glucocorticoid treatment. J Pediatr 86:438, 1975
32. Tyler DC, Murphy J, Cheney FW: Mechanical and chemical damage to lung tissue caused by meconium aspiration. Pediatrics 62:454, 1978
33. Murphy JD, Vawter GF, Reid LM: Pulmonary vascular disease in fatal meconium aspiration. J Pediatr 104:758, 1984
34. Williams EA: Resuscitation of the newborn. Guy's Hospital Gazette 80:536, 1966
35. Daily WJ, Smith PC: Mechanical ventilation of the newborn infant. I. Curr Probl Pediatr 1:1, 1971
36. Blaikley JB, Gibberd GF: Asphyxia neonatorum: Its treatment by tracheal intubation. Lancet 1:736, 1935
37. Hull D: Lung expansion and ventilation during resuscitation of asphyxiated newborn infants. J Pediatr 75:47, 1969
38. Boon AW, Milner AD, Hopkin IE: Lung expansion, tidal exchange, and formation of the functional residual capacity during resuscitation of asphyxiated neonates. J Pediatr 95:1031, 1979
39. Vyas H, Milner AD, Hopkin IE, Boon AW: Physiologic responses to prolonged and slow-rise inflation in the resuscitation of the asphyxiated newborn infant. J Pediatr 99:635, 1981
40. Milner AD, Vyas H, Hopkin IE: Efficacy of facemask resuscitation at birth. Br Med J 289:1563, 1984
41. Kouwenhoven WB, Langworthy OR: Cardiopulmonary resuscitation: An account of forty-five years of research. Hopkins Med J 132:186, 1973
42. Surks SN, Ladner W: Closed-chest cardiac massage in the stillborn. JAMA 180:142, 1962
43. Moya F, James LS, Burnard ED, Hanks EC: Cardiac massage in the newborn infant through the intact chest. Am J Obstet Gynecol 84:798, 1962
44. Thaler MM, Stobie GH: An improved technic of external cardiac compression in infants and young children. N Engl J Med 269:606, 1963
45. Todres ID, Rogers MC: Methods of external cardiac massage in the newborn infant. J Pediatr 86:781, 1975
46. David R: Technique of cardiopulmonary resuscitation in neonates. Pediatrics (In press)
47. Roberts RJ: Drug Therapy in Infants: Pharmacologic Principles and Clinical Experience. WB Saunders, Philadelphia, 1984
48. Oberhansli-Weiss I, Heymann MA, Rudolph AM, Melmon KL: The pattern and mechanisms of response to oxygen by the ductus arteriosus and umbilical artery. Pediatr Res 6:693, 1972
49. Tsang RC, Chen I, Hayes W, et al: Neonatal hypocalcemia in infants with birth asphyxia. J Pediatr 84:428, 1974
50. Salsburey DJ, Brown DR: Effect of parenteral calcium treatment on blood pressure and heart rate in neonatal hypocalcemia. Pediatrics 69:605, 1982
51. Mirro R, Brown DR: Parenteral calcium treatment shortens the left ventricular systolic time intervals of hypocalcemic neonates. Pediatr Res 18:71, 1984
52. Schanne FAX, Kane AB, Young EE, Farber JL: Calcium dependence of toxic cell death: A final common pathway. Science 206:700, 1979
53. Changaris DG, Purohit DM, Balentinc JD, et al: Brain calcification in severely stressed neonates receiving parenteral calcium. J Pediatr 104:941, 1984
54. Hughes WG, Ruedy JR: Should calcium be used in cardiac arrest? Am J Med 81:285, 1986
55. DiSessa TG, Leitner M, Ti CC, et al: The cardiovascular effects of dopamine in the severely asphyxiated neonate. J Pediatr 99:772, 1981
56. Fanaroff AA, Martin RJ (eds): Behrman's Neonatal-Perinatal Medicine, 3rd Ed. The CV Mosby, St. Louis, 1983

57. Schleien CL, Dean JM, Koehler RC, et al: Effect of epinephrine on cerebral and myocardial perfusion in an infant animal preparation of cardiopulmonary resuscitation. Circulation 73:809, 1986
58. Lindemann R: Resuscitation of the newborn: Endotracheal administration of epinephrine. Acta Paediatr Scand 73:210, 1984
59. Bucciarelli RL, Nelson RM, Egan EA, et al: Transient tricuspid insufficiency of the newborn: A form of myocardial dysfunction in stressed newborns. Pediatrics 59:330, 1977
60. Vannucci RC, Nardis EE, Vannucci SJ: Cerebral metabolism during hypoglycemia and asphyxia in newborn dogs. Biol Neonate 38:276, 1980
61. Blomstrand S, Hrbek A, Karlsson K, et al: Does glucose administration affect the cerebral response to fetal asphxyia? Acta Obstet Gynecol Scand 63:345, 1984
62. Gardiner M, Smith M-L, Kågström E, et al: Influence of blood glucose concentration on brain lactate accumulation during severe hypoxia and subsequent recovery of brain energy metabolism. J Cereb Blood Flow Metab 2:429, 1982
63. LaGamma EF, Itskovitz J, Rudolph AM: Effects of naloxone on fetal circulatory responses to hypoxemia. Am J Obstet Gynecol 143:933, 1982
64. Young RSK, Hessert TR, Pritchard GA, Yagel SK: Naloxone exacerbates hypoxic-ischemic brain injury in the neonatal rat. Am J Obstet Gynecol 150:52, 1984
65. Segal S, Anyan WR, Hill RM, et al (American Academy of Pediatrics Committee on Drugs): Naloxone use in newborns. Pediatrics 65:667, 1980
66. Fisher DJ: Acidaemia reduces cardiac output and left ventricular contractility in conscious lambs. J Dev Physiol 8:23, 1986
67. Hanashiro PK, Wilson JR: Cardiopulmonary resuscitation: A current perspective. Med Clin North Am 70:729, 1986
68. Corbet AJ, Adams JM, Kenny JD, et al: Controlled trial of bicarbonate therapy in high-risk premature newborn infants. J Pediatr 91:771, 1977
69. Graf H, Leach W, Arieff AI: Evidence for a detrimental effect of bicarbonate therapy in hypoxic lactic acidosis. Science 227:754, 1985
70. Grandin EH, Jarman GW: Practical Obstetrics. p. 194. Davis Company, London, 1895
71. LeGal YM: Effects of acute hemorrhage on some physiological parameters of the cardiovascular system in newborn pigs. Biol Neonate 44:210, 1983
72. Rodgers BM, Staroscik, RN, Reis RL: Effects of hemorrhage in fetal and newborn lambs. Surgery 71:51, 1972
73. Rowe MI, Arcilla R: Hemodynamic adaptation of the newborn to hemorrhage. J Pediatr Surg 3:278, 1968
74. Wallgren G, Barr M, Rudhe U: Hemodynamic studies of induced acute hypo- and hypervolemia in the newborn infant. Acta Paediatr (Stockholm) 53:1, 1964
75. Romero TE, Friedman WF: Limited left ventricular response to volume overload in the neonatal period: A comparative study with the adult animal. Pediatr Res 13:910, 1979
76. Setzer E, Ermocilla R, Tonkin I, et al: Papillary muscle necrosis in a neonatal autopsy population: incidence and associated clinical manifestations. J Pediatr 96:289, 1980
77. Cabal LA, Devaskar U, Siassi B, et al: Cardiogenic shock associated with perinatal asphyxia in preterm infants. J Pediatr 96:705, 1980
78. Rice CL: Selection of intravenous fluids for resuscitation. Prog Crit Care Med 2:99, 1985
79. Rackow EC, Falk JL, Fein IA, et al: Fluid resuscitation in circulatory shock: A comparison of the cardiorespiratory effects of albumin, hetastarch and saline solutions in patients with hypovolemic and septic shock. Crit Care Med 11:839, 1983
80. Horton J, Landreneau R, Tuggle D: Cardiac response to fluid resuscitation from hemorrhagic shock. Surg Gynecol Obstet 160:444, 1985
81. Gallagher TJ, Banner MJ, Barnes PA: Large volume crystalloid resuscitation does not increase extravascular lung water. Anesth Analg 64:323, 1985
82. Bove JR: Fresh frozen plasma: Too few indications—too much use. Anesth Analg 64:849, 1985
83. Barr PA, Bailey PE, Sumners J, Cassady G: Relation between arterial blood pressure and blood volume and effect of infused albumin in sick preterm infants. Pediatrics 60:282, 1977
84. Laptook A, Stonestreet BS, Oh W: The effects of different rates of plasmanate infusions upon brain blood flow after asphyxia and hypotension in newborn piglets. J Pediatr 100:791, 1982
85. Torphy DE, Minter MG, Thompson BM: Cardiorespiratory arrest and resuscitation of children. Am J Dis Child 138:1099, 1984
86. Willett LD, Nelson RM Jr: Outcome of cardiopulmonary resuscitation in the neonatal intensive care unit. Crit Care Med 14:773, 1986
87. Steiner H, Neligan G: Perinatal cardiac arrest: Quality of the survivors. Arch Dis Child 50:696, 1975

88. Scott H: Outcome of very severe birth asphyxia. Arch Dis Child 51:712, 1976
89. Thomson AJ, Searle M, Russell G: Quality of survival after severe birth asphyxia. Arch Dis Child 52:620, 1977
90. Hossmann K-A: Post-ischemic resuscitation of the brain: Selective vulnerability versus global resistance. p. 3. In Kogure K, Hossman K-A, Siesjo BK, Welsh FA (eds): Progress in Brain Research. Elsevier Science Publishers, Amsterdam, 1985
91. Svenningsen NW, Blennow G, Lindroth M, et al: Brain-oriented intensive care treatment in severe neonatal asphyxia. Arch Dis Child 57:176, 1982
92. Bass E: Cardiopulmonary arrest: Pathophysiology and neurologic complications. Ann Intern Med 103:920, 1985
93. Brain Resuscitation Clinical Trial I Study Group: Randomized clinical study of thiopental loading in comatose survivors of cardiac arrest. N Engl J Med 314:397, 1986
94. White BC, Winegar CD, Wilson RF, et al: Possible role of calcium blockers in cerebral resuscitation: A review of the literature and synthesis for further studies. Crit Care Med 11:202, 1983
95. Goldberg RN, Moscoso P, Bauer CR, et al: Use of barbiturate therapy in severe perinatal asphyxia: A randomized controlled trial. J Pediatr 109:851, 1986

2

New Treatment Methods in Neonatal Respiratory Distress Syndrome: Replacement of Surface Active Material

Walker A. Long
Ronald L. Sanders

Important new physiologic insights nearly always lead not only to explanations for previously unexplained diseases (or discoveries of new ones), but eventually also to new forms of therapy. The discovery of pulmonary surfactant is a case in point. This chapter considers the prospects for prevention and treatment of neonatal respiratory distress syndrome (NRDS) with surface-active material. First, the history of the discovery and characterization of pulmonary surfactant and the recognition of its role in idiopathic respiratory distress syndrome will be considered briefly. Second, the character and function of natural pulmonary surfactant will be reviewed. Third, the characteristics of an ideal pulmonary surfactant replacement will be considered. Fourth, the Food and Drug Administration's requirements for marketing any new drug will be examined, with special reference to factors influencing study designs in pulmonary surfactant replacement therapy. Fifth, the various surfactant types devised for replacement of surface active material NRDS will be discussed, contrasting each with a putative "ideal" surfactant. Sixth, the results from the initial clinical trials with each surfactant type will be considered. Finally, a brief summary and conclusions will be presented.

HISTORY OF THE DISCOVERY AND CHARACTERIZATION OF PULMONARY SURFACTANT

A comprehensive history of surfactant was elegantly presented by Comroe in 1977.[1–3] In the summary below, the critical references were pointed out by Comroe and, in an unpublished review, by Tooley.

In 1929, von Neergaard made the observation that it was easier to inflate lungs with liquid than with gas,[4] but this fundamental observation in lung physiology was lost until it was independently rediscovered by Gruenwald in 1947[5] and Radford in 1954.[6] Both Gruenwald[5] and Radford[6] independently showed that it was easier to inflate the lungs with liquid than with air, and correctly concluded that surface tension effects were involved. However, Radford incorrectly concluded that surface tension in the airways was probably the same as in the serum. Pattle,[7] noting that bubbles from lung extracts did not collapse, suggested that the surface tension in the airways was exceedingly low. Clements noted[8,9] a discrepancy between estimates of alveolar surface area made with histologic techniques on the one hand, and surface area calculations based on the assumption that the surface tension of the alveoli was the same as that of extracellular fluid on the other; he hypothesized that a substance existed in the airways that reduced surface tension and permitted easy lung inflation. In the 30 years since identifying and isolating this surface active material ("surfactant"), Clements and his colleagues have continued to make major contributions to research in pulmonary surfactant physiology.

In 1961, three groups reported that pulmonary surfactant was a lipoprotein.[10–12] The Clements group correctly recognized that the principal lipid moiety was dipalmitoyl lecithin.[12] The lipid composition of pulmonary surfactant was more fully reported by King and Clements in 1972,[13] and the importance of the surfactant apoproteins in adsorption was reported by King and co-workers in the following year.[14]

The type II alveolar cell was identified in 1954 by Macklin.[15] Also in 1954, Low identified lamellar inclusions in type II cells.[16] These lamellar inclusions were postulated to be the source of pulmonary surfactant by both Buckingham and Avery[17] and by Klaus et al. in 1962.[18] In the ensuing 23 years, the synthesis and release of surfactant has been characterized in fine detail (see below).

NEONATAL RESPIRATORY DISTRESS SYNDROME AND PULMONARY SURFACTANT DEFICIENCY

In 1947, Gruenwald differentiated lack of lung aeration in the newborn secondary to the aspiration of amniotic fluid.[5] Gruenwald also demonstrated in postmortem experiments that the placement of the surface active substance amyl acetate in the airways reduced the pressure required to inflate ateletatic human newborn lungs with air, but not with fluid.[5] In a prophetic concluding paragraph, Gruenwald said:

> The resistance to aeration is due to surface tension which counteracts the entrance of air, but has no effect on the aspiration of fluid. Surface active substances reduce the pressure necessary for aeration. This suggests that the addition of surface active substances to the air or oxygen which is being spontaneously breathed in or introduced by a respirator might aid in relieving the initial atelectasis of newborn infants.[5]

In 1959, Avery and Mead observed that lungs of newborns succumbing to neonatal respiratory distress syndrome had abnormally high surface tensions, and suggested that pulmonary surfactant was deficient.[19] Not long thereafter, the first attempt at pulmonary surfactant replacement in vivo was reported.[20]

ACCELERATION OF PULMONARY MATURITY

In studies of the onset of labor, Liggins reported in 1969 that fetal injection of steroids enhanced lung aeration in 6 of 10 lambs spontaneously delivered between 117 and 123 days gestation.[21] Lambs of this gestational age are extremely premature, and are virtually never are able to establish good lung aeration. Liggins' observations were subsequently confirmed by many others. Three years later, Liggins and Howie[22] followed with the first controlled clinical trial of maternal betamethasone administration for the prevention of NRDS; they demonstrated a reduction in NRDS in infants delivered more than 24 hours after maternal betamethasone treatment. Two hundred eighty-two women less than 37 weeks pregnant were entered in the study. Seventy-seven percent of these delivered more than 24 hours after betamethasone administration. NRDS occurred among 9 percent of the treated group and 26 percent of the control group. In infants of less than 32 weeks gestation, the incidences of NRDS in the treated and control groups were 12 percent and 70 percent, respectively. Mortality was 3.2 percent in the treated group, and 15.0 percent in the control group. Many subsequent studies have confirmed and refined the observations of Liggins and Howie, including a collaborative NIH study of 698 women that documented a reduction in RDS from 18 to 12.6 percent ($P<0.05$).[23] However, antenatal steroids are not the sole answer to the prevention of NRDS, for three reasons. First, no benefit of prenatal betamethasone treatment could be documented until after 24 hours had elapsed.[22] Unfortunately, in many premature labors, delivery cannot be delayed by 24 hours. Second, steroids appear to benefit female but not male infants.[23] The use of steroids in all relevant cases would therefore still leave half the population at significant risk for NRDS. Third, Caucasion infants show little benefit.[23] Nevertheless, prenatal steroids, although not a panacea, are now well accepted as useful and without significant hazard in the prevention of NRDS.[24]

Acceleration of pulmonary maturity has also been noted in some studies after maternal beta-agonist administration,[25–27] which is not surprising because beta agonists have been shown to have an important role in the regulation of surfactant secretion.[28–30] However, other investigators have not found beta agonists to stimulate surfactant release.[31] In 1973, Kero and co-workers reported that none of 26 premature infants whose mothers were treated prenatally with isoxsuprine developed NRDS, and that maternal isoxsuprine administration in 12 subsequent premature labors also appeared to prevent NRDS (0 of 12).[25] Bergman et al. looked retrospectively at 33 babies; only 1 of 24 babies of mothers receiving terbutaline developed NRDS.[26] In a randomized, controlled study, Boog et al. found NRDS to occur in 5 of 29 infants born to ritodrine-treated mothers and 12 of 34 infants born to control mothers.[27] However, other studies have failed to confirm that prenatal beta-agonist administration prevents RDS, and prenatal beta-agonist administration carries significant maternal hazards, including pulmonary edema and death.

Because acceleration of pulmonary maturity cannot entirely solve the problem of NRDS in premature infants, increasing interest has been focused on the use of surface active materials for either the treatment or prevention of NRDS.

CHARACTER AND FUNCTION OF NATURAL PULMONARY SURFACTANT

Chemical Composition

Pulmonary surfactant is a complex mixture of lipids and proteins which associate together to form membraneous structures with a density in the range of 1.03 to 1.10, depending upon the method of isolation. The complex is readily differentiated

Table 2.1. Lipid Composition (%) of Surfactant in the Adult Rat Lung. Comparison of Surfactant Isolated in Lavage Fluid, by Density Gradient Centrifugation, and in Lamellar Bodies[50]

	Lavage Fluid[155] (%)	Density Gradient Centrifugation[34] (%)	Lamellar Bodies[50] (%)
Lipid composition			
Phospholipid	89.6	78.7	
Neutral lipid	10.4	21.3	
Phospholipid composition			
Phosphatidylcholine			
Phosphatidylethanolamine	81.0	68.8	70.2
Sphingomyelin	4.6	9.8	11.7
Phosphatidylglycerol	2.3	5.0	1.6
Phosphatidylserine +	5.0	6.7	11.7
phosphatidylinositol	5.0	6.1	3.0
Others	2.0	3.6	

from the serum lipoproteins by its surface tension properties and composition. The complex is approximately 10 percent protein and 90 percent lipid.[32] The lipids are mainly phospholipids (78 to 90 percent), in proportions that are unique to the lung (Table 2-1). Phosphatidylcholine comprises 68 to 80 percent of the phospholipids, with approximately half of the phosphatidylcholines containing only saturated fatty acids, mainly palmitate, attached to the glycerol backbone. Thus, dipalmitoyl phosphatidylcholine (DPPC) is the predominant lipid species in pulmonary surfactant. Pure DPPC alone can produce the very low surface tensions characteristic of pulmonary surfactant (i.e., 0 to 10 mN/M), but does not produce surface films with the rapid spreading, adsorption, and stability properties characteristic of natural surfactant.[33]

The second important lipid in pulmonary surfactant is phosphatidylglycerol (PG). It represents 5 to 12 percent of the total phospholipid composition.[34] Like phosphatidylcholine, PG also contains a large percentage of saturated fatty acids. The role of PG in pulmonary surfactant is unknown at present. PG also produces low surface tensions, like DPPC, but the amount of PG present is too low to make a significant contribution to the surface tension properties of the overall surfactant complex. PG has been suggested as being important for the stabilization of tubular myelin[35] and the interconversion of pulmonary surfactant forms,[32] because PG in association with calcium promotes membrane fusion, but this is unproven. Although PG is currently the best indicator of fetal lung maturity [an infant can have a high lecithin/sphingomyelin (L/S) ratio and still be at risk for RDS, but if PG is present in the amniotic fluid, the risk of RDS is low,[36]], it is unnecessary for good pulmonary surfactant function.[37,38]

The other lipids in the pulmonary surfactant complex[32] (Table 2-1) are normal membrane components (i.e., phosphatidylethanolamine, phosphahatidylserine, phosphatidylinositol, and sphingomyelin), although they are present in lower percentages than would be found in membrane fractions of other organs. This is especially true of phosphatidylethanolamine, which usually constitutes less than 10 percent of the surfactant phospholipids, but may constitute 20 to 30 percent of the membrane phospholipids in other mammalian tissues.

While numerous proteins have been found in pulmonary surfactant, most of them are derived from serum. After removal of the serum proteins by immunoadsorption, it is still possible to identify in pulmonary surfactant a variety of proteins ranging in molecular weight from 6K to 250K.[32,33,39,40] By amino acid analysis, sequence analysis, or both, all of the pulmonary surfactant-associated proteins of 36Kd and above seem to contain a homology to collagen. Most studies of the proteins have been centered on the 10 to 11K and 34 to 36K species[33,41,42,43] as being unique to surfactant, with the 34K protein being the most abundant protein. In vivo labeling studies suggest that the 11K protein is a metabolic product of the 34K protein[41]; however, studies with isolated type II cells demonstrate that the two proteins are secreted with different time courses.[42] In addition, antisera to the 6Kd and 36Kd proteins[44] and sequence analysis (J. Clements, personal communication) suggest that the two proteins are distinct entities. The uniqueness of the 34K protein to pulmonary surfactant can be questioned with the recent demonstration that it may be made in bronchial Clara cells in addition to type II cells.[45] The gene for the 34K protein has been cloned from human DNA[46–48] and can be expressed in vitro. Cloning may provide very pure protein for examination of the role of the pulmonary surfactant proteins with the phospholipids in studies of pulmonary surfactant function and in pulmonary surfactant replacement (see below). Recently, a 6K protein was identified in human pulmonary surfactant[40]; this protein may prove to be extremely interesting, since a mixture of it and DPPC appear to have the same surface tension properties as natural pulmonary surfactant.[40]

Pulmonary Surfactant Forms (Morphology)

Pulmonary surfactant exists in at least four distinct forms that can be demonstrated with the electron microscope. The alveolar lining film is a thin monolayer between the alveolar fluid and the alveolar air space. This monolayer is the functionally important form of pulmonary surfactant that stabilizes the alveolar structure during breathing. The monolayer is also the most difficult form to visualize because of disruption during its fixation; as a result, the monolayer is rarely seen as a continuous film. Below the lining layer, loose myelin figures (common myelin), tubular myelin figures, and a homogeneous matrix can be visualized, especially in alveolar corners, where the fluid layer is thickest. The common myelin figures can be described as swollen, irregularly shaped liposomes. They are the lightest of the isolated forms of pulmonary surfactant,[49,50] and readily form surface films.[51] A preparation lighter than common myelin has been reported, containing small unilamellar vesicles,[52,53] but the significance of this fraction is unclear since it was not very surface active[52] and contained low amounts of surfactant apoproteins.[53] The tubular myelin figures are unique structures. They consist of membranes that form a square lattice (Fig. 2-1), with material inside the lattice pattern having a tubular configuration. Tubular myelin is the most dense of the four forms of pulmonary surfactant,[49,51] and may contribute to surface-film formation,[53,54] although it may not be highly surface active by itself.[55,56] Tubular myelin may be an intermediate form of extracellular surfactant during transformation of the latter from lamellar body form to alveolar lining film,[52,54] or an extracellular storage form for excess surfactant. Increases in the amount of tubular myelin are associated

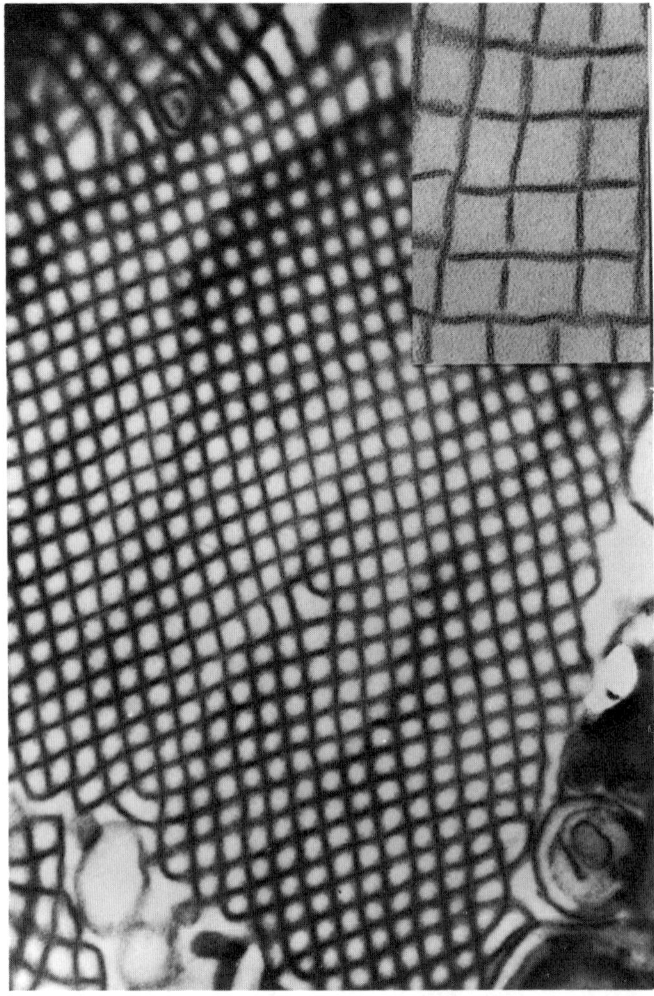

Fig. 2.1. This field of tubular myelin cut in cross-section was selected for its uniform quadratic lattice structure. However, close examination of the membranes and intersections demonstrates that considerable variation still exists in the architecture of this unique structure. 80,000 ×. Inset: higher magnification portion of tubular myelin selected for variation in the intersections. Membranes may appear continuous through the intersection, or may be discontinuous or offset. 151,000 ×. (Sanders RL, Hassett RJ, Vatter AE: Isolation of lung lamellar bodies and their conversion to tubular myelin figures in vitro. Anat Rec 198:485, 1980.)

with decreases in pulmonary function during constant tidal volume ventilation.[57,58] Inside the type II cell, the pulmonary surfactant is stored in the lamellar body, an organelle the size of a mitochrondrion (~ 1μ diameter), consisting of a distinct outer membrane with tightly packaged membranes (lamellae) inside. The lamellar body is intermediate in density between the common myelin and tubular myelin,[49,50] does not readily participate in surface film formation,[51,55] and is very unstable after isolation.[50] Lamellar bodies disrupt to form common myelin, and in the presence of calcium, also give rise to tubular myelin.[50] Calcium also promotes the formation of a surface-active film from the lamellar bodies[55] and an isolated surfactant fraction.[54]

Regulation of Synthesis and Secretion

The synthesis and secretion of pulmonary surfactant follows the general pattern seen in other secretory cells. Synthesis of both the lipid and protein components occurs in the rough endoplasmic reticulum of the type II cell. Both lipid and protein are transported through the Golgi system to the lamellar body, where they are stored until secretion.[59] Although the newly synthesized lipids and proteins may traverse the same route, it is not known when the various lipids and proteins associate into the pulmonary surfactant lipoprotein complex. The phosphatidylcholine molecule is predominantly synthesized by the cytidyl triphosphate pathway (Kennedy pathway),[60,61] with possible regulation by the phosphorylcholine cytidylyltransferase and choline phosphotransferase enzymes.[62,63] The actual DPPC moiety may come from a combination of de novo synthesis[63–65] and acyl rearrangement[63,66] of a phosphatidylcholine containing an unsaturated fatty acid, with the relative contribution of the two mechanisms being uncertain at the present time. After release from the type II cell, pulmonary surfactant may be taken back up by the type II cell and recycled through lamellar bodies for resecretion.[67–70]

Numerous agents have been shown to affect pulmonary surfactant synthesis in the developing fetus. The most notable are glucocorticoids. As mentioned earlier, they have been shown to accelerate maturation of the fetal lung,[21] with earlier pulmonary surfactant production, and to increase the survival of premature infants.[22] Glucocorticoids increase the activities of choline phosphotransferase,[71] phosphorylcholine cytidylyltransferase,[72] and the acyl rearrangement enzymes.[71,73] Cytoplasmic and nuclear glucocorticoid receptors have been demonstrated in the lung,[74,75] and a possible binding site for these receptors on the genome for the 34K apoprotein has been reported.[46] Glucocorticoids may act on the type II cell via a fibroblast pneumocyte factor (FPF) released by fibroblasts in response to glucocorticoids. This FPF accentuates the type II cell response to glucocorticoids and accelerates maturation in vivo.[76] However, glucocorticoid receptor binding to the genome for the apoprotein suggests that there is also a direct effect of glucocorticoids on pulmonary surfactant synthesis. Thyroid hormones, thyrotropin releasing hormone, estrogens, and epithelial growth hormone have also been shown to accelerate fetal development.[76–78] However, their mechanisms of action are not yet known.

As also mentioned earlier, the secretion of pulmonary surfactant from the type II cell is stimulated by β-adrenergic compounds[79–81] as well as by A23187[80] and tetradecanolyphorbol acetate,[79,82] with Ca^{2+} and/or cAMP serving as second messengers in the response. Adrenergic regulation of pulmonary surfactant secretion has been well demonstrated in vivo[83] and with isolated type II cells.[79,80,82,84] Pilocarpine stimulates pulmonary surfactant release in vivo,[85] but it is believed to act on the lung by an indirect mechanism, since the stimulation in vivo is blocked by propranolol[86] and does not occur in vitro.[84]

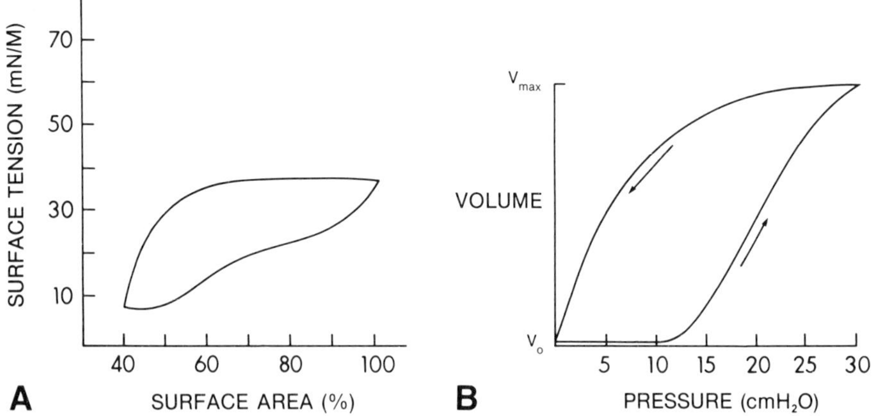

Fig. 2.2. Comparison of hysteresis curves produced by (**A**) compression of surfactant on a Langmuir trough and (**B**) pressure-volume curve of isolated intact lungs. (**A**) Surfactant is layered onto a saline subphase, allowed to equilibrate to constant surface tension, and then compressed to 40 percent of original area. Surface tensions less than 10 mN/m are to be expected at minimum area for pulmonary lavage fluid and isolated surfactant fractions. (**B**) Pressure-volume relationship upon expansion with air and collapse between the degussed state V_o and maximum volume V_{max}.

Surface Active Properties

The term surfactant is derived from the fact that the material removed from the alveoli produces very low surface tensions when measured under dynamic conditions on a Langmuir trough.[8,9] Surface tensions approaching 0 mN/m are not uncommon. It has become common to require surfactant substances isolated from the lung to produce interfacial surface tensions of 10 mN/m or less at 37°C in order for them to qualify as an effective pulmonary surfactant. The usual method for testing this is to layer the surface active material onto a saline hypophase, allow a period of time for film equilibration, and then begin cyclic compression and expansion of the film. Lung lavage fluid and purified pulmonary surfactant preparations are both capable of producing these low surface tensions when spread as aqueous suspensions, as are lipid extracts of pulmonary surfactant and pure DPPC when the latter are spread from organic solvents. In addition to low surface tension, these films exhibit a large hysteresis between the compression and expansion sides of the γ versus area isotherms (Fig. 2-2**A**). This hysteresis is very similar to the one seen in pressure/volume (P/V) curves of air-filled lungs (Fig. 2-2**B**), and was part of the basis for the original suggestion that surfactant is important for normal lung compliance.[8]

While pure DPPC can produce the very low surface tensions required of pulmonary surfactant, it apparently cannot serve the function of pulmonary surfactant by itself. The gel-liquid crystal transition temperature (41°C) of DPPC is above body temperature. It is difficult to make uniform dispersions of DPPC in water, and once formed, they generate surface films very slowly.[33] Consequently, it is necessary to spread DPPC monolayers from an organic solvent. The DPPC films occupy a smaller molecular area and are more rigid and more stable than natural pulmonary surfactant films. In contrast, the lipid mixture of natural pulmonary surfactant displays a broad phase transition between 15 and 42°C, and the surfactant lipoprotein complex rapidly participates in film formation from aqueous dispersions. Thus, lipids other than DPPC are needed in surfactant to increase the fluidity, and proteins are needed to promote dispersibility and adsorption.

Other Effects

Pulmonary surfactant was postulated to aid in the clearance of fluid from the lung of the neonate and to keep the adult lung dry as an "anti-edema" factor.[87,88] However, this function of pulmonary surfactant has received little attention and remains to be proven. The high degree of saturation of pulmonary surfactant lipids, and of lung lipids in general, may be somewhat of a protective mechanism for the lung against the damaging effects of high oxygen tension. Saturated fatty acids neither oxidize nor give rise to reactive oxygen species as easily as unsaturated fatty acids. Pulmonary surfactant may be important in the function of alveolar macrophages by aiding in phagocytosis[89–91] and in the killing of bacteria,[90] although this is disputed.[92] The fact that the 34K surfactant protein has collagen-like regions that are homologous to complement protein C1q and mannose binding protein (MBP) of the liver suggests that there may be additional functions of surfactant,[46,93] possibly as a primitive immune protectant.

Surfactant Inhibitors

It has long been known that plasma proteins would interfere with the behavior of pulmonary surfactant films on the Langmuir trough, although this effect was considered to be nonspecific because proteins like albumin also interfere. Recently, a protein was identified in plasma which inhibits pulmonary surfactant function in vitro and which can be demonstrated in the airways of premature lambs with NRDS.[94] A similar protein has also been demonstrated in the airways of patients with adult respiratory distress syndrome (ARDS).[95] Thus, conditions that alter the permeability of the pulmonary vasculature and permit proteins to enter the airspaces might introduce surfactant inhibitors to the airspaces, further compromising lung function. In addition, it has been shown that atelectasis and decreased lung compliance can be caused by constant volume ventilation with no positive end expiratory pressure (PEEP), and that this effect is reversed by periodic deep breaths.[57,58] Constant volume ventilation also caused a greater amount of this extracellular surfactant to be associated with tubular myelin. It was suggested that increases in tubular myelin lead to increased surface tension in the alveoli, which results in alveolar collapse.[57] This might represent a functional and rapidly reversible inhibition of pulmonary surfactant, due to its being in an inappropriate form.

CHARACTERISTICS OF AN IDEAL PULMONARY SURFACTANT REPLACEMENT

Formulation

The ideal formulation for a replacement for pulmonary surfactant would have four simple qualities. First, the formulation should permit easy, sterile manufacture in quantity, from readily available substances whose chemistries and toxic effects are well characterized. This first requirement is clearly more easily met by totally synthetic surfactants, which do not contain proteins isolated from biologic sources.

Second, the formulation should have no special storage requirements such as refrigeration or avoidance of light, and should have a long shelf-life (greater than 3 years) at room temperature. Again, this second requirement is more easily met by totally synthetic surfactants not containing biologic materials (proteins are more likely to degrade at room temperature).

Third, the formulation should permit easy administration, in doses adequate to rapidly improve lung function in surfactant-deficient lungs. The point here is that it should be possible to deliver sufficient quantities of surface-active material to line the entire lung in minutes. Intratracheal administration of liquid surfactant formulations can provide large quantities of surface-active materials to the airways in minutes. Such liquid "bolus" administrations have been documented to achieve good pulmonary distributions when administered within minutes of birth, although patchy distributions were noted when liquid surfactant administration was delayed until one-half hour of age.[96] In contrast, homogeneous pulmonary distributions of powdered surfactant formulations probably require aerosol administration, and the transfer capacity of aerosolization and breathing precludes achieving large doses in short periods of time.

Fourth, the formulation should be ready to use, and not require special handling, such as vortexing, prior to administration. Unfortunately, any currently conceivable pulmonary surfactant replacement is bound to have large quantities of DPPC, which is subject to low-grade hydrolysis if the surfactant is formulated as a liquid and stored at room temperature. One approach, which has been taken by Ross Laboratories with the semisynthetic Surfactant TA, is to leave the formulation as a liquid but to store it in the cold to retard hydrolysis. Cold storage is required for many drugs used in modern therapeutics, and is certainly an acceptable approach, but the ideal pulmonary surfactant replacement would be stored at room temperature. Room temperature storage would permit routine stocking of the surface-active material on every delivery room cart for immediate use in premature infants born unexpectedly, as well as storage on the shelf in many Third World dispensaries, where refrigeration, much less modern obstetric and neonatal care, does not yet exist.

Even if the problem of low grade DPPC hydrolysis during liquid storage at room temperature could be overcome, liquid surfactant formulations present a second problem in that they are suspensions, not solutions. As a result, the lipids settle out over time, and resuspension by vortexing or some other physical process is required prior to administration. Another approach, which has been taken by Burroughs Wellcome Co. (Research Triangle Park, NC) with the synthetic surfactant EXOSURF (Burroughs Wellcome Co.), is to remove the water after manufacture (i.e., formulate the surface-active material as a lyophilized powder), and then reconstitute the material immediately prior to administration. Formulating the surface-active material as a lyophilized powder and reconstituting it at the time of use is simpler than formulating it as a liquid, storing it in the cold, and vortexing it prior to use. Although formulation of the surface active material as a lyophilized powder does not meet the ideal of off-the-shelf use, reconstitution at the bedside is quick and simple. As long as DPPC remains a major component of pulmonary surfactant replacements, lyophilized formulations will probably be closest to the ideal formulation.

Pharmacokinetics/Dynamics

An ideal replacement for pulmonary surfactant would have a half-life several times that of exogenously administered human pulmonary surfactant, so that only one administration would be required to prevent or treat NRDS. Retreatment with up to a total of five administrations in the first 48 hours of life has been required in studies with amniotic fluid-derived human pulmonary surfactant.[97] Studies with various other natural and semisynthetic surfactants similarly suggest that retreatment is often necessary. The factors controlling the biologic half-life of exogenously administered natural and semisynthetic surfactants are incompletely known, but it is possible that surfactant inhibitors[94,95] are responsible for loss of biologic effect (i.e., need for retreatment). Thus, another characteristic of an ideal pulmonary surfactant replacement might be resistance to surfactant inhibitors, which would effectively prolong the surfactant's biologic half-life. Whether synthetic surfactants have a longer biologic half-life than natural or semisynthetic surfactants, and whether synthetic surfactants are less susceptible to surfactant inhibitors, remain unknown. However, the fact that synthetic surfactants are designed to replace deficient or ineffective endogenous pulmonary surfactant without the use of proteins may permit longer biologic half-lives than those observed with natural or semisynthetic pulmonary surfactants, because the pulmonary surfactant apoproteins are likely to be the keys to uptake of natural pulmonary surfactants from the airways,[98,99] and may be the targets of surfactant inhibitors. In addition, pulmonary surfactant apoprotein appears to turn off secretion of pulmonary surfactant by isolated type II cells;[98] and turning off endogenous pulmonary surfactant secretion would prolong the time a given natural or semisynthetic pulmonary surfactant would have to function, and effectively shorten its biologic half-life.

The effects of exogenously administered surface-active materials on the synthesis, release, and reuptake of endogenously produced natural pulmonary surfactant might also be very important. Although animal experiments can provide useful background information on these issues,[100–103] answers to these questions in humans can in fact really be answered only in humans. Significant advances in the technology for measuring pulmonary surfactant synthesis, release, and reuptake will have to occur before they can be adequately addressed. For example, to conduct such studies, one must be able to distinguish each component of exogenously administered surface-active material from each component of endogenously produced pulmonary surfactant. Using several different isotopes to radiolabel the various lipids and apoprotein moieties (either in exogenous surface active material or endogenously, in the patient, or most accurately in both) so as to distinguish components of exogenous surface active material from components of endogenous pulmonary surfactant would be unacceptable in critically ill neonates with NRDS; these infants should have a long life ahead of them if the surface-active material is effective. Similarly, administering radioactive exogenous surface-active material to healthy premature infants in order to conduct metabolic studies is not justfiable. Until new technologies are developed, pharmacokinetic and pharmacodynamic questions about exogenous surface active materials will remain unanswered in the premature neonate. However, if significant reductions in the current morbidity and mortality of NRDS can be documented with surfactant replacement therapy, the surfactant replacements proven to be effective will be approved and used in clinical practice without having answers to the pharmacokinetic and pharmacodynamic questions posed above.

Toxicologic Effects

Any ideal replacement for pulmonary surfactant would obviously be totally non-toxic. Unfortunately biologic systems are such that gargantuan doses of even the most inert substances are likely to cause toxicity if they are given for a long enough time. The questions asked in toxocologic studies must have biologic relevance if the studies are to be of value.

Although the toxic effects of various chemicals on the pulmonary surfactant system have recently been summarized,[104] very little has been published on the toxic effects of excessive amounts of surface-active materials on the lungs. Characterizing the toxicologic profile of surface-active materials intended for human use is important for two major reasons. First, the toxicologic effects of a new drug are not necessarily extensions of its pharmacologic effects; indeed, in toxicologic testing deleterious effects not even anticipated from extensive pharmacologic testing are often identified. It is for this reason that most new drugs fail in toxicology testing before ever reaching clinical trials. Second, identification of the therapeutic index of a new drug (the ratio of the pharmacologic dose to the toxic dose) can be reassuring when dosing schedules are being devised for subsequent clinical trials.

On the other hand, absence of significant toxicity in animals at doses far above those required to produce desired pharmacologic effects is no guarantee that toxicity will not occur in human studies.

In general, toxicologic studies are designed to mimic but exaggerate the intended clinical use of a drug. Thus, if a new drug is intended for oral use, toxicity studies of the orally administered compound are conducted with doses several times higher than those intended for clinical use, and dosing is continued for periods several times longer than anticipated in clinical practice. However, characterizing the toxicologic profiles of surface-active materials intended for human use is not a simple matter, since these agents will be administered intratracheally. If the surface-active material is to be administered as a liquid, intratracheal administration of increasing liquid volumes in attempts to achieve high doses will eventually drown both the group of subjects being given the surface-active material and the vehicle control group. Further, attempts to exaggerate the dosage by the repetition of intratracheal doses, either by several administrations per day or by daily intratracheal administrations for long periods of time, are far from ideal, since both repetitive endotracheal intubations and chronically implanted tracheal catheters are likely to cause histopathology in the airways.

If the surface-active material intended for human testing is to be administered as an aerosol, other constraints limit achievable doses. Even the most efficient aerosolization systems can suspend only small quantities of a compound, with the effect that doses can be increased only by prolonging the periods of exposure.

However, even the most resilient animal species can rarely tolerate more than 4 hours per day of restraint and aerosol administration.

Despite these caveats, toxicologic studies with various surface-active materials have been and are being performed by several laboratories around the world. Performing the in vitro and in vivo toxicologic studies outlined below appears to be sufficient to establish an adequate safety profile to justify trials in premature infants with NRDS.

In vitro

Only modest in vitro toxicology testing is necessary for surface-active material being considered for human trials. Documenting that the material has no mutagenic effects in standard assays such as the Ames test is sufficient.

In vivo

Rather extensive in vivo formal toxicologic trials of an exogenous surface active material are necessary, if not for the initiation of clinical trials, then certainly for eventual FDA approval of a given surface-active material's use in humans. Given the dosing constraints outlined above, exaggerated doses should be administered to animals of the same species in which pharmacologic testing is to be done, so that toxic and pharmacologic effects can be directly compared.

Pharmacologic Effects

Human pulmonary surfactant is often cited as the "gold standard" for pulmonary surfactant replacements. However this concept is not particularly useful, for several reasons. First, human pulmonary surfactant is certainly not the "gold standard" for the premature rabbit pup,[105,106] the premature lamb,[96,107–109] the premature monkey,[110] or the premature baboon[111]—the four standard premature animal models of NRDS. Yet it is in these models that pharmacologic testing is conducted with most surface-active materials. Second, the presence of normal quantities of the "gold standard" in the airways might not be enough to ward off NRDS in certain situations, such as in infants with surfactant inhibitors. Third, there are few materials in either the natural or man-made worlds that a bright and creative human mind will not eventually improve upon. Calling human pulmonary surfactant a "gold standard" tends to inhibit the extension of human inventiveness to an area that could use some improvements. For example, human pulmonary surfactant might possibly perform better if it had a longer half-life and were resistant to inhibitors. Indeed, it is probable that pulmonary surfactant substitutes superior to natural human pulmonary surfactant will be invented.

In vitro

At present, investigators devising replacements for natural pulmonary surfactant are studying products (natural, semisynthetic, or synthetic) that can closely mimic the natural surfactant by in vitro testing methods. When tested on a Langmuir trough or in a pulsating bubble apparatus, it is commonly held that a good surfactant substitute should produce a minimum surface tension of less than 10 mN/M at 37°C, should exhibit hysteresis between the compression and expanison sides of the γ/A isotherm, should spread rapidly from aqueous dispersions, and should form stable films (e.g., stable bubbles in the shake test).

However, it must be kept in mind that these are arbitrary criteria based on how natural pulmonary surfactant behaves in vitro. The only absolute criteria for a surfactant replacement product are that it safely and effectively improve lung stability and function in vivo. The lung, and particularly the alveolar surface, is like a black box. There are numerous proteins, lipids, and other compounds present, especially so in the sick infant, as well as a very active metabolic machinery that must modify whatever product is administered. Therefore, the way in which the product behaves in vivo may be different from the way it behaves in vitro. Such considerations may be particularly important in the future if new compounds are discovered that are as surface active as DPPC but are more dispersible.

In addition to rapidly spreading and rapidly reducing surface tension to low values on repetitive compression in instruments designed to measure surface-tension effects, an ideal replacement for natural pulmonary surfactant should be able to restore pulmonary compliance and end-expiratory volumes to normal in isolated, surfactant-depleted lungs ventilated with normal pressure patterns.

In vivo

Pharmacologic testing of surface-active materials in vivo must be performed in models in which pulmonary surfactant is deficient or inactivated. Most testing is done in premature rabbits,[105,106] lambs,[96,107–109] monkeys,[110] or baboons,[111] but adult animal models in which surfactant is washed out of the airways by repeated lavage are also useful.[112,113] There are many different ways to measure the effects of a given surface-active material on the function of pulmonary surfactant-deficient lungs, but most of these effects are directly or indirectly related to the surface-active material's restoration of functional residual capacity to normal. Once alveolar collapse during expiration is prevented and functional residual capacity is restored, inflation is much easier (compliance is improved), and gas exchange is enhanced. A listing of various endpoints useful in documenting beneficial effects of surface-active material in pharamacologic testing is found in Table 2-2.

Table 2.2. Measurements Useful in Pharmacologic Testing of Surface-Active Materials

Functional residual capacity
Lung compliance
Blood gases (pH, PaO_2, $PaCO_2$)
Alveolar/arterial PO_2 gradients
Lung water measurements
Lung epithelial protein leak measurements
Lung injury measurements
Pulmonary blood flow measurements
Systemic blood flow measurements
Systemic oxygen transport
Survival

Clinical Effects

The clinical effects of an ideal replacement for pulmonary surfactant in the prevention or treatment of NRDS should be a function both of the effectiveness of the surface-active material in reducing surface tension and of the contribution of surfactant deficiency to the pathophysiology under treatment. For example, polio vaccine is ineffective after the virus is replicating in the anterior horn cells. Similarly, an ideal pulmonary surfactant replacement may be of little value in NRDS after 24 to 48 hours of high oxygen concentrations and high ventilator pressures, because ductal shunt and oxygen- and ventilator-induced lung damage may be the predominant pathophysiology late in the course of NRDS. Severe histologic damage has been observed shortly after birth in premature animals mechanically ventilated with high oxygen concentrations.[114]

Thus, the most dramatic clinical effects of an ideal pulmonary surfactant replacement are likely to be observed in studies of its early administration, whether this early administration is a prophylactic one at birth to infants at risk of developing NRDS, or a rescue treatment given as soon as infants develop respiratory difficulty.

Physiologic endpoints

In any case, improvements in the clinical outcome of NRDS after the administration of surface-active material will be a function of surfactant-induced improvements in lung volumes, pulmonary compliance, and gas exchange. Perhaps the single best clinical measure of a surface-active material's efficacy would be its effect on functional residual capacity (lung volume at end expiration) with normal transpulmonary pressure, or conversely the reduction of end-inspiratory and end-expiratory pressures needed to maintain normal lung volumes. The high alveolar surface tensions in surfactant-deficient lungs result in alveolar collapse during expiration (low functional residual capacity). The reinflation of collapsed alveoli during inspiration requires a greatly increased work of breathing (low compliance). As a result of alveolar collapse during expiration, and poor alveolar inflation during inspiration, the exchange of oxygen and carbon dioxide between pulmonary capillary blood and alveolar air is markedly impaired. Reductions in arterial oxygen tensions and elevations in arterial carbon dioxide tensions result. Other laboratory measures of the efficacy of pulmonary surfactant have included chest radiographs[115] and tracheal fluid analyses.[116]

Thus, an ideal surfactant replacement would restore functional residual capacity to normal, and as a result greatly improve pulmonary compliance and gas exchange. Improvements in functional residual capacity, pulmonary compliance, and gas exchange should be obvious after the administration of surface-active material to surfactant deficient infants if the surfactant replacement is any good. However, accurate measurements of functional residual capacity in sick premature neonates are not simple. Measurements of pulmonary compliance are less difficult, but far from routine in most nurseries. In general, pilot trials with various surface-active materials have enthusiastically reported improvements in arterial oxygen tensions and reductions in FiO_2 and ventilator support, because these measurements are easy to make, but such changes naturally follow from surfactant-induced improvements in functional residual capacity.

Morbidity and mortality

As a result of its effects on functional residual capacity, an ideal pulmonary surfactant replacement would obviously prevent death and reduce morbidity from NRDS. Death is the clearest and most important endpoint for any clinical trial, but the incidence of the death in NRDS has been greatly reduced by modern neonatal care. As a result, proof of a reduced incidence of death in NRDS can require large scale clinical trials. In Tables 2-3 and 2-4 below, the sample sizes required to prove 10, 20, 30 and 40 percent reductions in death at various gestational ages (power = 0.9) are provided. These calculations assume that all deaths occur directly or indirectly from NRDS, and that the prevention or early treatment of NRDS with an effective surfactant replacement would prevent death; as a result, the calculations are obviously underestimates of the actual sample sizes needed to prove reductions in the incidence of death. Nevertheless, it is obvious that relatively large scale trials are required to prove modest but important reductions in death after pulmonary surfactant replacement therapy. Reduction in death may be fairly easy to prove in extremely premature infants (Table 2-3), but mortality may not be as closely linked to pulmonary surfactant deficiency in this weight group, where death from intraventricular hemorrhage is more common.

Reductions in mortality in infants between 700 and 1350 g would be difficult to prove, but reductions in morbidity should be provable (Table 2-4), because survival with complications is more frequent. However, bronchopulmonary dysplasia (BPD) is probably the only major complication of prematurity about which there is widespread agreement for a close pathophysiologic linkage to NRDS. Thus, it appears that an effective pulmonary surfactant replacement is more likely to reduce the incidence of BPD than the incidence of patent ductus arteriosus, necrotizing enterocolitis, retrolental fibroplasia, or intraventricular hemorrhage. Other measures of morbidity, including days on the ventilator, days in level III care,

Table 2.3. Number of Infants <700 g in Each Group Required to Detect Reduction in NRDS and Its Complications (Two-tailed Test, Power = 0.90)

Complication	Incidence (%) in Control Group	% Reduction in Surfactant Group			
		10	20	30	40
NRDS	80	597	164	78	45
Cardiopulmonary destruction	87	397	116	58	35
IVH	60	1429	361	160	89
Death	57	1604	402	177	99
PDA	30	4756	1149	491	265
BPD	30	4756	1149	491	265

NRDS—Neonatal respiratory distress syndrome; cardiopulmonary destruction—absence of life or the presence of BPD on day 28; PDA—patent ductus arteriosus; IVH—intraventricular hemorrhage; BPD—bronchopulmonary dysplasia.

Stated sample size requirements were obtained by requiring that a two-sided test for equality of proportions with a 0.05 level of significance and a power of 0.90 for detecting the indicated differences.

Computational formula is the (uncorrected for continuity) version found in Fliess, *Statistical Methods for Rates and Proportions*, 2nd Ed., John Wiley and Sons, New York, 1981, p. 41.

Table 2.4. Number of Infants > 700 g and < 1350 g in Each Group Required to Detect Reduction in NRDS and Its Complications (Two-tailed Test, Power = 0.90)

Complication	Incidence (%) in Control Group	% Reduction in Surfactant Group			
		10	20	30	40
NRDS	60	1429	361	160	89
PDA	40	3093	755	326	177
IVH	30	4756	1149	491	265
BPD	20	8084	1937	822	440
Death	10	18066	4301	1814	965
Intact cardiopulmonary survival	70	833	188	73	34

NRDS—Neonatal respiratory distress syndrome; intact cardiopulmonary survival—presence of life and absence of BPD on day 28; PDA—patent ductus arteriosus; IVH—intraventricular hemorrhage; BPD—bronchopulmonary dysplasia.

Stated sample size requirements were obtained by requiring that a two-sided test for equality of proportions with a 0.05 level of significance and a power of 0.90 for detecting the indicated differences.

Computational formula is the (uncorrected for continuity) version found in Fliess, *Statistical Methods for Rates and Proportions*, 2nd Ed., John Wiley and Sons, New York, 1981, p. 41.

days to regain birthweight, and costs per survivor, should show marked reductions after effective pulmonary surfactant replacement therapy, but calculations to predict the sample sizes necessary to prove such reductions are more difficult, given the wide variance in the control group.

UNITED STATES FOOD AND DRUG ADMINISTRATION REQUIREMENTS FOR PULMONARY SURFACTANT APPROVAL

IND

In the United States, clinical investigations of new pharmacologic agents are tightly regulated by the Food and Drug Administration (FDA). Prior to the human administration of any investigational drug, the FDA requires the sponsors of the investigation to file a request for an exemption called an Investigational New Drug Application (IND). The IND has to provide justification for human studies with the drug. INDs contain standards for the drug's manufacture, proof of sterility and lack of pyrogenicity; documentation of the desired pharmacologic effect in animals; documentation of an acceptable toxicologic profile and a wide safety margin in animals; and the protocol to be followed in the first human study. The investigators identified by the sponsor for conduct of the study must sign statements promising to abide by the federal rules of clinical investigation. These include obtaining approval of the protocol from the local institutional review board, obtaining informed consent from each patient, strict accounting for all investigational drug used, strict adherence to the protocol, and immediate sponsor notification of all serious adverse events.

After the IND is filed, the FDA has 30 days to reject the IND or request more information. If the sponsor has not heard from the FDA in 30 days, the sponsor is free to let the investigators start the study. Subsequently, additional protocols for new studies can be filed under the original IND.

The investigations are divided into four phases. Phase I studies are usually safety studies in normal volunteers, or pilot or feasibility studies in small groups of patients. Phase II studies are efficacy studies, and are usually randomized, controlled, parallel, and blinded. Phase III studies are large scale safety studies, designed to detect significant adverse reactions of low incidence. Phase IV studies are post-marketing surveillance studies, designed to provide additional safety data.

Factors important in the design of studies to gain FDA approval for a new medication include the severity of the illness to be treated, the characteristics and size of the population suffering from the illness, the magnitude of benefit expected to be derived from the drug, and the toxicologic profile of the drug in animals. First, the severity of the illness to be treated is an important factor in study design. If the drug is to be used symptomatically for the alleviation of minor, self-limited illnesses, such as the common cold, very large numbers of patients are necessary to provide adequate proof of a wide safety margin. On the other hand, if the drug is to be used to cure an invariably fatal disease, such as rabies, safety is almost irrelevant. NRDS would appear to lie somewhere in between these two extremes, for although few patients die in developed countries, NRDS remains a significant cause of morbidity. The number of patients necessary to demonstrate adequate safety for a given surfactant in NRDS will be larger for prophylactic use than for rescue use, for prophylactic use will entail treating some infants who would not develop the disease.

Second, the size and characteristics of the target patient population have to be taken into account in designing studies, as discussed above (Tables 2-3, and 2-4). If the disease is rare (primary pulmonary hypertension is an example), classical, randomized, parallel blinded studies may not be possible, and other designs, such as cross-over or withdrawal, may have to be used to establish efficacy. Patient recruitment should not be a problem in NRDS, and randomized parallel designs can therefore be used to establish efficacy.

Blinding is a more difficult issue. In neonates, the placebo effect will not be a problem, since the subjects won't know what they receive, but caretaker bias will be a significant problem once a given patient enters a study with an open design. On the other hand, placebo administraton may be difficult to justify. It would be far better to avoid caretaker bias, by using true double-blinding. One way in which this could be accomplished would be for a drug administration team to administer drug to the treatment group and nothing to the control group. The drug administration team should be well informed on the importance of blinding, and not participate in patient care.

Third, the expected degree of response to the drug is important. As with the introductions of insulin and penicillin, a new drug treatment for rabies would need only a very few survivors to prove its efficacy. On the other hand, given the high incidence of maternal group B streptococcal vaginal colonization (30 percent) and the low incidence of group B streptococcal pneumonia in newborns (0.1 percent), the demonstration that maternal penicillin prophylaxis reduces the incidence of group B streptococcal pneumonia in the newborn by 50 percent would require the randomization of approximately 47,070 mothers per group. Proof of reduction of NRDS by surfactant treatment again lies somewhere between the cases of rabies and group B strep infections. If a power of 0.9 (90 percent chance of getting the right answers from the study) and a 50 percent incidence of NRDS in infants of less than 1250 g weight are assumed, proving a reduction in the incidence of NRDS to 10 percent with surfactant prophylaxis would require the randomization of only

25 patients per group. A similar study size was apparently adequate to demonstrate the efficacy of amniotic fluid-derived human pulmonary surfactant in the study of Hallman et al.[117] However, the fact that eight patients were excluded from efficacy analysis in that study[117] presumably would invalidate the results during FDA review. In any case, quite dramatic but non-miraculous effects would be harder to detect; a reduction of NRDS from a 50 percent to 30 percent incidence (a 40 percent improvement) would require the randomization of 111 patients per group. Since the FDA requires at least two "pivotal" studies demonstrating efficacy at $p<0.05$ (so that the odds are less than 1 in 400 that both studies suggest a benefit that does not exist), the randomization of a minimum of 444 patients in two studies would be required to establish a 40 percent improvement in the incidence of NRDS.

Fourth, the formulation and toxicologic profile of a given surfactant may dictate certain features of study design, including method of administration (liquid, aerosol, powder), dosage intervals (single, continuing, multiple), and safety endpoints (local airway inflammatory reactions,[104] serum antibody titers).

Finally, very few new drugs are approved by the FDA simply because they produce improvements in laboratory measurements. For example, the demonstration that a new inotrope can cause sustained reductions in left ventricular end diastolic pressure and sustained improvements in cardiac output in patients with congestive heart failure is inadequate for FDA approval even though the congestive heart failure may be refractory to all other approved therapies. To gain FDA approval, a new inotrope must not only be demonstrated to have the expected hemodynamic effects, but also be demonstrated to have some clinical impact, such as a sustained increase in exercise tolerance or survival. Similarly, improvements in functional residual capacity, pulmonary compliance, and gas exchange are to be expected after the administration of any adequate pulmonary surfactant replacement to infants with NRDS; however, demonstrating of improvements in clinical outcome is a different and a more difficult matter.

NDA

Since 1962, *New Drug Applications* (NDAs) have been required for all investigational drugs that the sponsor would like to market. The NDA must account for every patient who received the investigational agent and document adequate safety. Clear efficacy must be established in at least two different "pivotal" studies, and no patient may be excluded retrospectively from efficacy analysis. The FDA review of the NDA always takes months, and usually years. The average cost of bringing a new drug through the FDA approval process is $50 million.

COMMERCIAL SPONSORSHIP

The FDA is an impartial and expert reviewing body that would presumably approve any NDA demonstrating reliable and sterile manufacture of a safe and effective new drug, no matter who the sponsor was. However, the magnitude of effort required to gain FDA approval is such that commercial sponsorship will be a virtual necessity for each surface active material marketed in the United States. (Except in rare circumstances, FDA approval must be obtained before any new drug can be sold.) Universities simply do not have the resources or expertise to manufacture drugs under sterile conditions on a large scale, or to conduct the required toxicologic testing under the code of Good Laboratory Practices. Further, although many universities do have expertise in the design and conduct of large scale multicenter trials, few have the resources to fund such studies on the bet that the drug being studied will provide safe and effective therapy for the disease being treated. Thus, surface-active materials lacking commercial sponsorship may have great scientific interest, but it is unlikely that they will ever be available for routine clinical use.

The question then becomes: Why do certain surface active materials have commercial sponsorship (see below) and others not? The answer is that any pharmaceutical firm developing a pulmonary surfactant replacement has to bet large sums of money that the surface-active material it is studying has certain advantages over other competing materials, and that these advantages will lead to FDA approval (and eventual recovery of the large financial investment the firm has made). Apparently, for one reason or another, the surface-active materials considered below that lack commercial sponsorship are not currently seen by the pharmaceutical industry as having sufficient advantages over other known surface-active materials to warrant sponsorship.

TYPES OF PULMONARY SURFACTANT REPLACEMENTS

Natural Surfactants

Three types of natural pulmonary surfactant are being tested. Human surfactant, isolated from pooled amniotic fluid,[97,117] should have high efficacy, but its production depends on the availability of amniotic fluid, and its use carries the theoretical risk of infection, including herpes, AIDS, and cytomegalovirus. Studies of amniotic fluid-derived human pulmonary surfactant are apparently being conducted without commercial sponsorship, although substantial financial support has been received from the FDA under the Orphan Product Law. Natural pulmonary surfactant harvested from cow[118] and pig[119] lungs may have an efficacy near that of human surfactant, and should be less expensive to produce, but the introduction of foreign proteins into the lungs of premature infants may have unexpected effects. It appears that heterologous pulmonary surfactants are also being studied without commercial sponsorship.

Semisynthetic Surfactants

The addition of certain chemicals to natural cow or pig surfactant may enhance batch uniformity,[120] efficacy, or yield without greatly increasing costs. However, the potential problem of foreign protein administration to the premature infant remains, since a protein component is present in all preparations containing natural surfactant. The protein component indeed appears to be crucial for function of the semisynthetic Surfactant TA,[40,120,121,122] and is, in fact, the 5 kD bovine apoprotein.[40] Tokyo Tanabe Pharmaceutical (Tokyo, Japan) is developing Surfactant TA in Japan in collaboration with Akita University. Under a license from Tokyo Tanabe, Abbott Laboratories (Chicago, Illinois) is sponsoring European trials with Surfactant TA, and Ross Laboratories (Columbus, Ohio), a subsidiary of Abbott Laboratories, is sponsoring American trials of Surfactant TA.

Synthetic Surfactants

Synthetic surfactants[106,108] have relatively low production costs, lack biologic hazards, and have long shelf-lives. However, the efficacy of synthetic surfactants is markedly dependent on their chemical composition. Even the best currently available synthetic surfactants may not be as efficacious as human pulmonary surfactant. The only synthetic surfactant known to have commercial sponsorship is EXOSURF, which was invented by John Clements, M.D. Pursuant to an agreement with the University of California, Burroughs Wellcome, Co. is developing EXOSURF. Large scale clinical trials are underway at several academic institutions in the United States and Canada. For a brief summary of EXOSURF, see Appendix A.

Genetically Engineered Human Pulmonary Surfactant

In the long run, it is possible that human pulmonary surfactant produced by genetic engineering will eventually become the standard surfactant for replacement therapy. Several groups have isolated surfactant apoproteins,[44,123–125] and at least two groups have cloned apoprotein genes.[46–48] Human pulmonary surfactant produced by genetic engineering should provide effective and safe surface active material of reproducible composition, using pure, pathogen-free components. However, much work remains to be done on the number of proteins to employ and the optimum lipid and protein proportions. In addition, the production of genetically engineered human surfactant is likely to be relatively expensive.

California Biotechnology Inc. (Mountain View, California), a small but highly effective genetic engineering firm, has licensed the European patent rights for its recombinant lung surfactant protein to Byk Gulden Lomberg Chemische Fabrik (Konstanz, West Germany). In the United States, California Biotechnology is apparently developing its recombinant lung surfactant protein on its own, and has recently received three substantial Small Business Innovative Research grants from the NIH to further study its discovery. Presumably, California Biotechnology is combining its recombinant lung surfactant protein with DPPC and perhaps other lipids to form an effective pulmonary surfactant replacement. However, clinical trials with California Biotechnology's genetically engineered human surfactant appear to be some distance off. In the interim, it appears that either a synthetic surfactant[106,108] or a semisynthetic surfactant[40,120–122] will be the first surfactant replacement approved by the FDA for use in the United States.

CLINICAL TRIAL RESULTS

Excluding three early trials of aerosolized DPPC,[20,126,127] and one trial of aerosolized DPPC plus PG,[128] at least 32 reports[97,117–119,129–154] have been published describing pulmonary surfactant replacement therapy with at least 10 different surface active materials[119,129,130,132,137,142,143,145,147,148] in approximately 1,660 treated and control patients (Tables 2-5 and 2-6). Surface active material has been administered both as prophylaxis (immediately after birth in premature infants at high risk of developing NRDS, in attempt to prevent the disease) (Table 2-6) and as rescue therapy (in infants with established NRDS) (Table 2-5). Both approaches have validity, and both approaches are subject to criticism. It

Table 2.5. Summary of Publications on NRDS Treatment with Surface Active Materials in Neonates

	Reference	Author	Year	Design	Blinded	Dose	Total No. Patients
Natural surfactants							
Human	129	Hallman	1983	Uncontrolled	No	60 mg/kg	5
	117	Hallman	1985	Randomized controlled	No	60 mg (3cc) minimum, or 60 mg/kg	53
Bovine	130	Smyth	1981	Uncontrolled	No	8 ml	3
	131	Smyth	1983	Uncontrolled	No	8 ml (200 mg)	6
Porcine	119	Berggren	1984	Uncontrolled	No	1.5 ml (120 mg)	4
Semisynthetic							
Bovine	132	Fujiwara	1980	Uncontrolled	No	120 mg/kg ~10 cc	10
	133	Fujiwara	1981	Uncontrolled	No	(6–8 cc/kg)	22
	134	Fujiwara	1984	Randomized controlled	No	Not stated	30
	135	Fujiwara	1984	Controlled, not randomized	No	~120 mg/kg (3–4 ml/kg)	42
	136 152	Anderson Raju	1986	Randomized controlled	Yes	100 mg/kg (3.3 cc)	30
	151	Gitlin	1987	Randomized controlled	No	100 mg/kg (3.3 ml/kg)	41
Porcine	137	Kobyashi	1981	Uncontrolled	No	50 mg	1
	138	Ohta	1981	Uncontrolled	No	—	1
	139	Nohara	1983	Uncontrolled	No	10–44 mg	6
Synthetic	140 141	Wilkinson Wilkinson	1982 1985	Randomized controlled	No	25 mg	24
	142	Friedman	1982	Uncontrolled	No	25–50 mg/kg	3
	143	Milner	1983	Uncontrolled	No	25 mg × 2	10
	144	Weintraub	1985	Uncontrolled	No	25–75 mg (1–3 cc)	22
Totals	20	Publications					313

NRDS, neonatal respiratory distress syndrome; BPD, bronchopulmonary dysplasia; PIE, pulmonary pressure; L/S, lecithin/sphingomyelin ratio; PDA, patent ductus arteriosus; IVH, intraventricular hem-

No. Surfactant	No. Control	No. Excluded	Entry Criteria	Results	Remarks
5	0	0		↑ PaO_2 ↓ FiO_2	Lasted 8–15 hrs.
25	28	8	< 1500 g < 10 hrs of age on ventilator Severe NRDS	↓ death or BPD ↓ PIE ↓ pneumothorax ↓ FiO_2 > 3 for > 30 days	9 retreated
3	0	0	Severe NRDS	↑ PaO_2 ↓ FiO_2	Transient CXR clearing
6	0	0	Not stated	↑ a/A gradient CXRs improved	lasted up to 24 hours
4	0	0	Severe NRDS	Gas exchange ↑	CXRs improved
10	0	0	NRDS	↑ PaO_2 ↓ $PaCO_2$	9 developed PDA, 8 survived
19	3	0	NRDS	↑ PO_2/FiO_2 ↓ FiO_2	↑ PDA
20	10	0	NRDS	↓ A/aPO_2 gradient CXRs cleared ↓ MAP	Early CXRs appeared better ↑ PDA
37	5	6	NRDS	↓ MAP ↓ FiO_2	↑ PDA
17	13	0	750–1750 g NRDS MAP ≥ 8 a/A PO_2 ratio ≤ .25 < 6 hrs age	↑ survival without BPD ↓ FiO_2 ↓ A/a gradient ↓ pneumothorax ↓ PIE	↑ PDA
18	23	0	> 1000 < 1500 g on mech. ventilation FiO_2 > 0.4 NRDS < 8 hours old	↓ pneumothorax ↓ days in O_2 ↓ days FiO_2 > 0.4	↓ Small study Very high MAP at start, 1.5 cc intratracheal NaCl to controls
1	0	0	NRDS	CXRs improved ↑ PaO_2/FiO_2 ratio ↓ $PaCO_2$	surfactant CK interstitial emphysema
1	0	0	—	—	
6	0	0	NRDS	↑ PaO_2 in 4/6 CXRs improved	surfactant CK lasted 1–21 hrs
12	17	0	NRDS < 32 wks	No effect × ↑ L/S	Morley's surfactant as a powder Type II error
3	0	0	NRDS	CXRs cleared in 2/3	4 components including DPPC & cholesterol 2 airleaks, 1 PDA, IVH
10	0	0	NRDS	No change in compliance or blood gases	Morley's surfactant as a powder
22	0	0	NRDS ≥20 cm PIP FiO_2 ≥ .6	↓ A/a gradient ↓ $PaCO_2$ ↓ PIP	7:3 DPPC:PG 8 died 3–6 hrs. improvement 7 treated twice 3 treated thrice
219	99	14			

interstitial emphysema; CXR, chest radiography; MAP, mean airway pressure; PIP, peak inspiratory orrhage; DPPC, dipalmitoyl phosphatidyl choline; PG, phosphatidylglcerol.

Table 2.6. Summary of Publications on Prophylactic Use of Surface Active Material in Neonates

Surfactant	Reference	Author	Year	Design	Blinded	Dose
Natural						
Human	97	Merritt	1986	Controlled randomized	Yes	60 mg (3 cc)
Bovine	118	Enhorning	1985	Controlled randomized	+/−	< 29 wks: 75 mg (3 cc) 27–29 wks: 100 mg (4 cc)
	145	Kwong	1985	Controlled randomized	Yes	90 mg (3 cc)
	146	Shapiro	1985	Controlled randomized	Yes	90 mg (3 cc)
Semisynthetic Bovine	147	Halliday	1984	Controlled randomized	Yes	33 mg (3–5 cc)
Synthetic	148	Morley	1981	Controlled, not randomized	Yes	25 mg (1 capsule)
	140 141	Wilkinson	1982	Randomized controlled	No	25 mg
	149	Morley	1985		Yes	25–50 mg
	150	Milner	1984	Controlled randomized	No	25 mg (1 cc) po 25 mg (1 cc) tracheal
	153	Morley	1987	Controlled randomized	Yes	100 mg in 1 cc
	154	Ten Centre Study Group	1987	Controlled randomized	Yes	100 mg (1 cc)
Total	12	Publications				

makes sense to attempt to prevent NRDS by the prophylactic administration of surface active material, given the fact that serious lung damage has been observed as early as 30 minutes after birth in premature animal NRDS models[114]; on the other hand, prophylactically treating all infants at substantial risk of developing NRDS with surface active material will entail administration of the material to a segment of the population not destined to develop NRDS. Any adverse effects of prophylactic treatment discovered in infants who do not have a deficiency of pulmonary surfactant will have to be far outweighed by the benefits proven in sur-

Total No. Patients	No. Surfactant	No. Control	No. Excluded	Entry Criteria	Results	Remarks
64	31	29	4	24–29 wks LS < 2.0 or immature profile	↓ Death ↓ BPD ↓ pneumothorax ↓ PIE ↓ time NICU	22 retreated
72	39	33	0	< 30 weeks	↓ Death ↓ IVH ↓ PIE ↓ pneumothorax	Higher no. males in control group
27	14	13	0	24–28 wks	↓ NRDS at 48 hrs ↓ FiO_2 ↓ ventilatory support	Saline control
32	16	16	0	25–29 wks	↓ Severity of NRDS at 12 and 24 hrs only	Saline control
100	49	51	0	25–33 wks	Inconclusive	9:1 DPPC:serum lipoprotein
58	22	33	3	< 34 wks	↓ Death	More males in control group 7:3 DPPC: PG powder
32	16	16	0	< 32 weeks resuscitated	No effect × ↑ L/S	Morley's surfactant
129	Not stated	Not stated	Not stated	< 35 weeks gestation requiring intubation at birth	↓ Death from 20% to 3%	7:3 DPPC: PG powder
22	10	6	6	< 34 weeks required intubation	No effect on lung mechanics	Morley's surfactant
463*	243*	220*	—	25–34 wks	↓ Mortality < 30 weeks	Morley's surfactant
328*	159*	149*	20	25–29 wks	↓ Mortality ↓ IVH ↓ Ventilator hours	Morley's surfactant
1,347	599	566	33			Saline control

Abbreviations same as Table 2.5.
* Overlapping patients.

factant-deficient infants for prophylactic treatment to be justified. Similarly, it makes sense to give surface-active material as rescue treatment to infants with established NRDS, since the absence or ineffectiveness of natural pulmonary surfactant is thought to be responsible for the disease; however, the administration of surface-active material only after NRDS is well established is likely to be far less effective than either prophylactic or early rescue administration, given the damaging effects of high oxygen concentrations and mechanical ventilation in the premature lung.[114]

DPPC

The first published report of surfactant replacement was by Robillard et al. in 1964[20]; nebulized DPPC appeared to have no dramatic effects on NRDS in 11 infants. The eight survivors were said to improve somewhat. Three years later, Chu et al.[126] reported nebulized DPPC to lack dramatic efficacy in NRDS in 15 infants who received 43 courses of therapy. Total lung compliance improved after 34 courses, but oxgenation and carbon dioxide exchange did not. Seven of 15 infants were thought to improve; 5 of the 15 survived. These early studies suggested that effective surfactant replacement therapy would require replacement with more than just the major lipid fraction of natural surfactant. In 1976, Shannon et al.[127] reported the aerosol administration of 20 ml of 1 percent DPPC to 20 infants three times at 8 hour intervals; the infants' A-a gradient improved, but their CO_2 exchange did not.

Natural Pulmonary Surfactants

The first preliminary report of natural pulmonary surfactant administration in NRDS appeared in 1981.[130] The first full reports appeared two years later.[129,131] In an uncontrolled study, a single dose of 8 ml of natural cow[131] surfactant isolated by lung lavage was administered to six infants with NRDS at an average of 15.5 hours after birth. Improvement was apparent for 2 to 4 hours, but waned. In another uncontrolled study,[129] human surfactant isolated from amniotic fluid was administered in doses of 60 mg/kg to five infants with severe NRDS; four of the five infants improved markedly. Five minutes after surfactant administration, the mean PaO_2 increased from 69 to 239 mmHg.[129] Within 1 hour, the FiO_2 was reduced from a mean of 94 percent to 49 percent. These beneficial effects wore off within 8 to 15 hours.[129]

In 1985, Hallman et al.[117] reported a randomized, prospective trial of the treatment with amniotic-fluid-derived human pulmonary surfactant of established NRDS in 53 infants of less than 1500 g weight at birth and less than 10 hours of age, who required mechanical ventilation. Twenty-five infants received surfactant (60 mg minimum, 60 mg/kg if the birth weight was greater than 1 kg, dissolved in 3 cc 0.6 percent NaCl) and 28 infants served as controls. Eight infants were excluded from the efficacy analysis for one reason or another (three treated infants and five control infants). Surfactant was administered at an average of 5.1 hours after birth. Retreatment was performed in nine infants. Neither death nor bronchopulmonary dysplasia alone were significantly reduced by treatment with the amniotic fluid-derived human pulmonary surfactant, but the combined endpoint of death or bronchopulmonary dysplasia (BPD) did appear to be reduced. Death or bronchopulmonary dysplasia occurred in 6 of 22 surfactant-treated infants and 14 of 23 control infants ($P<0.019$). However, it remains unclear whether the combined endpoint of death or bronchopulmonary dysplasia was defined prospectively or retrospectively; if the latter is the case, reduction in death or BPD has not been adequately demonstrated. In any case, only one of 22 treated and 7 of 23 control infants developed pneumothorax ($P<0.025$); and none of 22 treated and 5 of 23 control infants developed pulmonary interstitial emphysema ($P<0.028$). No significant difference in the incidence of intraventricular hemorrhage could be documented. Assuming that the exclusion of the eight patients didn't bias the results, these findings are good evidence that amniotic fluid-derived human pulmonary surfactant can improve the outcome of established NRDS. However, other studies will have to confirm these results, and the optimum dosages and treatment schedules will have to be determined.

In 1986, Merritt et al.[97] reported a randomized, prospective trial of prophylactic administration of amniotic fluid-derived human pulmonary surfactant in 60 infants born at 24 to 29 weeks gestation. Thirty-one infants received human surfactant, 29 infants served as controls. Mortality was reduced from 52 percent to 16 percent ($p<0.001$); there was a trend toward a reduction in bronchopulmonary dysplasia (31 percent vs 16 percent), and significantly fewer cases of pulmonary interstitial emphysema ($P<0.001$) and pneumothorax ($p<0.01$). The duration of neonatal intensive care was also substantially reduced. The curious finding in this study was the very high death rate in the control group, (52 percent); a control group death rate of 10 percent to 20 percent might be expected in most nurseries with a patient population whose average birth weight was 964 g. In any case, this study constitutes impressive evidence that the prophylactic administration of an effective surfactant replacement should have beneficial effects in extremely premature infants at high risk of NRDS.

In 1985, only transitory reductions in respiratory support were reported for the prophylactic administration of cow lung surfactant by Shapiro et al.[146] and by Kwong et al.,[145] but the studies were relatively small, with 32 and 27 patients, respectively. Kwong et al. did demonstrate a reduction in NRDS at 48 hours of age (2 of 14 treated infants, 7 of 13 controls, $P = 0.03$).

Thus, both bovine and amniotic fluid-derived human pulmonary surfactants also appear to hold significant promise in the treatment of NRDS. However, production of amniotic fluid-derived human pulmonary surfactant on a scale sufficient to supply the population at large would be an arduous task. Amniotic fluid from 212 mothers was required to isolate enough surfactant to treat 25 babies in Hallman and co-workers' 1985 report.[117] Further, even the possibility of transmitting an occult maternal infection such as AIDS will force the preparation of equivalent alternatives.

Semisynthetic Surfactants

The leading semisynthetic surfactant was discovered by Fujiwara, and is now known as Surfactant TA. TA stands for the collaboration of Tokyo *T*anabe Pharmaceutical and *A*kita University. In 1979, Fujiwara et al.[132] published an uncontrolled study of semisynthetic surfactant administration (10 ml, 105 mg//kg) (cow lung surfactant with added DPPC and PG) to 10 infants with NRDS at a mean of 12.3 hours after birth. The infants' arterial oxygenation improved markedly; the FiO_2 was decreased a mean of 81 percent within 3 hours. The mean arterial PO_2 increased from 45 to 212 mmHg; the mean arterial PCO_2 fell from 50 to 33 mmHg. However, this dramatic improvement was transitory, and although 8 of 10 infants survived, 9 of 10 developed a significant patent ductus arteriosus. Other publications on Surfactant TA have followed.[133–136,151,152] Supplemental PG was removed from Surfactant TA in about 1984.[135] In a preliminary report published in 1986, Anderson and colleagues described the first blinded controlled rescue trial of Surfactant TA administration; 30 infants were studied, 17 of whom were randomized to Surfactant TA.[136] The full report appeared recently.[152] Surfactant TA improved the survival rate, pneumothorax and pulmonary interstitial emphysema, as well as the FiO_2 and A-a ratio; the risk of patent ductus arteriosus was increased.[152] In an unblinded but randomized and controlled trial of Surfactant TA in 41 babies less than 8 hours of age with established NRDS, and FiO_2 above 0.4, and receiving mechanical ventilation, 18 of whom received Surfactant TA and 23 of whom served as controls, pneumothorax and days on oxygen were significantly reduced, but other endpoints, including BPD and death, were not affected. One advantage of current Surfactant TA over natural surfactants appears to be improved batch-to-batch uniformity in chemical content and surface-tension-reducing properties.[120]

Surfactant CK is another Japanese semisynthetic surfactant,[137–139] but surfactant CK is derived from pig lung rather than cow lung. Calcium chloride ($CaCl_2$) is added to natural pig surfactant to create surfactant CK.[135–137] Initial uncontrolled studies of this product appear to indicate beneficial effects.[135–137]

In 1984, Halliday and colleagues[147] reported a randomized, controlled trial of another semisynthetic surfactant (a mixture of DPPC and serum lipoprotein in a 10 : 1 ratio), administered at birth to prevent NRDS in 100 babies of less than 34 weeks gestation. By chance, the two groups were not equivalent; L/S ratios below 2 were present in 24 percent of the treatment group and 51 percent of the control group. Doses of 5 cc were administered intratracheally (30 mg DPPC, 3 mg protein). No benefit could be documented, but with a sample size of 50 subjects per group, the study had just over a 50 percent chance of detecting reduction in the incidence of NRDS from 50 percent to 30 percent. In any case, the physicochemical properties of the surfactant were not ideal, and no testing in animal models of NRDS was done beforehand to prove its efficacy.

Thus, at least Fujiwara's semisynthetic Surfactant TA appears to hold significant promise in the management of NRDS. Large scale, prospective, randomized, controlled studies of Surfactant TA are underway in Europe and North America.

Synthetic Surfactants

The first study of synthetic surfactant in the treatment of established NRDS was an uncontrolled trial carried out by Ivey et al.,[128] who gave a 9 : 1 mixture of DPPC/PG to six babies a total of 18 times. The infants' FiO_2 decreased 6 percent, and the PaO_2 increased 17 percent. In 1981, Morley et al.[148] were the first to report a prophylactic trial of surfactant replacement therapy in NRDS; a dry synthetic surfactant powder was used. The study was controlled but not adequately randomized, because treatment depended upon whether the investigators were available at the time of delivery of an infant or not. Twenty-two infants received a single dose of 25 mg of surfactant, and 33 infants served as controls. The synthetic surfactant used (7 : 3, DPPC : PG) had the physiochemical properties similar to those of natural surfactant. Although the treatment group had a nearly equal sex distribution, there were 21 males and 12 females among the controls. Only infants between 27 and 29 weeks demonstrated dramatic benefit. No treated infants died, whereas 8 of 33 control infants died. In other reports, Wilkinson et al. could find no benefit of Morley's artificial surfactant administered either prophylactically (to 16 of 32 babies) or therapeutically (to 12 of 24 babies).[140,141] However, even if 43 babies per group had been randomized in each study, there still would have been only a 50 percent chance of detecting a reduction in the incidence of NRDS or its complications from 50 percent to 30 percent. Similarly, Milner, Vyas, and Hopkin[143] could demonstrate no immediate improvement in pulmonary compliance after administration of Morley's surfactant to 10 infants with established NRDS. Later, these same investigators also looked at the prophylactic administration of Morley's surfactant[150] in 22 babies (15 treated, 7 saline controls). Again, no improvement in total respiratory system compliance could be demonstrated.[150] In preliminary accounts of a 341-baby trial in which Morley's surfactant was administered prophylactically at birth, reductions in NRDS and mortality were apparently observed.[151] A full report has not yet been published.

Weintraub et al. reported an uncontrolled study of a synthetic identical in composition to Morley's[144]; transient improvements in gas exchange were seen. Another uncontrolled study of a synthetic surfactant with a different composition was also published in preliminary form in 1982[142]; chest radiographs of the subjects were said to improve.

Thus, in early trials, synthetic surfactants do not appear to be as promising in NRDS as natural and semisynthetic surfactants, but each synthetic surfactant will have to be judged on its own merits, and rigorously designed and executed studies of sufficient power to detect important but less than miraculous effects will have to be completed. As mentioned above, large scale clinical trials with the promising synthetic surfactant EXOSURF[106,108] (Appendix A) are underway.

Genetically Engineered Human Pulmonary Surfactant

Initial clinical trials with genetically engineered surfactants are probably still 2 or 3 years away, but as discussed above, the rationale for and likelihood of success with gentically engineered human pulmonary surfactants are strong.

CONCLUSION

Studies of the replacement of surface active material indicate that pulmonary surfactant replacement will be a dramatic advance (but not a panacea) in the evolving management of NRDS. Few drugs have been tested in children before being tested in adults, and probably none have been given initially to newborns. Nevertheless, pulmonary surfactant replacement therapy in NRDS holds such promise, and NRDS carries such morbidity that the FDA could reasonably be expected to accord pulmonary surfactant substitutes fairly high priority at all stages of review. Pulmonary surfactant replacements should be available in the United States for routine clinical use in NRDS by 1990.

APPENDIX A: EXOSURF: A SYNTHETIC SURFACTANT

History

Natural pulmonary surfactant, a combination of lipids and protein, exhibits not only surface-tension-reducing properties, but also rapid spreading and adsorption. The major fraction of the lipid component of natural surfactant is dipalmitoylphosphatidylcholine (DPPC), which composes up to 70 percent of natural surfactant by weight. Phosphatidylglycerol, which is a useful biochemical marker for surfactant, has been shown to be unnecessary for good surfactant function. Although DPPC by itself markedly reduces surface tension, DPPC alone is ineffective in NRDS because DPPC spreads and adsorbs poorly. The rapid spreading and adsorption necessary for normal natural surfactant function are conferred by the apoproteins. EXOSURF is a totally synthetic surfactant patented by John Clements, M.D., in 1982. Since alcohols spread rapidly on the surface of water, Dr. Clements postulated that adding an alcohol to the major lipid fraction of natural surfactant, dipalmitoylphosphatidylcholine (DPPC), might create an effective synthetic surfactant. In this sense, the alcohol constituent of EXOSURF serves the same function as the apoprotein moieties of natural surfactant.

Composition

EXOSURF is a 13.5 : 1.5 : 1 mixture of DPPC, hexadecanol (cetyl alcohol), and tyloxapol [formaldehyde polymer with oxirane and 4-(1,1,3,3,-tetramethylbutyl) phenol].

Formulation

EXOSURF has been formulated as a sterile, lyophilized powder stored under vaccuum. Each 10 cc vial contains:

DPPC	108 mg
Hexadecanol	12 mg
Sodium chloride	46.75 mg
Tyloxapol	8 mg

When reconstituted with 8 cc sterile water, the EXOSURF suspension contains 13.5 mg/cc DPPC, 1.5 mg/cc hexadecanol, and 1 mg/cc tyloxapol in 0.1 N NaCl. The reconstituted EXOSURF suspension has an osmolality of 190 mOsm/liter.

Biophysics

EXOSURF rapidly lowers surface tension with a time constant of 0.7 seconds, reproducibly gives low surface tension on compression (from 0 to 10 mN/m), and generates extremely stable surface films (foam test stability beyond 8 days).

Toxicology

Formal toxicology studies have been completed in three species. EXOSURF had no significant pulmonary or systemic toxicity in rabbits, rats, or monkeys.

Pharmacology

In lungs excised from premature rabbit pups,[106] in a premature rabbit model of NRDS,[106] and in a premature lamb model of NRDS,[108] EXOSURF significantly improved lung volumes and compliance. Gas exchange was also significantly improved in both premature rabbits[106] and premature lambs.[108] Neither the amount nor distribution of lung water were affected by the EXOSURF treatment of premature rabbit pups.[106] The extent of lung injury in premature rabbit pups undergoing mechanical ventilation was significantly reduced by EXOSURF treatment.[106] In premature lambs neither systemic blood flow or pulmonary blood flow, nor ductal shunting, were affected by EXOSURF treatment.[108] Survival was significantly better in both premature rabbits[106] and premature lambs treated with EXOSURF.[108]

Neither EXOSURF nor its components appeared to have significant irritancy potential in rat models of inflammation.

Clinical Trials

Studies of both EXOSURF prophylaxis at birth to prevent RDS (single dose, 5 cc/kg), and EXOSURF treatment of established RDS (two doses, totaling 5 cc/kg, administered over 1 minute), are currently being conducted.

REFERENCES

1. Comroe J: Premature science and immature lungs. I. Some premature discoveries. Am Rev Respir Dis 116:127, 1977
2. Comroe J: Premature science and immature lungs. II. Chemical warfare and the newly born. Am Rev Respir Dis 116:311, 1977
3. Comroe J: Premature science and immature lungs. III. The attack on immature lungs. Am Rev Respir Dis 116:497, 1977
4. von Neergaard K: New concepts about a basis of breathing mechanism. The power of retraction of the lung dependent on surface tension in alveoli. Zeit fdges Ext Med 66:373, 1929
5. Gruenwald P: Surface tension as a factor in the resistance of neonatal lungs to aeration. Am J Obstet Gynecol 53:996, 1947
6. Radford EP, Jr: Method for estimating respiratory surface area of mammalian lungs from their physical characteristics. Proc Soc Exp Biol Med 87:58, 1954
7. Pattle RE: Properties, function and origin of the alveolar lining layer. Nature 175:1125, 1955
8. Clements JA: Dependence of pressure-volume characteristics of lungs on intrinsic surface active material. Am J Physiol 187:592, 1956
9. Clements JA: Surface tension of lung extracts. Proc Soc Exp Biol Med 95:170, 1957
10. Pattle RE, Thomas LC: Lipoprotein composition of the film lining the lung. Nature 189:844, 1961
11. Buckingham S: Studies on the identification of an antiatelectasis factor in normal sheep lung. Am J Dis Child 102:521, 1961
12. Klaus MH, Clements JA, Havel RJ: Composition of surface-active material isolated from beef lung. Proc Natl Acad Sci USA 47:1858, 1961
13. King RJ, Clements JA: Surface-active materials from dog lung. II. Composition and physiological correlations. Am J Physiol 223:715, 1972
14. King RJ, Klass DJ, Gikas EG, Clements JA: Isolation of apoproteins from canine surface active material. Am J Physiol 224:788, 1973
15. Macklin CC: The pulmonary alveolar mucoid film and the pneumonocytes. Lancet 266:1099, 1954
16. Low FN: The electron microscopy of sectioned lung tissue after varied duration of fixation in buffered osmium tetroxide. Anat Rec 120:827, 1954
17. Buckingham S, Avery ME: Time of appearance of lung surfactant in the foetal mouse. Nature 193:688, 1962
18. Klaus M, Reiss OK, Tooley WJ, et al: Alveolar epithelial cell mitochondria as source of the surface-active lung lining. Science 137:750, 1962
19. Avery ME, Mead J: Surface properties in relation to atelectasis and hyaline membrane disease. Am J Dis Child 97:517, 1959
20. Robillard E, Alaire Y, Dagenais-Perusse P, et al: Microaerosol administration of synthetic beta-gamma-dipalmitoyl-L-alpha-lecithin in the respiratory distress syndrome: A preliminary report. Can Med Assoc J 90:55, 1964
21. Liggins GC: Premature delivery of foetal lambs infused with glucocorticoids. J Endocrinol 45:515, 1969
22. Liggins GC, Howie RN: A controlled trial of antepartum glucocorticoid treatment for prevention of the respiratory distress syndrome in premature infants. Pediatrics 50:515, 1972
23. Collaborative group on antenatal steroid therapy: Effect of antenatal dexamethasone administration on the presentation of respiratory distress syndrome. Am J Obstet Gynecol 141:276, 1981

24. Avery ME: The argument for prenatal administration of dexamethasone to prevent respiratory distress syndrome. J Pediatr 104:240, 1984
25. Kero P, Hirvonen T, Talimaki I: Prenatal and postnatal isoxsuprine in respiratory distress syndrome. Lancet 2:198, 1973 (Letter)
26. Bergman B, Hedner T: Antepartum administration of terbutaline and the incidence of hyaline membrane disease in preterm infants. Acta Obstet Gynecol Scand 57:217, 1978
27. Boog G, Brahim M Ben, Gandar R: Beta-mimetic drugs and possible prevention of respiratory distress syndrome. Br J Obstet Gynaecol 82:285, 1975
28. Ekelund L, Enhorning G: Pulmonary surfactant release in fetal rabbits as affected by enprofylline. Pediatr Res 19:1000, 1985
29. Ekelund L, Enhorning G: Glucocorticoids and β-adrenergic-receptor agonists: Their combined effect on fetal rabbit lung surfactant. Am J Obstet Gynecol 152:1063, 1985
30. Corbet AJ, Kolni HW, Perreault T, et al: Development of β-adrenergic control of phospholipid secretion in rabbit lung. J Appl Physiol 58:2011, 1985
31. Hallman M, Teramo K, Sipinen S, Raivio K: Effects of betamethasone and ritodrine on the fetal secretion of lung surfactant. J Perinat Med 13:23, 1985
32. Sanders RL: The composition of pulmonary surfactant. p. 193. In Farrell PM (ed): Lung Development: Biological and Clinical Perspectives. Vol. 1. Academic Press, New York, 1982
33. King RJ: The surfactant system of the lung. Fed Proc 33:2238, 1974
34. Sanders RL: Major phospholipids in surfactant. p. 211. In Farrell PM (ed): Lung Development: Biological and Clinical Perspectives. Vol 1. Academic Press, New York, 1982
35. Sanders RL, Longmore WJ: Phosphatidylglycerol in rat lung. II. Comparison of occurrence, composition and metabolism in surfactant and residual lung fractions. Biochemistry 14:835, 1975
36. Bustos P, Kulovich MV, Gluck L, et al: Significance of phosphatidylglycerol in amniotic fluid in complicated pregnancies. Am J Obstet Gynecol 133:899, 1979
37. Beppu OS, Clements JA, Goerke J: Phosphatidylglycerol-deficient lung surfactant has normal properties. J Appl Physiol 55:496, 1983
38. Hallman M, Enhorning G, Possmayer F: Composition and surface activity of normal and phosphatidylglycerol-deficit lung surfactant. Pediatr Res 19:286, 1985
39. Sahu SC, Lynn WS: A high molecular weight alveolar glycoprotein in human amniotic fluid. Lung 157:71, 1980
40. Takahashi A, Fujiwara T: Proteolipid in bovine lung surfactant: Its role in surfactant function. Biochem Biophys Res Commun 135:527, 1986
41. King RJ, Martin H, Mitts D, Holmstrom FM: Metabolism of the apoproteins in pulmonary surfactant. J Appl Physiol 42:483, 1977
42. King RJ, Martin M: Intracellar metabolism of the apoproteins of pulmonary surfactant in rat lung. J Appl Physiol 48:812, 1980
43. Katyal SL, Amenta JS, Singh G, Silverman JA: Deficient lung surfactant apoproteins in amniotic fluid with mature phospholipid profile from diabetic pregnancies. Am J Obstet Gynecol 148:48, 1984
44. Whitsett JA, Hull WM, Ohning B, et al: Immunologic identification of pulmonary surfactant protein of molecular weight = 6000 daltons. Pediatr Res 20:740, 1986
45. Walker SR, Williams MC, Benson B: Immunocytochemical localization of the major surfactant apoproteins in type II cells, Clara cells, and alveolar macrophages of rat lung. J Histochem Cytochem 34:1137, 1986
46. White RT, Damm D, Miller J, et al: Isolation and characterization of the human pulmonary surfactant apoprotein gene. Nature 317:361, 1985
47. Floros J, Phelps DS, Taeusch HW: Biosynthesis and in vitro translation of the major surfactant-associated protein from human lung. J Biol Chem 260:495, 1985
48. Floros J, Steinbrink R, Jacobs K, et al: Isolation and characterization of cDNA clones for the 35-kDa pulmonary surfactant associated protein. J Biol Chem 261:9029, 1986
49. Gil J, Reiss OK: Isolation and characterization of lamellar bodies and tubular myelin from rat lung homogenates. J Cell Biol 58:152, 1973
50. Sanders RL, Hassett RJ, Vatter AE: Isolation of lung lamellar bodies and their conversion to tubular myelin figures in vitro. Anat Rec 198:485, 1980
51. Paul GW, Sanders RL, Hassett RJ: Kinetics of film formation and surface activity of lamellar bodies (LB), extracted lipids (EL), tubular myelin figures (TMF) and alveolar surfactant (AS) from rat lung. Fed Proc 36:615, 1977
52. Magoon MW, Wright JR, Baritussio A, et al: Subfractionation of lung surfactant. Implications for metabolism and surface activity. Biochim Biophys Acta 750:18, 1983
53. Wright JR, Benson BJ, Williams MC, et al: Protein composition of rabbit alveolar surfactant subfractions. Biochim Biophys Acta 791:320, 1984

54. Benson BJ, Williams MC, Sueishi K, et al: Role of calcium ions in the structure and function of pulmonary surfactant. Biochim Biophys Acta 793:18, 1984
55. Paul GW, Hassett RJ, Reiss OK: Formation of lung surfactant films from intact lamellar bodies. Proc Natl Acad Sci USA 74:3617, 1977
56. Massaro D, Clerch L, Massaro GD: Surfactant aggregation in rat lungs: Influence of temperature and ventilation. J Appl Physiol 51:646, 1981
57. Thet LA, Clerck L, Massaro GD, Massaro D: Changes in the sedimentation of surfactant in ventilated excised rat lungs. J Clin Invest 64:600, 1979
58. Massaro D, Clerch L, Temple D, Baier H: Surfactant deficiency in rats without a decreased amount of extracellular surfactant. J Clin Invest 71:1536, 1983
59. Chevalier G, Collet AJ: In vivo incorporation of choline-^{3}H, leucine-^{3}H, and galactose-^{3}H in alveolar type II pneumocytes in relation to surfactant synthesis. A quantitative radioautographic study in mouse by electron microscopy. Anat Rec 174:289, 1972
60. Weinhold PA: Biosynthesis of phosphatidylcholine during prenatal development of the rat lung. J Lipid Res 9:262, 1968
61. Farrell PM, Epstein MF: Lecithin synthesis in the fetal and neonatal primate lung as measured in vitro. Pediatr Res 8:356, 1974
62. Post M, Batenburg JJ, Schuurmans EA, et al: The rate-limiting step in the biosynthesis of phosphatidylcholine by alveolar type II cells from adult lung. Biochim Biophys Acta 712:390, 1982
63. van Golde LMG: Synthesis of surfactant lipids in the adult lung. Annu Rev Physiol 47:765, 1985
64. Hendry AT, Possmayer F: Pulmonary phospholipid biosynthesis: Properties of a stable microsomal glycerophosphate acyl-transferase preparation from rabbit lung. Biochim Biophys Acta 369:156, 1974
65. Ide H, Weinhold PA: Cholinephosphotransferase in rat lung. The in vitro formation of dipalmitoylphosphatidylcholine and general lack of selectivity using endogenously generated diacylglycerol. J Biol Chem 257:14926, 1982
66. Hallman M, Raivio K: Studies on the biosynthesis of disaturated lecithin of the lung: The importance of the lysolecithin pathway. Pediatr Res 8:874, 1974
67. Jacobs H, Jobe A, Ikegami M, Conway D: The significance of reutilization of surfactant phosphatidylcholine. J Biol Chem 258:4159, 1983
68. Moxley MA, Corpus VM, Westrich D, et al: Evidence of the direct incorporation of pulmonary surfactant into alveolar type II epithelial cells in primary culture. Fed Proc 44:1606, 1985
69. Moxley MA, Longmore WJ: Reutilization of surfactant phosphatidylcholine by isolated adult type II cells in culture. Fed Proc 45:1666, 1986
70. Hallman M, Epstein BL, Gluck L: Analysis of labeling and clearance of lung surfactant phospholipids in rabbit. Evidence of bidirectional surfactant flux between lamellar bodies and alveolar lavage. J Clin Invest 68:742, 1981
71. Oldenborg V, van Golde LMG: The enzymes of phosphatidylcholine biosynthesis in the fetal mouse. Effect of dexamethasone. Biochim Biophys Acta 489:454, 1977
72. Rooney SA, Gross I, Gassenheimer LN, Motoyama EK: Stimulation of glycerophosphate phosphatidyltransferase activity in fetal rabbit lung by cortisol administration. Biochim Biophys Acta 398:433, 1975
73. Possmayer F, Casola F, Chan F, et al: Glucocorticoid induction of pulmonary maturation in the rabbit fetus. The effect of maternal injection of betamethasone on the activity of enzymes in fetal lung. Biochim Biophys Acta 574:197, 1979
74. Giannopoulos G: Glucocorticoid receptors in the lung. I. Specific binding of glucocorticoids to cytoplasmic components of rabbit fetal lung. J Biol Chem 248:3876, 1973
75. Giannopoulos G, Mulay S, Solomon S: Glucocorticoid receptors in lung. II. Specific binding of glucocorticoids to nuclear components of rabbit fetal lung. J Biol Chem 248:5016, 1973
76. Smith BT, Bogues WG: Effects of drugs and hormones on lung maturation in experimental animals and man. Pharmacol Ther 9:51, 1980
77. Hitchcock KR: Lung development and the pulmonary surfactant systems: Hormonal influences. Anat Rec 198:13, 1980
78. Gross I: Regulation of fetal lung maturation: Initiation and modulation. p. 51. In Raivio KO, Hallman N, Kouvalaineu K, Valimaki I (eds): Respiratory Distress Syndrome. Academic Press, London, 1984
79. Dobbs LG, Geppert E, Williams MC, et al: Metabolic properties and ultrastructure of alveolar type II cells isolated with elastase. Biochim Biophys Acta 618:510, 1980
80. Dobbs LG, Gonzalez RF, Marinari LA, et al: The role of calcium in the secretion of surfactant by rat alveolar type II cells. Biochim Biophys Acta 877:305, 1986
81. Mason RJ, Cott GR, Robinson PC, et al: Pharmacology of alveolar Type II cells. Prog Resp Res 18:279, 1984

82. Dobbs LG, Mason RJ: Stimulation of secretion of disaturated phosphatidylcholine from isolated alveolar type II cells by 12-0-tetradecanoyl-13-phorbol acetate. Am Rev Respir Dis 118:705, 1978
83. Oyarzun MJ, Clements JA: Control of lung surfactant by ventilation, adrenergic mediators and prostaglandins in the rabbit. Am Rev Respir Dis 117:879, 1978
84. Dobbs LG, Mason RG: Pulmonary alveolar type II cells isolated from rats. Release of phosphatidylcholine in response to adrenergic stimulation. J Clin Invest 63:378, 1979
85. Goldenberg VE, Buckingham S, Sommers SC: Pilocarpine stimulation of granular pneumocyte secretion. Lab Invest 20:147, 1969
86. Corbet AJ, Flax P, Rudolph AJ: Role of autonomic nervous system controlling surface tension in fetal rabbit lungs. J Appl Physiol 43:1039, 1977
87. Pattle RE: The lining layer of the lung alveoli. Br Med Bull 19:41, 1963
88. Pattle RE: Surface lining of the lung alveoli. Physiol Rev 45:48, 1965
89. Zelig BJ, Nerurkar LS, Bellanti JA: Chemotactic and candidacidal responses of rabbit alveolar macrophages during postnatal development and the modulating roles of surfactant in these responses. Infect Immun 44:379, 1984
90. O'Neill S, Lesperance E, Klass DJ: Rat lung lavage surfactant enhances bacterial phagocytosis and intracellular killing by alveolar macrophages. Am Rev Respir Dis 130:225, 1984
91. O'Neill S, Lesperance E, Kalss DJ: Human lung lavage enhances staphylococcal phagocytosis by alveolar macrophages. Am Rev Respir Dis 130:1177, 1984
92. Jonsson S, Musher DM, Goree A, Lawrence EC: Human alveolar lining material and antibacterial defenses. Am Rev Respir Dis 133:136, 1986
93. Drickamer K, Dordal MS, Reynolds L: Mannaose-binding proteins isolated from rat liver contain carbohydrate-recognition domains linked to collagenous tails. Complete primary structures and homology with pulmonary surfactant apoprotein. J Biol Chem 261:6878, 1986
94. Ikegami M, Jobe A, Jacobs H, Lam R: A protein from airways of premature lambs that inhibits surfactant function. J Appl Physiol 57:1134, 1984
95. Ikegami M, Kaneda M, Nozaki M: A protein inhibitor of surfactant in the airways of patients with adult respiratory distress syndrome. Am Rev Respir Dis 131:A135, 1985
96. Jobe A, Machiko I, Jacobs H, Jones S: Surfactant and pulmonary blood flow distributions following treatment of premature lambs with natural surfactant. J Clin Invest 73:848, 1984
97. Merritt TA, Hallman M, Bloom BT, et al: Prophylactic treatment of very premature infants with human surfactant. N Engl J Med 315:785, 1986
98. Wright JR, Wagner RE, Hamilton RL, et al: Uptake of lung surfactant subfractions into lamellar bodies of adult rabbit lungs. J Appl Physiol 60:817, 1986
99. Dobbs LG, Wright JR, Hawgood S: Surfactant apoproteins inhibit secretion of surfactant by rat alveolar Type II cells in culture. Am Rev Respir Dis 133:A118, 1986
100. Oguchi K, Ikegami M, Jacobs H, Jobe A: Clearance of large amounts of natural surfactants and liposomes of dipalmitoylphosphatidylcholine from the lungs of rabbits. Exp Lung Res 9:221, 1985
101. Jacobs HC, Ikegami M, Jobe AH, et al: Reutilization of surfactant phosphatidylcholine in adult rabbits. Biochim Biophys Acta 837:77, 1985
102. Ikegami M, Jobe A, Duane G: Liposomes of dipalmitoylphosphatidylcholine associate with natural surfactant. Biochim Biophys Acta 835:352, 1985
103. Jacobs H, Jobe A, Ikepami M, et al: Reutilization of phosphatidylcholine analogues by the pulmonary surfactant system. The lack of specificity. Biochim Biophys Acta 793:300, 1984
104. Haagsman HP, van Golde LMG: Lung surfactant and pulmonary toxicology. Lung 163:275, 1985
105. Obladen M, Kampmann W, Zimmerman I, Lachmann B: Artificial surfactant in preterm rabbits with and without respiratory distress syndrome: Difference of in vitro and in vivo activities. Eur J Pediatr 144:195, 1985
106. Tooley WH, Clements JA, Brown CL, et al: Lung function in prematurely delivered rabbits treated with a synthetic surfactant. Am Rev Resp Dis 136:347, 1987
107. Notter RH, Egan EA, Kwong MS, et al: Lung surfactant replacement in premature lambs with extracted lipids form bovine lung lavage: Effects of dose, dispersion technique, and gestational age. Pediatr Res 19:569, 1985
108. Durand DJ, Clyman RI, Heymann MA, et al: Effects of a protein-free, synthetic surfactant on the survival and pulmonary function of preterm lambs. J Pediatr 107:775, 1985
109. Jacobs H, Jobe A, Ikegami M, Jones S: Accumulation of alveolar surfactant following delivery and ventilation of premature lambs. Exp Lung Res 8:125, 1985
110. Hessler JR, Mantilla G, Kirkpatrick BV, et al: Asphyxia and hyaline membrane disease in neonatal monkeys. Am J Perinatol 2:101, 1985
111. Vidyasagar D, Maeta H, Raju TNK, et al: Bovine surfactant (surfactant TA) therapy in immature baboons with hyaline membrane disease. Pediatrics 75:1132, 1985

112. Berggren P, Curstedt T, Grossman G, et al: Surfactant replacement in experimental respiratory distress induced by repeated lung lavage. IRCS Medical Science 11:787, 1983
113. Berggren P, Lachmann B, Crustedt T, et al: Gas exchange and lung morphology after surfactant replacement in experimental adult respiratory distress syndrome induced by repeated lung lavage. Acta Anaesthesiol Scand 30:321, 1986
114. Nilsson R, Grossman G, Robertson B: Bronchiolar epithelial lesions induced in the premature rabbit neonate by short periods of artificial ventilation. Acta Pathol Microbiol Immunol Scand [A] 88:359, 1980
115. Edwards DK, Hilton SvW, Merritt TA, et al: Respiratory distress syndrome treated with human surfactant: Radiographic findings. Radiology 157:329, 1985
116. Merritt TA, Cochrane CG, Hallman M, et al: Reduction of lung injury by human surfactant treatment in respiratory distress syndrome. Chest 83:273, 1983
117. Hallman M, Merritt TA, Jarvenpaa A-L, et al: Exogenous human surfactant for treatment of severe respiratory distress syndrome: A randomized prospective trial. J Pediatr 106:963, 1985
118. Enhorning G, Shennan A, Possmayer F, et al: Prevention of neonatal respiratory distress syndrome by tracheal instillation of surfactant: A randomized clinical trial. Pediatrics 76:145, 1985
119. Berggren P, Curstedt T, Grossman G, et al: Gynnsam effekt av surfaktantbehandling vid IRDS. Lakartidningen 81:4180, 1984
120. Asakura S: Natural surfactant & Surfactant TA. Surface activity of various natural surfactant preparations and their effects on lung-thorax pressure-volume characteristics of premature newborn rabbits: Comparison with Surfactant TA. J Iwate Med Ass 37:563, 1985
121. Taeusch HW, Keough KMW, Williams M, et al: Characterization of bovine surfactant for infants with respiratory distress syndrome. Pediatrics 77:572, 1986
122. Tanaka Y, Takei T, Aiba T, et al: Development of synthetic lung surfactants. J Lipid Res 27:475, 1986
123. Katyal SL, Singh G: In vitro translation of rat lung surfactant apoprotein mRNA. Biochem Biophys Res Commun 127:106, 1985
124. Floros J, Phelps DS, Kourembanas S, Taeusch HW: Primary translation products, biosynthesis, and tissue specificity of the major surfactant protein in rat. J Biol Chem 261:828, 1986
125. Benson B, Hawgood S, Schilling J, et al: Structure of canine pulmonary surfactant apoprotein: cDNA and complete amino acid sequence. Proc Natl Acad Sci USA 82:6379, 1985
126. Chu J, Clements JA, Cotton E, et al: Neonatal pulmonary ischemia. I. Clinical and physiological studies. Pediatrics 40:709, 1967
127. Shannon DC, Bunnell JB: Dipalmitoyl lecithin in IRDS. Pediatr Res 10:467, 1976 (abstract)
128. Ivey HH, Roth S, Kattwinkel J: Use of nebulized surfactant in treatment of the respiratory distress syndrome (RDS) of infancy. Pediatr Res 10:462, 1976 (abstract)
129. Hallman M, Merritt TA, Schneider H, et al: Isolation of human surfactant from amniotic fluid and a pilot study of its efficacy in respiratory distress syndrome. Pediatrics 71:473, 1983
130. Smyth JA, Metcalfe IL, Duffty P, et al: Surfactant therapy in hyaline membrane disease. Pediatr Res 15:681A, 1981
131. Smyth JA, Metcalfe IL, Duffty P, et al: Hyaline membrane disease treated with a bovine surfactant. Pediatrics 71:913, 1983
132. Fujiwara T, Chida S, Watabe Y, et al: Artificial surfactant therapy in hyaline membrane disease. Lancet 1:55, 1980
133. Fujiwara T: Tracheal instillation of artificial surfactants for the treatment of hyaline membrane disease. Ann Nestlé 48:24, 1981
134. Fujiwara T, Konishi M, Chida S, et al: Exogenous surfactant therapy in infants with RDS: Comparison of early vs. late treatment. Pediatr Res 18:353A, 1984
135. Fujiwara T: Surfactant replacement in neonatal RDS. p. 479. In Robertson B, van Colde LMG, Batenburg JJ (eds): Pulmonary Surfactant. Amsterdam, Elsevier, 1984
136. Anderson M, Raju TNK, Vidyasagar D, et al: A double-blind study of surfactant TA (STA) therapy in <1250 g infants with severe hyaline membrane disease. Clin Res 34:978A, 1986
137. Kobayashi T, Kataoka H, Murakami S, et al: A case of idiopathic respiratory distress syndrome treated by a newly developed surfactant (surfactant CK). J Japan Med Soc Biol Interface 12:1, 1981
138. Ohta A, Muramatsu K, Oda T: A case of respiratory distress syndrome treated with surfactant CK. J Japan Med Soc Biol Interface 12;33, 1981
139. Nohara K, Muramatsu K, Oda T: Six cases of RDS treated with surfactant CK. J Japan Med Soc Biol Interface 14:173, 1983
140. Wilkinson AR, Jeffrey JA, Jenkins PA: Controlled trial of dry surfactant in preterm infants. Arch Dis Child 57:802, 1982 (Abstract)

141. Wilkinson A, Jenkins PA, Jeffrey JA: Two controlled trials of artificial surfactant: Early effects and later outcome in babies with surfactant deficiency. Lancet 2:287, 1985
142. Friedman Z, Doody M: Artificial surfactant (AS): A therapeutic trial in infants with hyaline membrane disease (HMD). Pediatr Res 16:287A, 1982
143. Milner AD, Vyas H, Hopkin EI: Effects of artificial surfactant on lung function and blood gases in idiopathic respiratory distress syndrome. Arch Dis Child 58:458, 1983
144. Weintraub Z, Sorokin Y, Flohr E, et al: Surfactant replacement therapy for respiratory distress syndrome. p. 311. In Jones CT, Nathanielsz PW (eds): The Physiological Development of the Fetus and Newborn. Academic Press, London, 1985
145. Kwong MS, Egan EA, Notter RH, Shapiro DL: Double-blind clinical trial of calf lung surfactant extract for the prevention of hyaline membrane disease in extremely premature infants. Pediatrics 76:585, 1985
146. Shapiro DL, Notter RH, Morin FC III, et al: Double-blind, randomized trial of a calf lung surfactant extract administered at birth to very premature infants for prevention of respiratory distress syndrome. Pediatrics 76:593, 1985
147. Halliday HL, McClure G, McCReid M, et al: Controlled trial of artificial surfactant to prevent respiratory distress syndrome. Lancet I:476, 1984
148. Morley CJ, Bangham AD, Miller N, Davis JA: Dry artificial surfactant and its effects on very premature babies. Lancet I:64, 1981
149. Morley CJ: The Cambridge experience of artificial surfactant. p. 279. In Clich J, Mathews T (eds): Perinatal Medicine. MTP Press Limited, Lancaster, England, 1985
150. Milner AD, Vyas GS, Hopkin IE: Effect of exogenous surfactant on total respiratory system compliance. Arch Dis Child 59:369, 1984
151. Gitlin JD, Soll RF, Parad RB, et al: Randomized controlled trial of exogenous surfactant for the treatment of hyaline membrane disease. Pediatrics 79:31, 1987
152. Raju TNK, Bhat R, McCulloch KM, Maeta H, Vidyasagar D, Sobel D, Anderson M, Levy PS: Double-blind controlled trial of single-dose treatment with bovine surfactant in severe hyaline membrane disease. Lancet 1:651, 1987
153. Morley CJ. The cambridge experience of artificial surfactant. p. 255. In Shang L (ed): Proceedings of the International Symposium on the Physiology and Pathophysiology of the Fetal and Neonatal Lung. MTP Press, Lancaster, England, 1987
154. Ten Centre Study Group: Ten centre trial of artificial surfactant (artificial lung expanding compound) in very premature babies. Br Med J 294:991, 1987
155. Harwood JL, Desai R, Hext P, et al: Characterization of pulmonary surfactant from ox, rat and sheep. Biochem J 151:707, 1975

3

New Treatment Methods in Neonatal Respiratory Failure: High-Frequency Oscillatory Ventilation

Robert H. Perelman

Previous advances in neonatal mechanical ventilators have been related to matching of strategies for ventilator use to the unique pulmonary derangements in neonates, and to the technical refinement of conventional ventilatory apparatus for its use in newborns. Enhanced understanding of the pathobiology of neonatal respiratory diseases has also led to some improvements in artificial ventilation. The common clinical goal of these investigative efforts has been to lessen the barotrauma and oxygen toxicity that are antecedent to bronchopulmonary dysplasia (BPD) or chronic lung disease. A less traditional approach to improving the efficacy and efficiency of mechanical respiratory support is high-frequency ventilation. Utilizing very small tidal volumes at extremely rapid rates ranging from 150 to 1,800 cycles per minute, investigators have been able to successfully maintain gas exchange in animals in a fashion that is at least equivalent to normal spontaneous breathing or conventional mechanical ventilation.[1–3] In addition to being a fascinating basic concept for in vitro and in vivo physiologic investigation, high-frequency ventilation (HFV) may have great clinical utility, since effective gas exchange at lower tidal volume and peak inspiratory pressure could reduce pulmonary interstitial emphysema, air leak syndromes, barotrauma, and hence BPD.[4] The potential benefits of HFV are enumerated in Table 3-1.

EARLY HISTORY OF HFV

Although the technique had been mentioned in the literature earlier,[5,6] clinical applications of HFV arose fortuitously from laboratory research conducted in the mid- to late 1960s. In a series of publications, Oberg and Sjostrand[7–9] described synchronous respiratory variations in blood pressure, which were confounding their canine studies involving the carotid sinus reflex. In an effort to alleviate this phenomenon, they ventilated at rates greater than 100/min through an endotracheal tube incorporating an insufflation catheter (i.e., a primitive jet ventilator). The dogs were ventilated adequately at these rapid rates, and lower airway pressures were achieved with minimal circulatory interference. At about the same time, Lukenheimer and co-workers[10] observed that oscillations in transtracheal pressure

Table 3.1. Potential Benefits of High-Frequency Ventilation

Effective gas exchange at low peak airway pressure
Reduced intrapulmonary pressure swings
Decreased barotrauma and/or decreased incidence of airleak syndromes
Conservation of lung surfactant phospholipids
Decreased hemodynamic compromise
Decreased fluctuation in intracranial pressure
Enhanced understanding of basic pulmonary physiology

improved gas exchange when superimposed on conventional mechanical ventilation. Here an electromagnetic vibrator (a primitive acoustic speaker) was attached to an endotracheal tube and adequate carbon dioxide elimination was achieved at frequencies between 23 and 40 Hertz (1Hz = 60 cps). Subsequently, Klain and Smith[11] obtained confirmatory data in bench models and laboratory animals, while the first clinical applications were documented by Carlon et al.[12] and Butler and colleagues.[13]

The next major advances date from the late 1970s, when numerous reports of high-frequency ventilation using piston, acoustic, or rotating-ball-valve designs confirmed the potential for adequate carbon dioxide elimination and oxygenation. The latter occurred at exceedingly rapid respiratory rates and tidal volumes of less than the dead space of the lungs and airways.

TECHNICAL ASPECTS OF HFV

Ventilation at supraphysiologic rates can be achieved by numerous techniques. There remain staunch proponents for each specialized apparatus, and some of the merits and detriments of each are listed in Table 3-2. As all of these techniques utilize very rapid ventilator rates; HFV remains a generic term comprising all of the aforementioned modalities. In consideration of this latter point and the broad technical, descriptive, and investigative literature surrounding each method of generating HFV, the ensuing discussion will in large part be limited to high-frequency oscillatory techniques (HFO). For completeness, the reader is referred to other recent reviews of HFV describing jet ventilators[14–17] and conventional positive pressure machines.[18–21]

Two types of ventilators are currently in use in clinical trials of very-high-frequency ventilation. The first generates high-frequency oscillations with a piston pump and variable-speed motor. The pump is connected to an endotracheal tube by low-compliance tubing, and the inlet for fresh gas flow is at the proximal end of the endotracheal tube. In this configuration, a small volume of gas in the patient circuit is oscillated back and forth. A low-pass filter or Starling resistor offers an exit port for bias gas flow and the carbon dioxide diffused from the lung. The low-pass filter is quite important to successful ventilation.[22] At high frequencies, impedance to flow through the filter is related predominately to inertia rather than resistance; therefore, the low-pass filter has low impedance to low-frequency flows (the fresh gas) and high impedance to high-frequency flows (the oscillations). These filters are not perfectly efficient, and generally are not easily adjusted; therefore,

Table 3.2. Pros and Cons Associated with Various HFV Techniques

	Advantages	Disadvantages
HFPPV	Conventional, readily available device Incorporates required clinical alarms and safety features	Decreasing tidal volume at very high rates Maximum rate is 1–2 Hz Potential for advertent PEEP
HFJV	Commercially available Incorporates safety features Broad clinical experience in adults Permits spontaneous breaths during use	Rate limit is approximately 15 HZ Passive exhalation Numerous reports of tissue injury (i.e., necrotizing tracheobronchitis) Delivered volume and pressure monitoring is difficult
HFFI and HFO	Not mechanically rate limited Active expiratory phase (HFO) Can be combined with IMV	Mechanisms of gas transport incompletely understood Ventilator and circuit design not uniform Not widely available Long term efficacy and safety unsubstantiated Delivered volume and pressure monitoring is difficult

HFPPV: high frequency positive pressure ventilation; HFJV: high frequency jet ventilation; HFFI: high frequency flow interrupter; HFO: High frequency oscillation.

some oscillatory volume is usually lost to the filter.[23] The volume loss depends upon the relative impedance of the patient's respiratory system and endotracheal tube, balanced against that of the filter. Thus, a "standard" filter may not be ideal for each patient, nor ideal at all times for any given patient with dynamic lung disease and changing pulmonary function. The importance of bias flow rate on gas transport during HFO has been assessed by Solway and co-workers[24] in anesthetized, paralyzed canines. At a fixed tidal volume of 40 ml (or 2 to 2.5 ml/kg), carbon dioxide removal rates were dependent on bias flow at all frequencies tested (2 to 12 Hz), and this dependence was most marked at bias flow rates below 10 L/min. Furthermore, tidal volume is also frequency-dependent in this system, and volume losses are probably related to compliance and resistance of the ventilatory system, the compression of gas, and leaks around an uncuffed endotracheal tube.[22] Emphasizing the latter, Brusasco et al.[25] have noted that changing the resistance to gas flow, gas compliance, and (or) gas inertance of the ventilator circuit components (i.e., connecting tubing, endotracheal tube, etc.) significantly alters the ratio of delivered tidal volume to stroke volume of the piston pump oscillator. Their data and that of others[26,27] highlight the importance of utilizing a consistent or fixed ventilatory circuit if comparability between experimental and clinical data from various investigations is to be expected.

In the second commonly used system for HFO, the high flow of a heated, humidified gas mixture is interrupted by a spinning ball valve or solenoid-like mechanism. Here the amplitude and resultant volume of the pulses necessarily decrease with increasing frequency at a fixed flow rate when the valve or switching mechanism is of fixed configuration. To compensate, the amplitude of pulses can be readily increased by increasing the flow of gas through the circuit. This system is technically not oscillatory, and the term flow interruptor is often used for it.

The flow interruptor-type ventilator is similar to a modified jet ventilator, but in contrast, the inspiratory pulse is delivered at some distance proximal to the patient's airway. Unlike piston-pump oscillators, the expiratory phase of the respiratory cycle is passive and dependent upon elastic recoil of the chest and lung tissue.

GAS EXCHANGE DURING HFO

The mechanisms by which these specialized machines provide for adequate gas exchange has yet to be determined conclusively. During either spontaneous breathing or standard mechanical ventilation, gas transport is classically described in terms of cyclic ventilation, wherein most of the fresh gas transport is achieved by bulk flow or convection through the airways, and mixing through the large alveolar compartment is by simple diffusion. The pressure required to move a tidal volume is dependent upon the dynamics of the respiratory system (i.e., resistance, compliance, etc.). On the other hand, HFV produces a pattern of flow that enhances gas mixing throughout the lung, producing a rate of gas exchange several orders of magnitude greater than that accounted for by simple diffusion alone.[4]

Because the tidal volumes during HFV were so small (often less than anatomic dead space), initial investigations concentrated on gas diffusion in efforts to explain equivalent or improved ventilation by the high-frequency technique. The term "augmented" or "facilitated" diffusion, coined by Fredberg[28] and Slutsky et al.,[3] considered the action of turbulent flow and diffusion. In classic experiments performed in the early 1950s, Taylor[29] showed that for laminar flow through rigid straight tubes, the effective diffusivity (or more simply, the radial spreading of molecules in a tubular system) increases as the square of the velocity and tube diameter. Similar results have been obtained by Scherer and co-workers[30] in a lung model with five generations of airways. Although these experiments are not exactly analogous to the clinical situation because they deal with steady unidirectional flow, they do emphasize the potential magnitude for augmented diffusion. In Scherer's study, at a velocity of 100 cm/sec, effective diffusivity was some 3,000 times as great as that for simple diffusion alone. In humans or experimental animals, oscillatory flow velocities have ranged from 100 to greater than 500 cm/sec.[2] In simplistic terms, at low tidal volume, when the rate of cycling of the ventilator is increased, the flow rate must necessarily increase in order to maintain the pulsed volume. At sufficiently high flow rates, the movement of gas down the airways becomes not only a result of molecular diffusion but also of turbulent mixing.

Gas transport during conventional mechanical ventilation does not present homogeneous gas mixtures to all alveolar surfaces, because of local differences in time constants, small airways, resistance, and tissue compliance. Recent evidence suggests that this may not be the case during HFO. Schmidt and associates[31] induced large regional differences in ^{133}Xe concentration and then demonstrated that sufficient mixing occurs during HFO to equalize the ^{133}Xe concentration throughout the lung fields. More specifically, they noted that at 15 Hz, mean clearance rates were significantly faster in basal non-dependent and basal-dependent portions of the lung than in apical non-dependent lung regions, indicating a cephalocaudal gradient in regional clearance rates. Additionally, when ^{133}Xe was infused during pulmonary perfusion without HFO, little interregional mixing resulted. However, following the institution of HFO, ^{133}Xe cleared immediately from basal-dependent regions and increased transiently in basal non-dependent regions prior to clearance. These findings tended to be greater at 30 Hz than at lower frequencies. The investigators concluded that a uniform distribution of ^{133}Xe during HFO may not represent truly uniform ventilation per unit of lung volume, but rather rapid interregional mixing, which abolishes differences in regional gas concentrations that may otherwise exist. Allen et al.[32] have also demonstrated substantial phase differences in alveolar pressure swings among peripheral alveolar locations in rabbits ventilated at frequencies above resonance. In a recent review, Slutsky[33] noted that "the implication of these findings is that during HFO it should be possible to redistribute gas flow within the lung by the appropriate choice of frequency and tidal volume."

Germane to the concept of rapid, complete interregional gas mixing are the findings of Lehr,[34] who promulgated the concept of "disco lung" when describing regional lung movements or undulations at the surface of the lung during HFO. In Lehr's work, small squares were precisely laid out on excised dog lungs, and the deformations they underwent during HFO were studied by stroboscopic photography. With the assumption that the change in the area of a given square reflected changes in the volume of the underlying lung, it was determined that volume changes of the parenchyma were twice as great at 30 Hz as at 1 Hz. The volume changes were attributed to "pendelluft" or out-of-phase flow between lung units, which enhances intra- and interregional gas mixing. The potentially significant contribution of convective gas mixing as described above to overall gas transport during HFO has recently been substantiated in a constructed physical model.[35]

Brusasco and co-workers[36] investigated the effects of varying tidal volume on the regional clearance of ^{133}Xe during HFO. Dogs were ventilated at frequencies of 5 to 60 Hz at tidal volumes of about two-thirds of their anatomic pulmonary dead space. Brusasco's group noted that the ^{133}Xe clearance rate was nearly uniform when the tidal volume was less than two-thirds of the anatomic dead space, and that the mean ^{133}Xe clearance for the lung increased with tidal volume at all frequencies. They concluded that HFV yields increased longitudinal conductance of gas along the airways, and probably increased interregional gas mixing between lung regions, leading to homogenization of ventilation. Additionally, by using gases of varying density, these investigators suggested that compression of gas was not sufficiently significant to change the tidal volume generated by a piston pump or that delivered to the lung at a frequency of up to 30 Hz.

The optimal frequency at which to deliver HFV remains indeterminate. In general, at a fixed tidal volume, carbon dioxide elimination increases with frequency until a critical frequency is reached, above which no further increases in elimination occur. The diminished effectiveness may be due to distention of the large airways, which in turn reduces the volume transmitted to the periphery.[37] The critical frequency is most likely determined by the mechanical properties of the lung. Above this critical frequency, however, additional CO_2 elimination appears to be mainly a function of tidal volume.[1,28]

Comparison of various investigations concerning alveolar ventilation during HFO (i.e., CO_2 elimination) are difficult, since equivalence in mean airway pressure, alveolar pressure, or lung volume between experimental protocols cannot be assumed. The delivered gas volume may be smaller than the stroke volume of an oscillator pump because of loss of gas through the bias exhaust or expansion of compliant tubing in the ventilator circuit. Additionally, the delivered volume may be larger than anticipated because of entrainment of gas or amplification of gas volume at the resonant oscillatory frequency. Indeed, in vitro and in vivo investigations have confirmed that pressures measured at the airway opening could underestimate alveolar pressure at resonant frequencies.[25,32,38–41] A simplified explanation has been offered by Brusasco et al.[25]: "To understand the phenomenon of resonance, consider the behavior of gas in a system consisting of a pump, tube, and bottle. At low oscillation frequencies the gas in the tube moves to-and-fro in phase with the pump piston, and the volume of gas delivered to the bottle equals the volume displacement of the piston. At higher oscillation frequencies the inertia of the gas requires large pressures to be developed by the pump to accelerate the gas. By virtue of its inertia, the gas continues its movement into the bottle, even when the piston is already moving in the opposite direction (phase lag). This phase lag causes rarification of gas in the pump and tube simultaneous with compression of gas in the bottle."

In a recent study utilizing excised canine lungs, Fredberg et al.[38] measured regional alveolar pressures during HFO (1 to 60 Hertz). At resonant frequencies, the ratio of alveolar pressure to pressure at the airway opening was 1.9, 2.9, and 4.8 at transpulmonary pressures of 5, 10, and 25 cmH_2O, respectively. Additionally, both the spatial homogeneity and temporal synchrony of alveolar pressure between sampled lung regions decreased with increasing frequency and increased with increasing transpulmonary pressure. Although the magnitude of alveolar pressure amplification was less, these data were corroborated by Allen at al.[32] in rabbits. The quantitative disparity was attributed to size-related differences in lung mechanical properties. Additionally, the effect may be accentuated by shifting from the supine to a lateral position.[39]

The above studies were conducted at quite low oscillatory flows and pressure amplitudes in order to preserve linearity, and hence interpretable physiologic data—an approach not consistent with current regimens for HFO in humans. However, Frantz et al. utilized more clinically analogous settings in close-chested adult rabbits ventilated at 2 to 37.5 Hz.[40] He measured dynamic and mean pressure at the airway opening, trachea, and alveoli, as well as the delivered tidal volume in vivo. Alveolar pressure swings (Fig. 3-1) and the delivered tidal volume fell with increasing frequency. Also, alveolar pressure swings were always lower than those at the airway opening or in the trachea. The clinical extrapolation derived from these data was to minimize alveolar pressure swings (and therefore potential barotrauma) during HFO by selecting the highest frequency at which adequate gas exchange could be achieved.

On the whole, in both experimental animals and human subjects, HFO results in a similar level of oxygenation to that achieved by conventional ventilators at comparable mean airway pressures or lung volumes.[22,23,42–44] The advantage of HFO appears to be that respiratory units may be held at pressures above closure while maintaining smaller phasic pressure–volume fluctuations than those that occur during conventional mechanical ventilation. Theoretically, the latter could decrease the incidence or severity of air leak syndromes and BPD. This potential

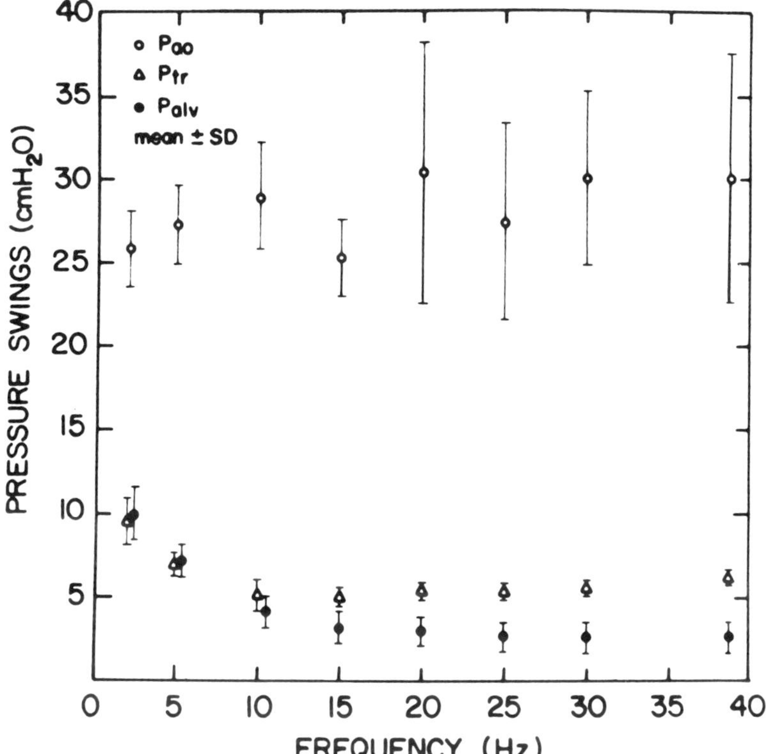

Fig. 3.1. Pressure swings at the airway opening (Pao, open circles), trachea (Ptr, open triangles), and alveoli (Palv, closed circles), plotted versus frequency during HFO in adult rabbits. Values are mean ± SD. (Frantz ID, Close RH: Alveolar pressure swings during high frequency ventilation in rabbits. Pediatr Res 19:162, 1985.)

clinical advantage, however, has yet to be demonstrated in large, prospective, randomized clinical trials.

In summary, the mechanisms responsible for gas transport during HFO are numerous and not mutally exclusive. Their interplay depends upon the geometric and mechanical properties of the lung, the anatomic position of a particular respiratory unit, and the presence of specific pathobiologic processes. However, the net result is a more efficient mixing of inspired gases. In a recent review, Chang[45] attributed successful HFO to five modes of gas transport (Fig. 3-2).

1. The direct ventilation of some alveoli by bulk convection, which always occurs when the tidal volume exceeds a certain low limit, and should provide the most efficient gas exchange for those alveoli that are ventilated in this manner.

2. Convection by out-of-phase HFO or high-frequency *pendelluft* as a result of imbalances of time constants between neighboring lung units, which tends to homogenize the conducting airways, serving as a "clearinghouse" for those lung units that have long time constants. It may also ventilate some alveoli otherwise not reached by the primary HFO tidal volume.

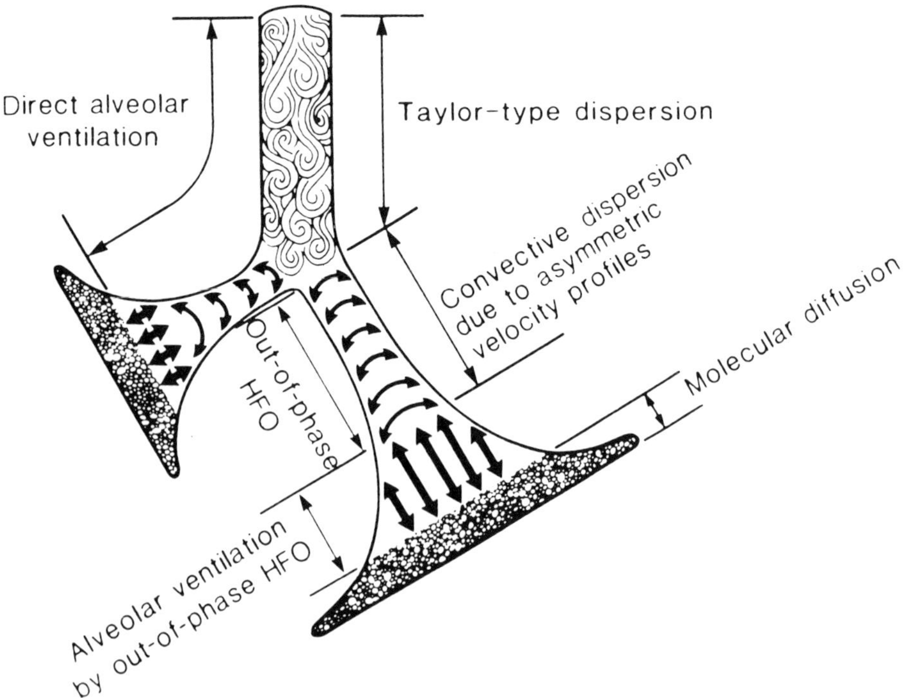

Fig. 3.2. Modes of gas transport during HFO and tentative sketch of their zones of dominance. (Chang HK: Mechanisms of gas transport during ventilation by high-frequency oscillation. J Appl Physiol 56:553, 1984.)

3. Convective exchange may occur in the large or medium airways in which inspiratory and expiratory velocity profiles are asymmetric.

4. Longitudinal dispersion by the interaction of axial convective velocities and lateral transport due to turbulent eddies, and secondary swirling motions, which may exist in the large and medium airways. This mode of transport must exist as long as there is oscillatory flow through the tracheobronchial tree, and is probably important in the trachea for CO_2 elimination.

5. Near the alveolar capillary membrane, molecular diffusion is expected to be the dominant form of gas transport, as in any type of ventilation.

PULMONARY PATHOLOGY AND SURFACTANT METABOLISM

In order to test the more general hypothesis that minimizing cyclic alveolar pressure swings would be beneficial to diseased lungs, Hamilton and associates[46] investigated the histologic differences in rabbit lungs ventilated with standard mechanical ventilation and HFO after the depletion of surfactant by repeated saline lavage. These studies revealed insignificant differences in pH or PCO_2 during 5 hours of meachnical ventilation. Though all of the animals had evidence of pneumonitis, pulmonary edema, and bronchoepiehtlial desquamation and necrosis, the epithelial damage was more severe in animals maintained on conventional ventilators. These abnormalities were also evident in lavaged but nonventilated animals, and absent in nonlavaged, nonventilated control animals. The major difference between the control and experimental groups was the finding of extensive alveolar hyaline membrane formation in the conventionally ventilated rabbits. The presence of hyaline membranes was assumed to represent alveolar damage resulting from the large volume and pressure swings generated by conventional mechanical ventilation. Additionally, the investigators speculated that the same trauma seen in conventional mechanical ventilation would lead to physical disruption of surfactant surface films at the alveolar air/liquid interface. Unfortunately, no surfactant phospholipid analyses were done. However, others have noted no adverse effects of HFO on pressure/volume measurements, surface balance experiments, or on whole-lung, lavage-fluid, or lamellar-body phospholipid concentrations.[42,43,47–49]

In addition to these data, tangential evidence lends credence to the hypothesis that ventilation at minimal tidal volumes may conserve pulmonary surfactant. Numerous investigators have shown that increased ventilation can influence pulmonary surfactant and the pressure-volume characteristics of isolated lungs.[50–56] Reduced compliance observed in hyperventilated lungs has been attributed to a decrease in surfactant. This conclusion is supported by the observed reduction in the surface tension-lowering capacity of lung extracts.[52,54] Faridy and co-workers[51] have suggested that ventilation enhances the movement of surfactants from alveoli into airways. Other studies,[50,54] utilizing radiolabelled phospholipid precursors, suggest that hyperventilation promotes the release, then inactivation, of surface-active material. One may speculate that by reducing the large-volume, cyclic expansion and compression of the surfactant lining the alveolar surface that might occur in conventional ventilation, low-pressure, low tidal volume, high-frequency ventilation may enhance surface film stability and lessen the bronchoalveolar pathology[57] reported after conventional mechanical ventilation.

APNEA ASSOCIATED WITH HFO

One curious observation made in animals and humans during early studies of HFV was the occurrence of prolonged apnea following the initiation of oscillations.[13,58–59] This was initially attributed to a prolongation of expiration (Hering-Breuer reflex) secondary to increases in mean lung volume during oscillatory ventilation. By measuring lung volume, airway pressure, and end-tidal CO_2, and by assessing the activity of respiratory muscles, Banzett et al.[60] showed that the phasic stimulation of upper airway stretch receptors by oscillation leads to an active inhibition of respiration that is independent of lung volume. These effects were abolished by vagotomy, and demonstrate that oscillatory ventilation produces apnea independent of, or perhaps in addition to, the Hering-Breuer reflex. In another study, Barnas and co-workers[61] compared the response of pulmonary afferents during HFV and conventional ventilation at a constant mean lung volume and end-tidal PCO_2. The average discharge of slowly adapting pulmonary stretch receptor (PSRs) increased during HFV. Rapidly adapting pulmonary stretch receptors (RARs) were generally silent during conventional ventilation and HFV at functional residual capacity and above, but increased greatly when HFV was applied at low lung volumes. The investigators concluded that the increased discharge of PSRs occurring during HFV is a sufficient explanation for the observed reflex lengthening of expiratory time, and that RAR discharge may be involved in augmented breaths (gasps or sighs) during HFV in some animals.

CARDIOVASCULAR AND OTHER HEMODYNAMIC EFFECTS OF HFO

Numerous experimental protocols have addressed cardiovascular or pulmonary hemodynamics during HFV. However, much is yet to be learned. In 1982, Thompson et al.[22] reported data comparing gas exchange and cardiac output during HFO or conventional mechanical ventilation in an adult canine model of acute lung injury. After inducing hemorrhagic pulmonary edema with oleic acid, they noted no difference in systemic arterial pressure, cardiac output estimated by thermodilution techniques, or pulmonary artery and capillary wedge pressures between the two modes of ventilation under normovolemic conditions. In general, the magnitude of deleterious cardiovascular effects induced by the particular method of ventilation depended on the extent to which elevated intrapulmonary pressures were transmitted to the pleural space.

More recently, Oguchi and associates[62] studied the hemodynamic status and left ventricular performance of premature lambs that were treated with autologous exogenous surfactant and subjected to ductus arteriosus occlusion at birth. Surfactant treatment permitted ventilation and survival during the experiment, while ductal occlusion eliminated the potential variable of a large left-to-right shunt. At the same mean airway pressure (no lung volumes were determined), blood pressure, left ventricular stroke volume, ejection fraction, cardiac output, and organ blood flows were equivalent for HFO and conventional mechanical ventilation. Additionally, the integrity of left atrial reflexes that influence the regulation of intravascular volume[63–65] are unaffected by HFO.[66]

While others have obtained similar results under a variety of experimental conditions,[67–70] Lucking and associates[71] have reported a significant, 19 percent increase in cardiac output and 32 percent decrease in pulmonary vascular resistance during HFO as compared to standard ventilatory techniques in a dog model of right ventricular dysfunction produced by ventriculotomy. When the arterial blood gases, core temperature, and ventricular preload were held constant, cardiac output increased from 1.16 ± 0.24 to 1.38 ± 0.28 L/min ($P<0.05$), and pulmonary vascular resistance decreased from 734 ± 257 to 554 ± 169 dyne · sec/cm^5 during HFO relative to conventional mechanical ventilation.

To date, published data about the effects of HFO on the pulmonary vascular response to hypoxia remain contradictory. Wetzel et al.[72] have reported that in isolated sheep lungs, HFO attenuated hypoxia-induced pulmonary vasoconstriction; they speculated that this may be secondary to enhanced prostacyclin (PGI_2) release. The latter hypothesis was based on the observation of the increased net rate of change in the concentration of 6-keto-prostaglandin $F_1\alpha$ (a measurable metabolite of prostacyclin) in the perfusate during hypoxia and ventilation with HFO as compared to conventional techniques. The experimental findings were abolished by pretreatment with indomethacin. On the contrary, Troug et al.[73] noted increased pulmonary artery pressures and pulmonary vascular resistance both during normoxic and hypoxic stimuli in premature, nonhuman primates ventilated by HFO. Additionally, Mitchell et al.[70] could detect neither the release of prostacyclin (as $PGF_1\alpha$) or of thromboxane (a potent pulmonary vasoconstrictor) into blood passing through the lung, nor differences in pulmonary vascular response to hypoxia/hypercapnia in neonatal piglets during HFO or conventional mechanical ventilation.

The potential effects of HFO on lung fluid balance, lymph flow, and protein clearance have been estimated in a limited number of recent investigations. In premature nonhuman primates, Troug and associates[42] noted increased total lung water 24 hours after birth in all animals with RDS as compared to controls. However, no differences occurred when the mode of ventilation was varied. Likewise, Frantz et al.[48] found no change in lung wet/dry ratios in healthy adult cats ventilated for 6 hours with HFO or conventional techniques. During in vivo experiments involving sheep and goats with chronic lung lymph fistulas, Jefferies and coworkers[74] demonstrated that short-duration HFO (e.g., 1 to 2 hours) does not impair lymphatic function under resting conditions, and that increases in water and protein clearance stimulated by air microembolization are preserved. However, the lymph collected in this study may not have indicated events occurring at the lung's microvascular membrane, since the collection sites were postnodal and could have contained lymph draining extrapulmonary sources.[75] In an open-chested dog preparation in which prenodal lymph flow was recorded, Martin et al.[75] reported that lymph flow and lung water increased by 68 percent and 20 percent, respectively, after HFO. As indicated by an analysis of lymph protein flux obtained at elevated left atrial pressures, the authors concluded that HFO did not alter microvascular permeability. To explain their findings, they hypothesized that HFO may decrease the perivascular interstitial fluid pressure surrounding the larger extra-alveolar vessels, resulting in the accumulation of small amounts of edema fluid in this region; lymph flow then increases by some unspecified manner.

Overall, it appears that HFO causes no major perturbations in cardiovascular or hemodynamic function, at least during normovolemia. Theoretically, ventilation at very high frequencies and low tidal volumes may be advantageous in protecting systemic venous return, right ventricular filling, and perhaps cardiac output, by minimizing intrathoracic phasic pressure swings.

It should be mentioned that most of the preceding research efforts varied with regard to the species studied (i.e., rabbits, monkeys, sheep, piglets, etc.), animal age (premature, newborn, or adult), experimental conditions (i.e., in vitro vs. in vivo, healthy vs. diseased lungs, etc.), and technical aspects of the mechanical ventilation used (i.e., mean airway pressure, lung volume, respiratory frequency, etc.). This is obviously important, since each variation may alter the results obtained. Therefore, the practical clinical and physiologic implications of these data remain unclear.

THE CLINICAL USE OF HFO

Although one must be cautious in generalizing from data accumulated in laboratory animal experiments to the clinical care of sick neonates, certain concepts seem applicable. A synthesis of animal investigations of HFO supports the contentions that:

1. HFO can support ventilation (e.g., CO_2 elimination) and oxygenation at a level equivalent to conventional mechanical ventilation.

2. For the most part, carbon dioxide elimination is dependent upon frequency and amplitude, while oxygenation is related to FiO_2 and mean airway pressure.

3. Sufficiency of ventilation and the clinical regimen employed may be directly related to the particular machine and circuit design or configuration utilized.

4. The delivered tidal volume and resistance to gas transport during HFO are related to endotracheal tube size.

5. A periodic recruitment maneuver (e.g., sustained inflation or sighing) may be required to counteract progressive atelectasis resulting from volume losses in an open-circuit system or as a component of the primary respiratory disease.

6. Potentially deleterious cardiovascular effects depend on lung volume and pressure transmission to the plural space.

7. Monitoring of pressures at the proximal airway opening may not reliably reflect those occurring at the midtracheal or alveolar level.

8. While very-high-frequency, low-tidal-volume ventilation may have significant potential for reducing pulmonary barotrauma, its true impact on the incidence of other morbidities common in ill neonates with respiratory failure, such as patent ductus arteriosis, CNS hemorrhage, or BPD is as yet unknown.

To date, no clinical trial has been done in which human neonates with RDS have been maintained on HFO without prior conventional mechanical ventilatory support. Although the following preliminary studies are imperfect, they represent the only non-anecdotal clinical data currently in print. In the first published clinical study, Marchack and associates[23] evaluated short-term HFO in eight neonates with severe RDS. The mean gestational age and birthweight for these infants were 33 weeks and 2.36 kg, respectively, and their age at the time of study ranged from 12 to 60 hours. All were initially ventilated by conventional techniques prior to the high-frequency, low-tidal-volume trial. The oscillatory frequency varied between 8 and 20 Hz, and the piston-pump-generated tidal volumes ranged from 5.7 to 12.7 ml/kg. The results suggest that short-term, very-high-frequency ventilation can provide gas exchange at least equivalent to conventional mechanical ventilation in neonates with RDS. Although many hypothetical advantages of HFV were cautiously proposed, only incomplete data were collected: the mean airway pressure was measured in only three infants; sequential, matched measures of ventilation were not reported; and the tidal volumes actually delivered could not be obtained.

The study reported by Frantz and co-workers[76] included 10 infants with RDS and 5 with extensive bilateral pulmonary interstitial emphysema (PIE). The neonates with RDS (mean gestational age = 33.4 weeks; mean birthweight = 1.9 kg) were less than 48 hours of age when the trial of HFV (with a flow-interrupter device) was conducted for a duration of 1 hour. All of the patients were paralyzed with pancuronium and initially ventilated with conventional techniques. The results demonstrated that the infants' arterial blood gas values were similar to those obtained during conventional ventilation, but the data reported for ventilator frequency and pressure were gathered at the time of the best combination of oxygenation and carbon dioxide elimination during HFV. Although peak proximal airway and tracheal pressures were equivalent during conventional ventilation, the peak tracheal pressures were considerably below the peak pressures in the proximal airway during HFV. Additionally, peak and mean tracheal pressures were lower during HFV than during conventional mechanical ventilation. Again, these data confirm the capacity of HFV to maintain gas exchange equivalent to that with conventional ventilation, but at lower distal airway pressures.

In the largest clinical study published to date, 27 neonates with respiratory disease complicated by PIE and persistent hypercarbia were considered for HFO.[77] Attempts to normalize arterial blood gases with conventional ventilation and hand bagging had failed in all. The gestational ages of the patients ranged from 25 to 34 weeks, and their birthweights from 0.55 to 2.0 kg. The mean duration of HFO (initiated at the same mean airway pressure and FIO_2 as in prior conventional mechanical ventilation) was 6.2 days (range; 1 to 30 days). Assignment to HFO was not randomized. Seven infants were removed from the study analysis because of documented septic shock before HFO treatment. Sixteen of the remaining study patients survived and experienced a resolution of PIE while on HFO, and 4 died of progressive chronic respiratory insufficiency. Although the timing of its occurence was not mentioned, 15 neonates required therapeutic intervention for pneuomothoraces. Additionally, all of the survivors "developed varying degrees of BPD." In concluding that HFO is an appropriate treatment for PIE, the authors speculated that the amount of air leaking into the interstitial space is reduced as a result of reduced phasic pressure swings in the distal airway.

A somewhat different experimental design, combining HFO with concurrent intermittent positive pressure ventilation (IMV), was used by Boynton et al.[78] to treat 12 critically ill neonates with respiratory failure. The technique, based on earlier studies,[79–80] was devised to sustain adequate lung volume during oscillation and to avoid atelectasis and progressive deterioration of oxygenation. In this unique approach, HFO-IMV was administered at the same mean airway pressure, IMV rate, and flow rate as the preceding IMV alone. The initial oscillatory frequency was approximately 20 Hz, with an amplitude sufficient to cause chest wall vibration. Subsequently, the major goal was to decrease the IMV rate and mean airway pressure. Improved oxygenation occurred in six patients, while all had a reduction in PCO_2. The authors reported mucus plugging of the endotracheal tube in four infants and increased secretions in three, which may have been a result of increased mucus production or coalescence of normal airway secretions. This observation has been addressed experimentally[81] and in a recent clinical review.[82]

CONCLUSION

Although positive-pressure ventilators have contributed significantly to the trend toward an improved outcome for preterm infants with respiratory failure secondary to surfactant deficiency (i.e., RDS) and other neonatal pulmonary disorders, pulmonary sequelae such as air-leak syndrome, barotrauma, and BPD remain as major contributors to prolonged hospitalization and late mortality in this population. Additionally, because of the experimental status of HFO, clinical trials thus far have essentially been rescue attempts for premorbid neonates. However, the preceding experience documents the potential utility of HFO in salvaging infants with respiratory failure unresponsive to conventional technology.

The safety and efficacy of HFO early in the course of neonatal respiratory disease are currently being assessed in an NHLBI-sponsored, randomized, multicenter clinical trial. This collaborative effort is designed to address major outcome criteria, including mortality and the incidence of BPD, but also co-morbidities such as CNS hemorrhage, patent ductus arteriosus, necrotizing enterocolitis, and air-leak syndromes. It should be mentioned that some morbidity may actually be increased by HFO. Although clinical enthusiasm for HFO persists, the technique may not prove to be a panacea but rather a worthwhile addition to current care for a select group of neonates with specific respiratory diagnoses. As noted by Froese and Bryan,[83] "We are left at present with the conviction that high-frequency ventilation is an intriguing phenomenon with wide-ranging theoretical and practical implications."

REFERENCES

1. Slutsky AS, Kamm RD, Rossing TH, et al: Effects of frequency, tidal volume, and lung volume on CO_2 elimination in dogs by high frequency (2–30 hz), low tidal volume ventilation. J Clin Invest 68:1475, 1981
2. Bohn DJ, Miyasaka K, Marchak BE, et al: Ventilation by high-frequency oscillation. J Appl Physiol 48:710, 1980
3. Slutsky AS, Drazen JM, Ingram RH, et al: Effective pulmonary ventilation with small-volume oscillations at high frequency. Science 209:609, 1980
4. Special Conference Report, High frequency ventilation for immature infants, Report of a Conference, March 2–4, 1982, Pediatrics 71:280, 1983
5. Henderson YH, Chillingworth FP, Whitney JL: The respiratory dead space. Am J Physiol 38:1, 1915
6. Briscoe WA, Forster RE, Comroe JH: Alveolar ventilation at very low tidal volumes. J Appl Physiol 7:27, 1954
7. Oberg PA, Sjostrand V: Studies of blood pressure regulation II. On-line simulation as a method of studying the regulatory properties of the carotid-sinus reflex. Acta Physiol Scand 75:287, 1969
8. Oberg PA, Sjostrand V: Studies of blood pressure regulation I. Common-carotid artery clamping in studies of the carotid sinus baroreceptor control of the systemic blood pressure. Acta Physiol Scand 75:276, 1969
9. Oberg PA, Sjostrand V: Studies of blood-pressure regulation III. Dynamics of antenatal blood pressure on carotid sinus nerve stimulation. Acta Physiol Scand 81:96, 1971
10. Lukenheimer PP, Rafflenberl W, Keller H: Application of transtracheal pressure oscillations as a modification of "diffusion of respiration." Br J Anaesth 44:627, 1972
11. Klain M, Smith RB: High frequency percutaneous transtracheal jet ventilation. Crit Care Med 5:280, 1977
12. Carlon GC, Kahn RC, Howland WS, et al: Clinical experience with high frequency jet ventilation. Crit Care Med 9:1, 1981
13. Butler WJ, Bohn DJ, Bryan AC, et al: Ventilation by high-frequency oscillation in humans. Anesth Analg 59:577, 1980
14. Pagani G, Rezzonico R, Marini A: Trials of high frequency jet ventilation in preterm infants with severe respiratory distress. Acta Pediatr Scand 74:681, 1985
15. Carlo WA, Chatburn RL, Martin RJ, et al: Decrease in airway pressure during high-frequency jet ventilation in infants with respiratory distress syndrome. J Pediatr 104:101, 1984
16. Boros SJ, Mammel MC, Coleman JM, et al: Neonatal high-frequency jet ventilaton: Four years' experience. Pediatrics 75:657, 1985
17. Trindade O, Goldberg RN, Bancalari E, et al: Conventional vs. high-frequency jet ventilation in a piglet model of meconium aspiration: comparison of pulmonary and hemodynamic effects. J Pediatr 107:115, 1985
18. Boros SJ, Campbell K: A comparison of the effects of high frequency-low tidal volume and low frequency-high tidal volume mechanical ventilation. J Pediatr 97:108, 1980

19. Heicher DA, Kasting DS, Harrod JR: Prospective clinical comparison of two methods for mechanical ventilation of neonates: Rapid rate and short inspiratory time versus slow rate and long inspiratory time. J Pediatr 98:957, 1981
20. Bland RD, Kim MH, Light MJ, et al: High frequency mechanical ventilation in severe hyaline membrane disease, an alternative treatment? Crit Care Med 8:275, 1980
21. Boros SJ, Bing DR, Mammel MC, et al: Using conventional infant ventilators at unconventional rates. Pediatrics 74:487, 1984
22. Thompson WK, Marchak BE, Froese AB, et al: High-frequency oscillation compared with standard ventilation in pulmonary injury model. J Appl Physiol 52:543, 1982
23. Marchak BE, Thompson WK, Dufty P, et al: Treatment of RDS by high-frequency oscillatory ventilation: A preliminary report. J Pediatr 99:287, 1981
24. Solway J, Gavriely N, Slutsky AS, et al: Effect of bias flow rate on gas transport during high-frequency oscillatory ventilation. Respir Physiol 60:267, 1985
25. Brosasco V, Beck KC, Crawford M, et al: Resonant amplification of delivered tidal volume during high-frequency ventilation. J Appl Physiol 60:885, 1986
26. Boynton BR, Mannino FL, Meathe EA, et al: Airway pressure measurement during high frequency oscillatory ventilation. Crit Care Med 12:39, 1984
27. Rossing TH, Solway J, Saari AF, et al: Influence of endotracheal tube on CO_2 transport during high-frequency ventilation. Am Rev Respir Dis 129:54, 1984
28. Fredberg JJ: Augmented diffusion in the airways can support pulmonary gas exchange. J Appl Physiol 49:232, 1980
29. Taylor G: Dispersion of soluble matter in solvent flowing slowly through a tube. Proc R Soc Lond, Series A, 219:186, 1953
30. Scherer PW, Shendalman LH, Greene NM, et al: Measurement of axial diffusivities in a model of the bronchial airways. J Appl Physiol 38:719, 1975
31. Schmid ER, Knopp TJ, Rehder K: Intrapulmonary gas transport and perfusion during high-frequency oscillation. J Appl Physiol 51:1507, 1981
32. Allen JL, Fredberg JJ, Keese DH, et al: Alveolar pressure magnitude and asynchrony during high-frequency oscillation of excised rabbit lungs. Am Rev Respir Dis 132:343, 1985
33. Slutsky AS: High frequency oscillations: Physiologic considerations. Med Instrum 19:199, 1985
34. Lehr J: Circulating currents during high frequency ventilation. Fed Proc 39:516, 1980, abstract
35. Isabey D, Harf A, Chang HK: Alveolar ventilation during high-frequency oscillation: Core dead space concept. J Appl Physiol 56:700, 1984
36. Brusasco V, Knopp TJ, Rehder K: Gas transport during high-frequency ventilation. J Appl Physiol 55:472, 1983
37. Rossing TH, Slutsky AS, Lehr JL, et al: Tidal volume and frequency dependence of carbon dioxide elimination by high-frequency ventilation. N Engl J Med 305:1375, 1981
38. Fredberg JJ, Keefe DH, Glass GM, et al: Alveolar pressure nonhomogeneity during small-amplitude high-frequency oscillation. J Appl Physiol 57:788, 1984
39. Simon BA, Weinmann GG, Mitzner W: Mean airway pressure and alveolar pressure during high-frequency ventilation. J Appl Physiol 57:1069, 1984
40. Frantz ID, Close RH: Alveolar pressure swings during high frequency ventilation in rabbits. Pediatr Res 19:162, 1985
41. Saari AF, Rossing TH, Solway J, et al: Lung inflation during high-frequency ventilation. Am Rev Respir Dis 129:333, 1984
42. Troug WE, Standaert TA, Murphy JH, et al: Effects of prolonged high-frequency oscillatory ventilation in premature primates with experimental hyaline membrane disease. Am Rev Respir Dis 130:76, 1984
43. Troug WE, Standaert TA, Murphy J, et al: Effect of high-frequency oscillation on gas exchange and pulmonary phospholipids in experimental hyaline membrane disease. Am Rev Respir Dis 127:585, 1983
44. Mansel JK, Gillespie DJ: Oxygenation during ventilation by high-frequency oscillation in dogs with acute lung injury. Crit Care Med 14:955, 1986
45. Chang HK: Mechanisms of gas transport during ventilation by high-frequency oscillation. J Appl Physiol 56:553, 1984
46. Hamilton PP, Onayemi A, Smyth JA, et al: Comparison of conventional and high-frequency ventilation: Oxygenation and lung pathology. J Appl Physiol 55:131, 1983
47. Mannino FL, McEvoy RD, Hallman M: Surfactant turnover in high frequency oscillatory ventilation. Pediatr Res 16:356A, 1982
48. Frantz ID, Stark AR, Davis JM, et al: High frequency ventilation does not affect surfactant, liquid or morphologic features in normal cats. Am Rev Respir Dis 126:909, 1982

49. Ennema JJ, Reijngoud DJ, Egberts J, et al: High-frequency oscillation affects surfactant phospholipid metabolism in rabbits. Respir Physiol 58:29, 1984
50. Egan EA, Nelson RM, MacIntyre B: Ventilation induced release of pulmonary surfactant in immature fetal goats. Pediatr Res 12:560, 1978
51. Faridy EE, Permutts S, Riley RE: Effect of ventilation on surface forces in excised dogs' lungs. J Appl Physiol 21:1453, 1966
52. Faridy EE: Effect of distension on release of surfactant in excised dogs' lungs. Respir Physiol 27:99, 1976
53. Faridy EE: Effect of ventilation of movement of surfactant in airways. Respir Physiol 27:323, 1976
54. Hildebran JN, Goerke J, Clements JA: Air inflation released phospholipids (PL) into the air-spaces of excised rat lungs. Fed Proc 34:387, 1975
55. McClenahan JB, Urtnowski A: Effect of ventilation on surfactant and its turnover rate. J Appl Physiol 23:215, 1976
56. Wyszogrodski I, Kyel-Aboagye K, Taeusch HW, et al: Surfactant inactivation by hyperventilation: Conservation by end-expiratory pressure. J Appl Physiol 38:461, 1975
57. Nilsson R, Gossmann G, Robertson B: Lung surfactant and the pathogenesis of neonatal bronchiolar lesions induced by artificial ventilation. Pediatr Res 12:249, 1978
58. Thompson WK, Marchak BE, Bryan AC, et al: Vagotomy reverses apnea induced by high-frequency oscillatory ventilation. J Appl Physiol 51:1484, 1981
59. England SJ, Onayami A, Bryan AC: Neuromuscular blockade enhances phrenic nerve activity during high-frequency ventilation. J Appl Ph,iol 56:31, 1984
60. Banzett R, Lehr J, Geoffroy B: High-frequency ventilation lengthens expiration in the anesthetized dog. J Appl Physiol 55:329, 1983
61. Barnas GM, Banzett RB, Reid MD, et al: Pulmonary afferent activity during high-frequency ventilation at constant mean lung volume. J Appl Physiol 61:192, 1986
62. Oguchi K, Baylen BG, Ikegami M, et al: Hemodynamic effects of high frequency ventilation in surfactant-treated preterm lambs. Biol Neonat 49:21, 1986
63. Peterson TV, Felts FT, Chase NL: Intravascular receptors and renal responses of monkey to volume expansion. Am J Physiol 244:55, 1983
64. Karim F, Mackay D, Kappagoda CT: Influence of cartoid sinus pressure on atrial receptors and renal blood flow. Am J Physiol 242:220, 1982
65. Ledsome JR, Linden RJ, O'Conner WJ: The mechanisms by which distension of the left atrium produces diuresis in anesthetized dogs. J Physiol 159:87, 1961
66. Rewa G, Man P, Kappagoda CT: A trial reflexed during high frequency oscillatory ventilation. Proc Soc Exp Biol Med 180:505, 1985
67. Armengol JA, Wells A, Man GC, et al: Hemodynamic and blood gas effects of high frequency oscillatory ventilation. Crit Care Med 9:192, 1981
68. Robertson HT, Coffey RL, Standaert TA, et al: Respiratory and inert gas exchange during high-frequency ventilation. J Appl Physiol 52:683, 1982
69. Vincent RN, Stark AR, Lang P, et al: Hemodynamic response to high-frequency ventilation in infants following cardiac surgery. Pediatrics 73:426, 1984
70. Mitchell JA, Green RS, Leffler CW: Effects of high frequency oscillatory ventilation compared to conventional ventilation upon pulmonary vascular prostanoid production in neonatal piglets. Prostag Leukot Med 17:107, 1985
71. Lucking SE, Fields AI, Saade M, et al: High frequency ventilation versus conventional ventilation in dogs with right ventricular dysfunction. Crit Care Med, 14:798, 1986
72. Wetzel R, Gordon J, Gregory TJ, et al: High-frequency ventilation attenuation of hypoxid pulmonary vasocontriction. Am Rev Respir Dis 132:99, 1985
73. Troug WE, Standaert TA: Effect of high-frequency ventilation on gas exchange and pulmonary vascular resistance in lambs. J Appl Physiol 59:1104, 1985
74. Jefferies AL, Hamilton P, O'Brodovich HM: Effect of high-frequency oscillation on lung lymph flow. J Appl Physiol 55:1373, 1983
75. Martin D, Rehder K, Parker JC, et al: High frequency ventilation: Lymph flow, lymph protein flux, and lung water. J Appl Physiol 57:240, 1984
76. Frantz ID, Werthammer J, Stark AR: High-frequency ventilation in premature infants with lung disease: Adequate gas exchange at low tracheal pressure. Pediatrics 71:483, 1983
77. Clark RH, Gerstmann DR, Null DM, et al: Pulmonary interstitial emphysema treated by high-frequency oscillatory ventilation. Crit Care Med 14:926, 1986
78. Boynton BR, Mannino FL, Davis RF, et al: Combined high-frequency oscillatory ventilation and intermittent mandatory ventilation in critically ill neonates. J Pediatr 105:297, 1984
79. Harf A, LeGall R, Chang HK: Mechanical ventilation with superimposed high frequency oscillation in the normal rat. Respir Physiol 54:31, 1983

80. El-Baz N, Faber LP, Doolas A: Combined high-frequency ventilation for management of terminal respiratory failure: A new technique. Anesth Analg 62:39, 1983
81. McEvoy RD, Davies NJH, Hedenstirrna G, et al: Lung mucociliary transport during high-frequency ventilation. Am Rev Respir Dis 126:452, 1982
82. Boynton RB: High frequency ventilation in newborn infants. Respir Care 31:480, 1986
83. Froese AB, Bryan AC: High frequency ventilation. Am Rev Respir Dis 123:249, 1981

4
Clinical Assessment and Management of Bronchopulmonary Dysplasia

Henry J. Rozycki
Alan R. Spitzer
William W. Fox

Bronchopulmonary dysplasia (BPD) represents one of the most difficult management problems in neonatology today. The evaluation and therapy of this disease are constantly undergoing revision and refinement. The following sections will present some of the most recent developments in the clinical management of BPD.

PULMONARY FUNCTION CHANGES IN BPD

The lung damage that underlies BPD is reflected in abnormalities in pulmonary function. Within the first week of life, measurements of pulmonary resistance are significantly higher in those infants who subsequently require prolonged oxygen therapy as compared to those who do not.[1] This increase in lung resistance is the predominant and persistent abnormality found in patients with BPD throughout the course of the disease.

By 1 month of age, lung compliance is lower than in normal infants and airways resistance remains very high, leading to a marked increase in the work of breathing.[2,3] Functional residual capacity (FRC) in these patients is near normal.[4] By 6 months of age, infants with BPD demonstrate the following abnormalities in their pulmonary functions: minute ventilation is increased due to an increase in respiratory rate with a normal tidal volume,[5] compliance continues to be below normal for age, and both inspiratory and expiratory resistance continue to rise.[1–5]

Over the next 6 months, however, pulmonary functions begin to improve. In mild cases, minute ventilation decreases as the respiratory rate declines.[1,2] but in infants who have persistently severe disease during this period, minute ventilation remains elevated.[5] In most series there is an improvement in lung compliance,[2–5] but Tepper et al.,[6] using a method that determined total respiratory system compliance, reported that in five infants with BPD, specific compliance was 53 percent of normal control compliance at 10 months of age.

Over the next 2 years of life, children who clinically recover from BPD have been shown to have normal FRC, normal minute ventilation, and normal compliance, but they continued to have a higher pulmonary resistance. Bancalari and Gerhardt[1] report that in 10 survivors followed for 24 months, resistance was 130 percent of normal.

Beginning around 18 months, other subtle changes in lung function begin to appear. Spirometric measurements reveal that maximal expiratory flow is reduced in children who receive prolonged mechanical ventilation compared with children born at the same gestational age who have little or no lung disease.[4] The few long term follow-up studies of pulmonary function show that by the time children born with BPD reach school age, all abnormalities except for the changes in forced expiratory flow have resolved.

BPD "SPELLS"

Almost every clinician caring for infants with BPD has seen BPD "spells." These episodes, which often resemble temper tantrums, can begin as early as 2 weeks of life, but are more common at 1 month. Two types of acute spells occur, one of which appears to be associated with obstructive airway disease and cyanosis of acute onset. These infants require removal from the ventilator and hand bagging, often with very high peak inspiratory pressures (up to 80 cmH_2O), and 100 percent inspired O_2 before a spell resolves. Following the spell, and depending on the severity and time needed to stop the symptoms, these infants usually require increased inspired O_2 concentrations and increased peak inspiratory pressures on the ventilator. We have observed this type of spell in infants with a tracheostomy, and the anatomic location of the obstruction may therefore sometimes be in the lower trachea, bronchi, or smaller airways.

A second type of BPD spell is primarily characterized by acute and severe cyanosis. These events are most commonly of sudden onset, and in a typical case the infant goes from being adequately oxygenated to deeply cyanotic within seconds. The rapidity of onset and severity of the cyanosis make it appear that this problem is initiated by acute changes in pulmonary vascular resistance resulting in right-to-left shunting. To resolve the spell, these infants must be ventilated or hyperventilated with 100 percent inspired O_2 and increased peak inspiratory pressure.

A third type of episode is a more chronic deterioration with a decreased PO_2 and increased PCO_2 for a period of 1 to 2 weeks. These episodes may be associated with intercurrent pulmonary infection. If the infection is viral, cultures will be negative. If bacterial infection is present, a leukens aspirate of the endotracheal tube or tracheostomy will reveal increased polymorphonuclear leukocytes and a predominant organism on culture.

In general, there is no specific treatment that works for all of these episodes. We have used theophylline and metaproterenol (Alupent) in most of our chronically ill infants with BPD, and check blood levels if spells persist. In addition, we have used epinephrine, isoproterenol, nebulized terbutaline, steroids, and morphine with no consistent improvement. In general, one should try to diagnose a treatable etiology such as an infection, and increase the peak inspiratory pressure by 3 to 5 cmH_2O or increase the FiO_2 by 5 to 10 percent to prevent these episodes.

The first two types of acute spells may have their onset when the infant is stimulated or suctioned. In certain infants, simply approaching the bed seems to trigger the spell. In this respect the spells resemble breath-holding episodes in older infants.

Most of these spells are associated with severe hypoxemia, and should be prevented if possible. If the spells are either frequent or severe, the weaning schedule must be interrupted, and respiratory support must be increased.

MECHANICAL VENTILATION AND BPD

While the use of conventional mechanical ventilation has dramatically reduced neonatal morbidity and mortality from respiratory distress syndrome (RDS), many problems still exist with this form of therapy. Babies still die of ventilatory failure with RDS, and with the increasing use of conventional mechanical ventilation to treat infants with birthweights as low as 400 to 500 g, BPD appears to be on the increase. Complications of BPD include prolonged hospitalization, late death, and neurologic and respiratory handicaps that may persist throughout life.

The exact factors that cause BPD are not clear, but oxygen toxicity and pulmonary barotrauma appear to be important predisposing factors. As many as 30 percent of infants requiring mechanical ventilation will develop varying degrees of BPD. In general, BPD is defined as an oxygen requirement at 1 month of life associated with clinical respiratory distress. Although a number of new therapies, such as the administration of surfactant, may reduce the ventilatory requirements of an individual infant, attention has also focused upon the type of ventilators being used to treat RDS in the premature baby. In general, currently used neonatal ventilators rely on convection and diffusion for gas exchange in the lungs and bronchi, much like what occurs during normal spontaneous breathing.

Mechanical ventilation with positive pressure has been implicated in the etiology of BPD. The clinician is faced with the necessity for administering high O_2 concentrations as well as increased peak respiratory pressures to premature infants to maintain life. In the past, there have been controversies about the efficacy of volume versus pressure ventilators for the prevention of BPD. In the mid 1970s, a method of ventilation was proposed advocating an inverse inspiratory-to-expiratory ratio and a square-wave flow pattern.[7] This method was initially reported to decrease the incidence of BPD, but no controlled trial has been done to show it has an advantage in preventing BPD.

By the late 1970s there was almost exclusive use of continuous-flow, time-cycled, pressure-limited ventilators. These machines are relatively inexpensive, easy to use, and reliable. The focus of operation with these machines was inspiratory pressure, and most clinicians tried to use the lowest peak inspiratory pressure possible to provide adequate ventilation. The real questions that are now arising concern the definition of adequate ventilation and adequate oxygenation for a neonate. Empirically, most clinicians define acceptable arterial PO_2 tension as 50 to 80 mmHg, PCO_2 as 40 to 50 mmHg, and pH as above 7.30. The PO_2 values given are selected to provide a safe cushion from sudden deterioration, or the "flip-flop" pattern of acute hypoxemia often seen during management of acute RDS. The high PO_2 limits are considered low enough to prevent retinopathy of prematurity from oxygen exposure. The PCO_2 values are chosen to provide adequate ventilation and prevent respiratory acidosis. The values for pH are accepted because animal studies indicate that at a pH below 7.25 there was a significant increase in pulmonary vascular resistance.

Now we must question if these arterial blood gas criteria are too stringent, especially for the very low birthweight infant. The overall incidence of BPD in high-risk nurseries is in the range of 20 percent, but in infants below 700 grams may be as high as 80 to 85 percent. The lungs in these very low birthweight infants are so immature that even short term exposrue to positive ventilation may be excessive and initiate chronic lung disease.

Since various types of conventional ventilation have not produced a significant decrease in BPD, the only alternative approach to investigate is either to use another ventilator concept (high-frequency ventilation is discussed later), or decide whether we are being too aggressive with blood gas criteria. One published study, by Rhodes et al.,[8] instituted a new set of arterial blood gas requirements that accepted lower values for PO_2 and pH and higher values for PCO_2. In this study PO_2 values as low as 35 mmHg were allowed before the inspired O_2 concentration was increased. The PCO_2 was not corrected unless pH values were below 7.2. All patients were transfused when Hgb levels were less than 14. Although neurologic follow-up was not reported, the overall incidence of BPD was 3.7 percent—a remarkably low level considering that there were 156 infants weighing less than 1500 g. It will be critically important to report follow-up data on infants treated with this regimen, because if the neurologic outcome is good, it could represent a breakthrough in mechanical ventilation of the very low birthweight infant.

Apparently, a variation of this approach was also used by one center, as recently reported in a review of eight tertiary care nurseries.[9] This center had a lower incidence of BPD. The center rarely uses endotracheal tubes, and apparently accepts much lower PO_2 and pH values and higher PCO_2 values during mechanical ventilation. A prospective, randomized clinical trial comparing ventilation with these new blood gas criteria to conventional ventilation will resolve this issue.

HIGH-FREQUENCY VENTILATION IN THE TREATMENT OF RDS AND PREVENTION OF BPD

The classical model of pulmonary gas exchange requires that tidal volume must exceed dead space volume in order for effective exchange of oxygen and carbon dioxide to occur. During the late 1950s, however, Emerson developed an airway vibrator capable of producing ventilation at up to 2,000 breaths per minute. The original intent of this device was to provide internal physiotherapy for patients suffering from chronic obstructive lung disease and cystic fibrosis. It was noted, however, that application of this therapy also resulted in adequate gas exchange, even though tidal volume was less than dead space ventilation. This form of therapy was subsequently developed further by groups working around the world in a variety of clinical situations (see Ch. 3 for more details).

Some of the earliest efforts related to treatment of RDS occurred at the Children's Medical Center of Boston, when Frantz et al.[10] reported a number of babies with lung disease treated with high-frequency ventilation. The frequency of ventilation in that therapy was 20 Hz (1,200 breaths per minute). Additional reports of oscillatory ventilation have also suggested that this form of therapy may be beneficial for the treatment of infants with severe RDS.[11] Furthermore, reports utilizing high-frequency jet ventilation have also been favorable, in that adequate gas exchange can occur at lower peak inflating pressures in infants treated with high-frequency ventilation as compared with conventional mechanical ventilation.[12]

Three distinct forms of high-frequency ventilation have evolved: high-frequency positive-pressure ventilation, high-frequency jet ventilation, and high-frequency oscillatory ventilation. The high-frequency positive pressure ventilator is simply a conventional mechanical ventilator capable of being used at rates of up to 150 breaths per minute in the neonate. Investigations by Bland[13] have suggested that rapid respiratory rates at decreased peak inflating pressures may be beneficial in decreasing the incidence of BPD in babies being treated for hyaline membrane disease. High-frequency jet ventilation is a specialized form of high-frequency ventilation, produced by the rapid delivery of small pulses of gas through a special injection cannula in the airway. Jet ventilation may be produced either distally with the jet entering into the endotracheal tube at a site near the carina, or proximally with the jet being delivered at the endotracheal tube adapter. With the use of jet ventilation, expiration is passive. Gas returns to the atmosphere through the periphery of the endotracheal tubes. High-frequency oscillatory ventilation, in contrast, is provided by devices that are piston activated or acoustically developed, and produce gas movement both into and out of the airway. A variation of the previous two types of ventilators is a device that operates through a rotating-ball-valve apparatus that interrupts flow at a preset frequency. These devices are called flow interrupters. In all cases, the intent of high-frequency ventilation is to produce adequate oxygenation and ventilation while minimizing potential pulmonary damage from either a high inspired oxygen concentration or pulmonary barotrauma.

At the present time, regardless of the type of high-frequency ventilation utilized, several statements can be made from established data. First, high-frequency ventilation does provide adequate oxygenation and ventilation for prolonged periods of time, in spite of the fact that the tidal volumes produced in general are near or below dead space volumes. In general, most patients can be ventilated at distal endotracheal pressures that are less than those required in the same patients upon conventional ventilation, so that pulmonary barotrauma can be reduced. What is not established, however, is the effect of this form of ventilation on the prevention of BPD. A large collaborative study has been undertaken by the National Institutes of Health at 10 major pediatric centers around the country in order to attempt to answer this question. Babies are randomized within 24 hours after birth to either conventional mechanical ventilation or high-frequency oscillation with a strict protocol, in order to determine the ability of high-frequency oscillatory ventilation to decrease the incidence of BPD at these centers.

At The Children's Hospital of Philadelphia during the past 4 years, a large number of patients have been treated with high-frequency jet ventilation (Bunnell Life Pulse, Salt Lake City, Utah) for a variety of respiratory diseases of the newborn. Of the 122 infants treated to date, 67 (54 percent) have survived. All of the cases in which this form of ventilation has been used been rescue efforts, involving infants who were failing with conventional mechanical ventilation or had significant air leaks at the time they were switched to high-frequency jet ventilation. All required high ventilatory rates and peak inspiratory pressures just to maintain life. It was, therefore, highly likely that the majority of these infants would not have survived without the use of this jet ventilator. The treatment began anywhere from 2 hours of life to as late as 3 months of life, when BPD was already established. The majority of infants were treated before 1 week of age. With high-frequency ventilation there was a mean reduction in mean airway pressure of 24.4 percent within 12 hours of the initiation of therapy, and a corresponding decrease in peak inflating pressure. At the same time, the $PaCO_2$ in treated patients decreased from a level of 45.3 $\pm$ 2.34 to 35.8 $\pm$ 1.8 mmHg ($P<0.01$) during the same time interval. Oxygenation increased from a level of 65.7 $\pm$ 3.81 to 82.6 $\pm$ 5.82 mmHg ($P<0.05$) by 12 hours after institution of high-frequency jet ventilaton.

The infants who have responded best to this form of therapy are premature infants of less than 2,000 g weight with RDS. The technique of high-frequency ventilation, however, also appears to be effective for treating other forms of neonatal respiratory disease, including meconium aspiration syndrome, persistent pulmonary hypertension of the newborn, group B streptococcal pneumonia, and pulmonary hypoplasia, including that related to congenital diaphragmatic hernia. The incidence of BPD in babies treated in these salvage attempts is high, with approximately 40 percent of babies developing BPD. To date, however, only three babies in this group of infants have remained chronically ventilator dependent for more than 6 weeks following treatment. Initial follow-up results on infants to 1 year of age in the group of survivors are also encouraging, in that the incidence of intraventricular hemorrhage appears to be less than that reported in babies treated with conventional mechanical ventilation. Follow-up data suggest that neurodevelopmental outcome in the large majority of babies who survive is within normal limits. Although much attention in the literature has focused on the acute complications related to jet ventilation (primarily necrotizing tracheobronchitis), in our experience there has been no significant clinical increase in this condition (see also Ch. 11). As a result, we feel that infants with lung disease unresponsive to conventional mechanical ventilation should be switched to high-frequency ventilation at the earliest possible time in order to lessen the likelihood of significant pulmonary barotrauma. Further work, however, must define the appropriate application of both jet ventilation and oscillatory ventilation in the treatment of RDS of the newborn, as well as BPD.

SURFACTANT ADMINISTRATION FOR THE TREATMENT OF RDS AND PREVENTION OF BPD

Since the observation in 1957 by Avery and Mead[14] that babies dying of RDS lacked a substance in the lungs, subsequently characterized as surfactant, much interest has focused on the administration of surfactant to prevent or decrease the severity of RDS. A notable early attempt was reported in October of 1967, by Drs. William Tooley and John Clements working at the Kandang Maternity Hospital in Singapore. Fifteen infants were treated with dipalmitoyl lecithin, with 5 infants surviving. The authors, however, felt that the results of their work did not appear to support the lack of pulmonary surfactant material as the primary problem in RDS. They focused instead on the pulmonary ischemia often seen in infants with RDS. As a result, they recommended the use of pulmonary vasodilitation as opposed to surfactant administration as the primary pharmacologic treatment for babies with RDS.[15]

Interest in surfactant replacement, however, was reinitiated by a report from Fujiwara et al.[16] in 1980, suggesting that artificial surfactant therapy given through endotracheal tubes in infants suffering from hyaline membrane disease improved oxygenation, decreased alveolar arterial oxygen gradients, reduced the required levels of inspired oxygen and peak respirator pressure, and reversed acidosis and systemic hypotension. The primary side effect noted in that study was the appearance of a patent ductus arteriosus in 9 of the 10 infants treated. This report, however, served to rekindle interest in the development of a replacement surfactant for the baby with RDS, primarily motivated by the increased incidence of BPD in nurseries throughout the country (see Ch. 2 for a more detailed discussion).

At present, it is believed that approximately 20 to 30 percent of babies under 1,500 g will develop BPD as determined by an increased inspired oxygen requirement at 30 days of age. Since it is thought that the combination of increased ventilatory support and inspired oxygen concentration is a major contributing factor to the development of BPD, the reduction of ventilatory support might be expected to decrease the number of children who have BPD. At present, a number of studies have been performed with both synthetic and naturally occurring surfactants that suggest some benefit from this mode of therapy (Tables 4-1 and 4-2). Some statements, however, can be made regarding the type of surfactant utilized to treat RDS. First, no synthetic surfactant that has been tested in humans has so far produced a significant, reproducible improvement in outcome.[17–19] This includes trials both to prevent the development of RDS and rescue trials in which infants with already established RDS are treated with synthetic surfactant.

In contrast, a series of human studies in which babies were treated with naturally occurring surfactant extracted from either bovine lung or human amniotic fluid have suggested that there is a definite improvement in treated infants both from the point of view of prevention of RDS[20–23] and that of rescue from RDS.[16,24–

Table 4-1. Recent Human Studies With Synthetic Surfactant

					Outcome	
Strategy	Study	Surfactant	N	RCT	Early Improvement[a]	Late Improvement[b]
Prevention	Morley 1981[17]	DPPC/PG 7:3	55	No	No	↓ Death
	Halliday 1984[18]	DPPC/HDL	100	Yes	No	No
	Wilkinson 1985[19]	DPPC/PG 7:3	24	Yes	No	No
Rescue	Wilkinson 1985[19]	DPPC/PG 7:3	24	Yes	No	No

RCT = randomized controlled trial; DPPC = dipalmitoyl phosphatidylcholine; PG = phosphatidyl glycerol; HDL = high density lipoprotein.

[a] Respiratory support or oxygenation during first week.

[b] Morbidity or mortality at 1 month.

(Adapted with permission of Ross Laboratories, Columbus, OH 43216, from Soll, RF: Ross Laboratories Special Conference, Three More Hot Topics in Neonatology, p. 87, 1986.)

Table 4-2. Human Studies With Natural Surfactants

Strategy	Study	Surfactant	N	RCT	Outcome: Early Improvement[a]	Outcome: Late Improvement[b]
Prevention	Enhorning 1985[20]	Bovine lung lavage extract	72	Yes	Yes	↓ Death
	Kwong 1985[21]	Bovine lung lavage extract	27	Yes	Yes	No
	Shapiro 1985[22]	Bovine lung lavage extract	32	Yes	Yes	No
	Hallman 1986[25]	Human amniotic fluid extract	60	Yes	Yes	↓ BPD/death
Rescue	Fujiwara 1980[16]	Enriched bovine lung extract	10	No	Yes	No
	Gitlin 1986[24]	Enriched bovine lung extract	41	Yes	Yes	No
	Hallman 1985[25]	Human amniotic fluid extract	53	Yes	Yes	↓ BPD/death
	Raju 1986[26]	Enriched bovine lung extract	30	Yes	Yes	↓ Death

[a] Respiratory support or oxygenation during first week.
[b] Morbidity or mortality at 1 month.
(Adapted with permission from Ross Laboratories, Columbus, OH 43216, from Soll, RF: Ross Laboratories Special Conference, Three More Hot Topics in Neonatology, p. 88, 1986.)

[26] However, the ultimate outcomes in the series of studies published to date have been somewhat equivocal. Some studies have demonstrated no alteration in incidence of BPD, while others have indicated that the incidence of BPD is decreased and the ultimate survival of babies with RDS is enhanced. Differences between synthetic surfactant and naturally occurring surfactant are not completely clear at the present time. A new surfactant developed synthetically by Clements and called EXOSURF, which is composed of dipalmitoyl phosphatidyl choline as well as hexadecanol and tyloxapol, has improved survival and pulmonary function when administered to preterm lambs.[27] Human studies of this synthetic preparation, however, have yet to be published. Continued work clearly needs to be done both with artificial and naturally occurring surfactant extracts. However, the results with natural surfactant are highly encouraging to date, and suggest that the future may see these agents used to treat infants with RDS, so that the incidence of chronic lung disease can be substantially decreased.

PHARMACOTHERAPY OF BPD

Over the last decade, there has been an increase in the use of bronchodilators in the management of BPD. The most commonly used bronchodilator, theophylline, has been shown to reduce the high pulmonary resistance found in infants with chronic lung disease.[28] Recent data have shown that as early as 2 weeks after birth and at 28 weeks postconception, sensitive methods can detect reactivity in the small bronchial airways.[29] Smooth muscle is present in premature infants and hypertrophied in those with BPD.[30] Intravenous theophylline improves compliance, lowers resistance, and shortens the duration of mechanical ventilation in a majority of infants with BPD. The mechanisms for this improvement are as yet unclear. Methylxanthines have a diuretic effect and so may reduce interstitial lung fluid (see below). In adults, theophylline improves diaphragmatic contractility.[2] However, given the hyperreactivity of the airways and their response to sympathomimetics, it is likely that theophylline acts predominantly as a bronchodilator.

A loading dose of 6 to 7 mg/kg over 20 minutes, followed by 1.1 to 1.5 mg/kg every 8 hours, will usually achieve the desired theophylline serum levels of 10 to 20 μg/ml. Serum levels should be monitored regularly to make certain that they remain in this range. Side effects including tachycardia, arrhythmia, jitteriness, diuresis, and seizures are rare. In infants requiring therapy for more than 6 months, the dosing interval may need to be shortened.

Another class of bronchodilators, sympathomimetic agents, have been shown to reduce airways resistance in infants with BPD.[31] Beta-2 agonists are the preferred drugs because of their reduced effects on the heart. These drugs can be used acutely in aerosol form[31] or subcutaneously[32] in the management of an acute bronchospastic episode, or chronically in an aerosol or enteral form. We have found that metaproterenol (Alupent), 0.3 to 1.0 mg/kg given orally every 8 hours, is useful when toxic reactions limit theophylline therapy.

The pathologic picture of BPD includes evidence of interstitial edema.[2] Lymphatic drainage is interrupted and there may be alterations in transendothelial hydrostatic forces from pulmonary hypertension, and in transendothelial permeability from oxygen or pressure trauma. It is not surprising, therefore, that diuretics have been used in the management of BPD. Furosemide, administered intravenously at a dose of 1 mg/kg to patients with BPD, caused an acute fall in airways resistance and a rise in compliance.[33] Patel et al.,[34] however, found that with the same dose they could not demonstrate a clinical effect on gas exchange. In spite of the lack of documented evidence regarding the usefulness of chronic furosemide administration in patients with BPD, the drug is commonly given for long periods of time at doses of 0.5 to 3.0 mg/kg intravenously or enterally twice daily. Side effects include hyponatremia, hypokalemia, metabolic alkalosis, and nephrolithiasis from hypercalciuria.[35]

Other, less potent diuretics have also been used and found to be effective. Kao et al.[36] performed a double-blind crossover study comparing placebo and a combination of chlorothiazide, 20 mg/kg, and spironolactone, 1.5 mg/kg, every 12 hours. The diuretics consistently caused a fall in pulmonary resistance and a rise in compliance. Diuretics may also allow the administration of a larger volume of fluid than would otherwise be tolerated, and so may allow for a larger number of calories to be given, an important consideration in the nutritional management of BPD.

CORTICOSTEROIDS FOR THE TREATMENT OF BPD

The chronic nature of BPD has resulted in a variety of pharmacologic approaches to this disease. Because of the well established anti-inflammatory effects of corticosteroids, several recent studies have attempted to show that glucocorticoids, and in particular dexamethasone, may substantially decrease requirements for ventilatory support and shorten hospitalization.[37–39] However, few prospective studies have demonstrated a clear benefit from use of glucocorticoids in the treatment of BPD. Mammel et al.[37] reported a double blind crossover study of dexamethasone in six infants. The infants were treated with intravenous dexamethasone for a 3-day period and showed a significant reduction in respiratory rate, peak inflating pressures, and inspired oxygen concentration. All six babies treated with dexamethasone were successfully extubated by 3 to 12 days after initiation of treatment. The authors, however, noted that infection occurred in five of the six infants, and two babies died of pneumonia while still on corticosteroids.

In a subsequent study by Avery et al.,[39] dexamethasone also acutely decreased ventilatory support. In this prospective controlled study there was a significant improvement in pulmonary compliance in 64 percent of the dexamethasone-treated group, while only 5 percent of the control group showed improvement ($P<0.01$). Weaning from the ventilator could be accomplished in the treated infants. Long term results from this study were not quite as favorable. Of the babies treated with dexamethasone, five of eight (63 percent) compared to six of eight untreated babies (75 percent) survived. The incidence of septicemia and hypertension was higher in the treated infants, although the numbers of patients in the study were insufficient for statistical analysis.

A number of other reports[40,41] in the medical literature, primarily in abstract form, also suggest short term benefits from the use of corticosteroids, although to date no one has clearly demonstrated a substantial alteration in ultimate outcome. Concerns still exist about the potential short term and long term complications related to the use of glucocorticoids. Hyperglycemia, hypertension, fluid retention, septicemia, and fluid and electrolyte imbalance have all been noted as acute complications. Long term effects on neurodevelopmental outcome and bone mineralization also are theoretical concerns with the use of these anti-inflammatory agents.

Our own personal experience with the use of corticosteriods in neonates with BPD has been variable. The ability to wean infants from the ventilator appeared to be enhanced in infants treated between 2 and 4 weeks of age with 0.5 mg of dexamethasone given daily in two divided doses. In babies treated at 2 to 5 months of age, however, with well-established BPD, a significant reduction in ventilatory support was commonly seen as measured by decreased FIO_2 and peak inflating pressure, but the effect was a transient one. In this group of babies treated for 7 days with dexamethasone, a significant rebound effect was noted approximately 2 to 4 weeks following the cessation of dexamethasone therapy, with deterioration to a level of ventilatory support similar to what the infant had prior to initiation of therapy. As a result, it is inappropriate at this time to recommend the use of this medication for the treatment of BPD, except in prospective controlled studies that examine both the acute and long term effects of the use of corticosteroids. Alternative dose schedules also need to be studied (long term, every other day, etc.). It does appear, however, that infants treated with steroids early in the course of BPD have a better result than those infants treated at a later stage of their illness. The mechanisms by which steroids might theoretically improve lung function are at present theoretical. Since bronchospasm is often a major part of the illness in these infants, relaxation of bronchospasm and a decrease in peribronchial edema may improve ventilation, improve compliance, and decrease ventilatory requirements. Other steroid-related effects may be important as well. These include a decrease in pulmonary hypertension, stabilization of cell and lysosomal membranes, decrease in synthesis of inflammatory agents such as prostaglandins and leukotrienes, enhancement of surfactant synthesis, and other nonspecific effects on while cell and inflammatory reactions within the lung. Again, however, it is important to emphasize that this therapy, at the present time, is experimental and cannot be advocated for all infants with BPD. It does appear, however, that early diagnosis and institution of treatment at an early phase of the disease are likely to produce the most significant benefit from the use of glucocorticoid therapy.

RECOVERY MANAGEMENT OF BPD

Once an infant develops clinical and radiographic evidence of BPD, management and therapy are aimed at two major goals. The first is to keep further lung damage to a minimum, and the second is to enhance the growth and repair of existing lung disease. Therefore, a balance between adequate support and minimal damage must be maintained.[5]

Arterial carbon dioxide levels in the range of 50 to 60 mmHg are acceptable when enough time has elapsed for renal compensation to occur such that the pH is above 7.30. Peak inspiratory pressure is reduced as much as possible, but these infants require between 20 and 30 cmH_2O, probably because their lung compliance continues to be poor. Once an optimal level of pressure is achieved, a weaning schedule can be started. Usually the rate is decreased by one breath/minute, and changes are made every day if tolerated. Occasional exacerbations, such as bronchospastic episodes, acute pulmonary edema, or intercurrent infections are aggressively treated, and if the ventilatory support must be escalated, the short term goal becomes to reduce that support to the pre-exacerbation level as soon as possible. When rates below 5 breaths/minute are achieved, a period on continuous positive airway pressure (CPAP) commonly precedes extubation. If an infant does not tolerate CPAP alone, a regimen of "sprinting" may be useful. Under this system, the ventilator breaths are turned off for a brief period each day, leaving the child on oxygen and CPAP alone. This may be for as little as 10 minutes twice per day. Gradually, the amount of time on CPAP is increased by 5- or 10-minute increments until the patient can tolerate an hour or two without an artificial breath. At this point, the "sprinting" time can be increased by larger increments until full CPAP is achieved.

Oxygen, while contributing to the pathogenesis of BPD, is an essential component in its therapy.[30] The pulmonary arterioles constrict in the presence of hypoxia, and this may worsen ventilation-perfusion mismatching as well as increase the risk of right ventricular overload.[42] The goal of oxygen therapy is to provide a neutral oxygen environment, by providing enough oxygen to eliminate the oxygen respiratory drive (which would use up too many calories), but as little as possible to reduce the dysplastic effects of high oxygen concentrations on the airways and lungs.

Usually the need for supplemental oxygen persists beyond the need for mechanical ventilation. Low-flow oxygen delivered by nasal cannula is an efficient method and allows more freedom of movement than a hood or tent. During periods of increased activity, such as during feeding, the concentration of inspired oxygen may need to be raised.[2] With the advent of improved home health care, patients with BPD who still require increased oxygen can go home to complete their recovery.[43]

Infants on chronic ventilator therapy require monitoring of pH, $PaCO_2$, and PaO_2. Each method of monitoring has its advantages and disadvantages. Maintaining indwelling arterial catheters for the complete course of therapy is probably the least advisable method, carrying with it a large thrombotic and infectious risk. Intermittent arterial punctures are painful and can cause abrupt decreases in arterial oxygen levels. Capillary blood is adequate for estimating arterial pH and PCO_2 levels but not for measuring PO_2. Transcutaneous oxygen sensors seem to decrease in effectiveness as the patients grow older. However, transcutaneous carbon dioxide monitors have been shown to correlate with arterial CO_2 tension in older BPD patients. Newer oxygen-saturation sensors, using the pulse oximetry method, are quite sensitive and maintain their effectiveness under most clinical conditions.[44]

With small decrements in inspired oxygen and mechanical ventilation, a regimen of once-daily determinations of transcutaneous oxygen or oxygen saturation and of transcutaneous CO_2 or capillary pH and CO_2 are usually sufficient to monitor the therapy. More invasive procedures should be reserved for intermittent correlations with noninvasive monitoring and for clinical exacerbations of BPD. Finally, growth is a sensitive indicator of adequate oxygen support. Frequently, an infant recovering from BPD will stop gaining weight after the inspired oxygen concentration has been decreased by 1 to 2 percent. Even if adequate calories are given, the extra work of breathing in relatively low inspired oxygen concentrations utilizes excessive calories.

Patients with BPD usually do not tolerate extra, or in some cases normal, fluid loads.[2] This often imposes restrictions on caloric delivery to these patients. At the same time, nutrition is a critical part of recovery management, providing the energy and substrate for lung growth and repair. The metabolic rate, as reflected by oxygen consumption, is higher in patients with BPD than in age-matched controls.[45] In our experience, growth can be achieved by providing at least 110 kcal/kg/day enterally, although this will vary from one individual to the next. Concentrated formula tube feedings at 150 cc/kg/day will provide this. Diuretic doses may have to be increased in order to deal with the fluid load. When maximal fluid levels are reached, addition of fat, carbohydrates, or both to the feeds may increase the caloric density without adding more volume. In adults, it has been shown that patients with chronic respiratory diseases tolerate fat supplementation better than carbohydrate, perhaps because of the lower respiratory quotient for fat (0.6 vs. 1.0).

Adult patients who remain ventilated for more than 1 week undergo elective tracheostomies.[46] For infants, the optimal timing for tracheotomy has not been established. Chronic tracheal intubation results in the development of granulation tissue and subsequent subglottic stenosis. This risk is related to length of intubation, frequency of reintubation, relative size of tube, and evidence of stridor.[47] We recommend tracheostomy if it becomes difficult to keep an orotracheal or nasotracheal tube in place, if it is noted that reintubation is difficult, or if by 3 months of age the prognosis for extubation is beyond about 2 weeks.

The presence of a foreign body in the airway predisposes the infant to infection. Weekly tracheal aspirates, sent for semiquantitative bacterial culture, aid in the rapid diagnosis and specific therapy of tracheitis and pneumonia. The appearance of a predominant organism in these cultures, the presence of a large number of neutrophils on Gram stain of the aspirates, a change in the quality or quantity of secretions, and a worsening of the respiratory status are all signs pointing to the presence of bacterial infection. Parenteral antibiotics chosen by the sensitivity pattern of the predominant organism are then indicated.

Viral infections also add to the morbidity and mortality of BPD. While at present only symptomatic support can be offered for infections caused by most viruses, an aerosol antiviral agent, ribavirin, is available to treat pulmonary infections caused by respiratory syncytial virus (RSV).[48] It is therefore important that during the peak season of RSV disease (winter), patients who undergo a worsening of their lung disease have nasal washings sent for serologic diagnostic testing and be started on ribavirin therapy. At present, the drug is contraindicated in patients on mechanical ventilation. However, protocols to determine how to overcome the problems of drug precipitation in the ventilator system are underway at several institutions.

HOME RESPIRATORY CARE

During the past 3 years at The Children's Hospital of Philadelphia, we have discharged home more than 15 infants requiring continuing respiratory care. A review of these 15 infants revealed that they had been hospitalized an average of 8.4 months (range 3.5 to 15 months). Thirteen of these infants had a previous diagnosis of RDS and BPD, and all had subglottic stenosis. Eight infants required a T-piece, O_2 therapy, and a tracheostomy, and five had CPAP with a tracheostomy. These babies required a mean of 13.8 months from hospital discharge to decannulation. Management of these infants has helped us develop a program for more efficient discharge while such infants still require continuing respiratory support. The four major components of the program consist of a hospital team, equipment administration, follow-up program, and community resources (Table 4-3).

There are several components of the hospital team, including the Nursing Service, Neonatology Unit, Biomedical Department, Respiratory Therapy Team, and Social Work Department. All of these groups of professionals must be integrated to provide the quality of care necessary to effect proper training of the patient's family and assure quality care at home. In addition, the medical equipment supplier plays an integral role in patient management after discharge. In most cases, the equipment distributor coordinates home visits and continuing respiratory therapy. The coordination of financial aspects of each case prior to discharge is essential. In our series, all infants had either Blue Cross or private insurance, and these companies all require lists of equipment, justification for therapy, and documentation of nursing or respiratory therapy requirements before authorization for outpatient care is given. Follow-up of these babies is divided between the tertiary care physicians and the private pediatrician. The private pediatrician provides well-baby care and manages common childhood illnesses. The tertiary care physician or team is available for respiratory-related problems. Finally, as in home apnea management programs, the utility companies must make provisions for back-up if there is a power failure.

Table 4-3. Neonatal Home Ventilation–Tracheostomy Care: Components of Program

Hospital Team
Nursing
Doctor
Biomedical
Respiratory therapy
Social work
Parents
Infant
Equipment
Equipment distributor
Administrative–financial
Follow-up
Private pediatrician
CHOP team
Community
Fire
Police
Electrical company

The most significant part of the organization of home respiratory care is a flow sheet outlining the role of every member of the care team. Our flow sheet includes the Family, Infant Development Team, Respiratory Therapy Team, Physicians, Nursing Service, and Social Services Department. It outlines all stages in training, financial arrangements, parent orientation, and other needs for 6 weeks prior to discharge of the patient. The major advantage of a written flow sheet is that each member of the team is accountable for training or coordination of the effort at specific times prior to discharge.

REFERENCES

1. Bancalari E, Gerhardt T: Functional alterations in the acute phase of bronchopulmonary dysplasia. p. 43. In Bronchopulmonary Dysplasia and Related Chronic Respiratory Disorders. Report of the Ninetieth Ross Conference on Pediatric Research. Ross Laboratories, Columbus, Ohio, 1985
2. Bancalari E, Gerhardt T: Bronchopulmonary dysplasia. Pediatr Clin North Am 33:1, 1986
3. Cunningham MD, Desai NS: Methods of assessment and findings regarding pulmonary function in infants less than 1000 grams. Clin Perinatol 13:299, 1986
4. Tepper RS: Chronic respiratory disturbances in bronchopulmonary dysplasia. p. 46. In Bronchopulmonary Dysplasia and Related Chronic Respiratory Disorders. Report of the Ninetieth Ross Conference on Pediatric Research. Ross Laboratories, Columbus, Ohio, 1985
5. Morray JP, Fox WW, Kettrick RG, Downes JJ: Improvement in lung mechanics as a function of age in the infant with severe bronchopulmonary dysplasia. Pediatr Res 16:290, 1982
6. Tepper RS, Pagtakhan RD, Taussig LM: Noninvasive determination of total respiratory system compliance in infants by the weighted-spirometer method. Am Rev Respir Dis 130:461, 1984
7. Reynolds EO, Taghizadeh A: Improved prognosis of infants mechanically ventilated for hyaline membrane disease. Arch Dis Child 49:505, 1974
8. Rhodes PG, Graves GR, Patel DM, et al: Minimizing pneumothorax and bronchopulmonary dysplasia in ventilated infants with hyaline membrane disease. J Pediatr 103:634, 1983
9. Avery ME, Hurd SS, Tooley WH: Is chronic lung disease in prematurely-born infants preventable? Pediatr Res 20:341A, 1986
10. Frantz ID, Werthammer J, Stark AR: High-frequency ventilation in premature infants with lung disease: Adequate gas exchange at low tracheal pressure. Pediatrics 71:483, 1983
11. Boynton BR, Mannino FL, David RF, et al: Combined high frequency oscillatory ventilation and intermittent mandatory ventilation in critically ill neonates. J Pediatr 105:297, 1984

12. Carlo WA, Chatburn RL, Martin RJ, et al: Decrease in airway pressure using high-frequency jet ventilation in infants with respiratory distress syndrome. J Pediatr 104:101, 1984
13. Bland RD, Kim MH, Light MJ, Woodson JL: High frequency mechanical ventilation in severe hyaline membrane disease: An alternative treatment? Crit Care Med 8:275, 1980
14. Avery ME, Mead J: Surface properties in relation to atelectasis and hyaline membrane disease. Am J Dis Child 97:517, 1957
15. Chu J, Clements JA, Cotton EK, et al: Neonatal pulmonary ischemia. I. Clinical and physiological studies. Pediatrics, 40:Suppl., 709–782, 1967
16. Fujiwara T, Maeta H, Chida S, et al: Artificial surfactant therapy in hyaline-membrane disease. Lancet 1:55, 1980
17. Morley CJ, Bangham AD, Miller N, Davis JA: Dry artificial lung surfactant and its effect on very premature babies. Lancet 1:64, 1981
18. Halliday HL, McClure G, Reid MM, et al: Controlled trial of artificial surfactant to prevent respiratory distress syndrome. Lancet 1:476, 1984
19. Wilkinson A, Jenkins PA, Jeffrey JA: Two controlled trials of dry artificial surfactant: Early effects and later outcome in babies with surfactant deficiency. Lancet 2:287, 1985
20. Enhorning G, Shennan A, Possmayer F, et al: Prevention of neonatal respiratory distress syndrome by tracheal instillation of surfactant: A randomized clinical trial. Pediatrics 76:145, 1985
21. Kwong MS, Egan EA, Notter RH, Shapiro DL: Double-blind clinical trial of calf lung surfactant extract for the prevention of hyaline membrane disease in extremely premature infants. Pediatrics 76:585, 1985
22. Shapiro DL, Notter RH, Morin FC, et al: Double-blind randomized trial of a calf lung surfactant extract administered at birth to very premature infants for the prevention of respiratory distress syndrome. Pediatrics 76:593, 1985
23. Merritt TA, Hallman M, Bloom BT, et al: Prophylactic treatment of very premature infants with human surfactant. N Engl J Med 315:785, 1986
24. Gitlin JD, Soll RF, Parad RB, et al: A randomized controlled trial of exogenous surfactant for the treatment of hyaline membrane disease. Pediatr Res 20:429A, 1986
25. Hallman M, Merritt TA, Jarvenpaa AL, et al: Exogenous human surfactant for treatment of severe respiratory distress syndrome: A randomized prospective clinical trial. J Pediatr 106:963, 1985
26. Raju T, Vidyasagar D, Bhat R, et al: A double blind study of surfactant TA (STA) therapy in <1250 g infants with severe hyaline membrane disease (HMD). Pediatr Res 20:438A, 1986
27. Durand DJ, Clyman RI, Heymann MA, et al: Effects of a protein-free, synthetic surfactant on survival and pulmonary function in preterm lambs. J Pediatr 107:775, 1985
28. Rooklin AR, Moomjian AS, Shutack JG, et al: Theophylline therapy in bronchopulmonary dysplasia. J Pediatr 95:882, 1979
29. Motoyama EK, Fort MD: Evidence of bronchial reactivity in premature infants with bronchopulmonary dysplasia. p. 53. In Bronchopulmonary Dysplasia and Related Chronic Respiratory Disorders. Report on the Ninetieth Ross Conference on Pediatric Research. Ross Laboratories, Columbus, Ohio, 1985
30. O'Brodovich HM, Mellins RB: Bronchopulmonary dysplasia. Unresolved neonatal lung injury. Am Rev Respir Dis 132:694, 1985
32. Kao LC, Warburton D, Platzker ACG, Keens TG: Effect of isoproterenol inhalation on airway resistance in chronic bronchopulmonary dysplasia. Pediatrics 73:509, 1984
32. Sosulski R, Abbasi S, Fox WW: Therapeutic value of terbutaline in bronchopulmonary dysplasia. Pediatr Res 16:309A, 1982
33. Kao LC, Warburton D, Sargent CW, et al: Furosemide acutely decreases airways resistance in chronic bronchopulmonary dysplasia. J Pediatr 103:624, 1983
34. Patel H, Yeh TF, Jain R, Pildes R: Pulmonary and renal responses to furosemide in infants with stage III–IV bronchopulmonary dysplasia. Am J Dis Child 139:917, 1985
35. Aranda JV, Chemtob S, Laudignon N, Sasyniuk BI: Furosemide and vitamin E: Two problem drugs in neonatology. Pediatr Clin North Am 33:583, 1986
36. Kao LC, Warburton D, Cheng MH, et al: Effect of oral diuretics on pulmonary mechanics in infants with chronic bronchopulmonary dysplasia: Results of a double-blind crossover sequential trial. Pediatrics 74:37, 1984
37. Mammel MC, Green TP, Johnson DE, Thompson TR: Controlled trial of dexamethasone therapy in infants with bronchopulmonary dysplasia. Lancet 1:1356, 1983
38. Donn SM, Faix RG, Banagale RC: Dexamethasone for bronchopulmonary dysplasia. Lancet 2:460, 1983
39. Avery GB, Fletcher AB, Kaplan M, Brudno DS: Controlled trial of dexamethasone in respirator-dependent infants with bronchopulmonary dysplasia. Pediatrics 75:106, 1985

40. Bonta BW, Otero L: Efficacy of dexamethasone (DXM) in management of progressive bronchopulmonary dysplasia (BPD). Pediatr Res 19:335A, 1985
41. Pomerance JJ, Puri A: Treatment of severe neonatal bronchopulmonary dysplasia with dexamethasone. Pediatr Res 16:359A, 1982
42. Halliday HL, Dumpit FM, Brady JP: Effects of inspired oxygen on echocardiographic assessment of pulmonary vascular resistance and myocardial contractility in bronchopulmonary dysplasia. Pediatrics 65:536, 1980
43. Pinney MA, Cotton EK: Home management of bronchopulmonary dysplasia. Pediatrics 58:856, 1976
44. Solimano AJ, Smyth JA, Mann TK, et al: Pulse oximetry advantages in infants with bronchopulmonary dysplasia. Pediatrics 78:844, 1986
45. Weinstein MR, Oh W: Oxygen consumption in infants with bronchopulmonary dysplasia. J Pediatr 99:958, 1981
46. Safar P: Cardiopulmonary-cerebral resuscitation. p. 9. In Shoemaker WC, Thompson WL, Holbrook PR (eds): Textbook of Critical Care. WB Saunders, Philadelphia, 1984
47. Sherman JM, Lowitt S, Stephenson C, Ironson G: Factors influencing acquired subglottic stenosis in infants. J Pediatr 109:322, 1986
48. Hall CB, McBride JT, Walsh EE, et al: Aerosolized ribavirin treatment of infants with respiratory syncytial viral infection: A randomized double-blind study. N Engl J Med 308:1443, 1983

5

Apnea of Prematurity: Current Theories of Pathogenesis and Treatment

Kenneth W. Klesh
Beverly S. Brozanski
Robert D. Guthrie

Apnea of prematurity (AOP) is among the most common, yet least well-understood, disorders of preterm infants. Despite a profusion of theories as to its pathogenesis and a literature replete with various effective or ineffective methods of treating it, AOP remains a perplexing condition for clinicians and a frustrating problem for parents awaiting an end to their infant's "A's and B's." In addition, the economic costs of prolonged monitoring for apnea, either in the hospital or at home, are substantial. Ongoing research promises to elucidate the basic mechanisms of abnormal respiratory control in these infants, and will provide a basis for more specific, effective therapy. Already there exists a new appreciation for the roles of brain stem neurodevelopment and of upper airway muscle coordination. It is the purpose of this chapter to review and to put into perspective current theories on the pathogenesis of idiopathic AOP, and to summarize recommendations for its treatment.

DEFINITION

Apnea is defined as cessation of respiratory airflow as a result of a central (no respiratory effort), obstructive (respiratory effort but no flow, usually secondary to upper airway obstruction), or mixed (central and obstructive) mechanism. While brief interruption of airflow may be normal, pathologic apnea is defined as a pause of 20 seconds or longer, or less if accompanied by cyanosis, bradycardia (less than 100 beats/minute), marked hypotonia, or sudden pallor.[1] This must be distinguished from periodic breathing, defined by Kelly and Shannon[2] as three or more respiratory pauses of greater than 3 seconds duration with less than 20 seconds of respiration between pauses. Such a pattern, generally unaccompanied by hypoxemia, is thought to be benign. On the other hand, apnea of prematurity or periodic breathing with pathologic apnea in a preterm infant may result in significant developmental morbidity, though well-controlled long term studies of this are lacking. Idiopathic AOP, a developmental phenomenon which usually ceases by 37 weeks postconceptual age, is distinct from apnea of infancy, the onset of which occurs at an older age. Further, apnea is among the most common nonspecific symptoms of concurrent illness in the preterm infant, and there are many clinical conditions such as sepsis, intraventricular hemorrhage, and hypoglycemia in which apnea is an associated finding.

INCIDENCE

The true incidence of AOP remains to be determined. A generally accepted definition of AOP has only recently been adopted; pauses in respiration for as little as 10 seconds, though probably representing uncomplicated periodic breathing, were frequently considered apneic spells in many early investigations. Additionally, early studies of the incidence of AOP did not consistently distinguish between unexplained episodes (idiopathic) and those secondary to identifiable illness, nor did they employ monitoring techniques to specifically detect absence of air flow.

It has been estimated that 25 percent of infants born at less than 37 weeks gestation manifest apnea.[3] The incidence of idiopathic AOP increases with decreasing gestational age, emphasizing the importance of immaturity in its pathogenesis. At 34 to 35 weeks gestation, the incidence is 7 percent, whereas approximately 50 percent of infants at 30 to 31 weeks gestation become apneic.[4] The majority of infants less than 28 to 29 weeks gestation develop apnea,[5] with episodes classically beginning on the second day of life and peaking in incidence later in the first week.

Most studies of neonatal apnea have utilized respiratory impedance monitoring, which fails not only to distinguish between obstructed and unobstructed respiratory efforts, but which also may fail to detect an obstructive episode altogether unless the event is accompanied by absence of chest/abdominal movement (mixed apnea) or bradycardia. However, even among those studies that employ monitoring of the heart rate, thoracic breathing movement, and airflow, the reported incidence of the various types of AOP varies widely. Guilleminault in 1975[6] reported that all apneas detected in 11 premature infants were of a central type, and Korner[7] later found that in 8 apneic preterm infants, obstructive and mixed episodes comprised only 3 percent and 5 percent, respectively, of the recorded events. A recent investigation by Mathew and colleagues[8] indicated a much higher incidence of upper airway obstruction in nine preterm infants, with 94 of 102 episodes having an obstructive component. In a much larger population, Dransfield and Fox[9] found that of 433 idiopathic apneic episodes in 76 preterm infants, 55 percent were central, 12 percent were obstructive, and 33 percent were mixed. Sixty-eight percent of the infants demonstrated some degree of obstructive apnea while 32 percent had central apnea only. Of additional importance, bradycardia did not occur in any infant unless accompanied by apnea, though the authors did concede the existence of other causes of isolated bradycardia in preterm infants, such as vagal stimulation and arrhythmia. Thus recent evidence proves that AOP includes central, obstructive, and mixed events, though one form may predominate in a given infant.

PATHOGENESIS

Current theories of the pathogenesis of idiopathic apnea of prematurity focus on the hypothesis that a relative immaturity of brain stem respiratory control centers accounts for this disorder. It is known that fetal breathing movements occur in utero as early as 20 weeks gestation, and that the apnea which occurs commonly in preterm infants usually disappears through natural development by 37 weeks postconceptual age. Thus the complex synaptic interconnections among the respiratory pattern generator, respiratory premotor and motoneurons, peripheral and central chemoreceptors, and the various mechanoreceptors of the lung, chest wall, and airways evolve over a normal developmental timespan to form a regular pattern of breathing (Fig. 5-1). Apnea can certainly still occur in full-term infants (and in

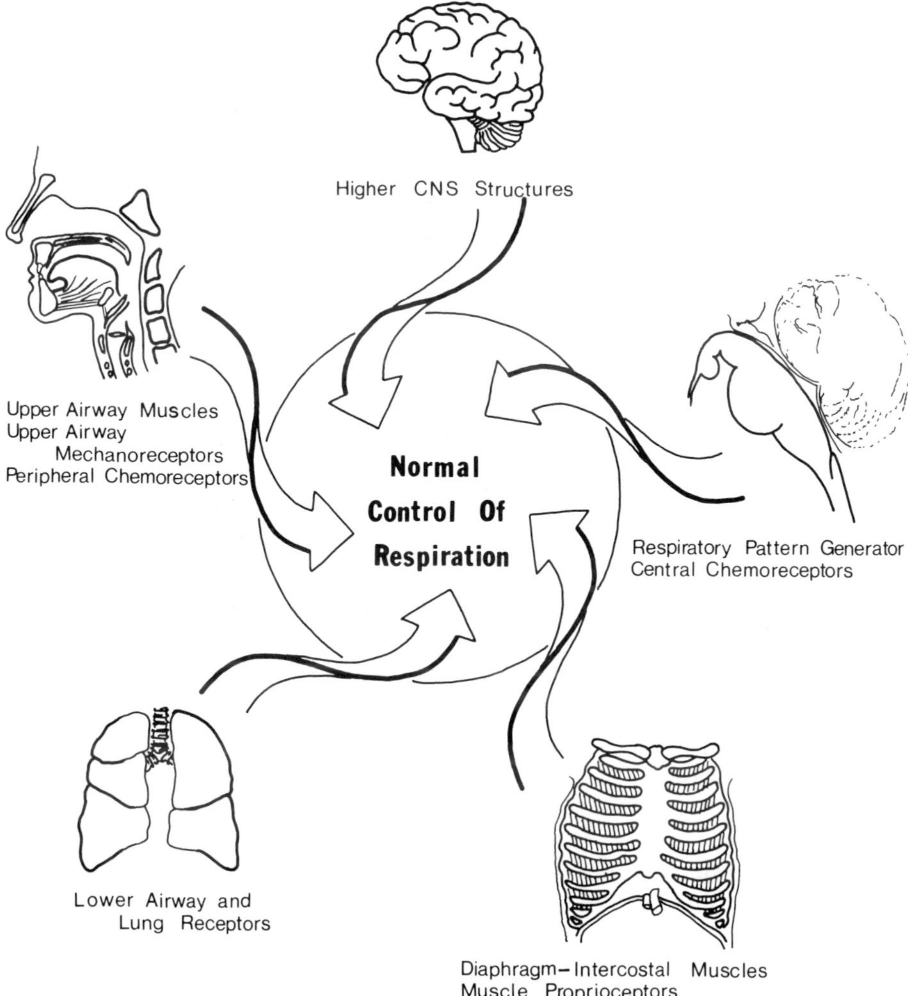

Fig. 5.1. Factors influencing the normal control of respiration.

adults), but usually does so with an identifiable cause. An understanding of the mechanisms involved in generating a normal central respiratory pattern may clarify our theories concerning the failure of many preterm infants to maintain a regular breathing pattern.

Theories of Central Respiratory Pattern Generation

Despite the fact that various groups of brain stem respiratory neurons have been identified and their anatomy, function, and interconnections characterized, the mechanism of normal respiratory rhythmogenesis remains unknown. Two classes of models for the respiratory pattern generator have been proposed: a network oscillator model and a pacemaker-driven oscillator model. In the former, according to von Euler,[10] mechano- and chemoreceptor inputs are processed through a *central inspiratory activity* (CIA) *integrator,* which is thought to reside in the ventrorostral medulla. The CIA integrator generates the respiratory rhythm with input from a *timing integrator,* a neuronal pool that may be located in an area distinct from the CIA integrator. The onset of inspiratory activity occurs as the result of both an abrupt release of inhibitory drive from an *on-off* switch center to the CIA integrator, and a subsequent progressive excitation of inspiratory premotor neurons by the CIA integrator. This on-off switch center receives and integrates input from pulmonary stretch receptors, chest wall proprioceptors, and chemoexcitatory and inhibitory afferents. Inspiration is also terminated by the on-off switch, which in this case is triggered by inspiratory-related activity of the CIA integrator and by afferent input from pulmonary stretch receptors.

More recently, Feldman and colleagues[11] have proposed that the respiratory pattern generator is a *pacemaker-driven oscillator.* In this hypothetical model, rhythmic activity is generated by a neural *pacemaker* in the brain stem network of respiratory neurons at locales yet unknown, but which functions as a sine wave generator or a gate to turn the circuitry on and off. The brain stem respiratory pattern generator in this new model is thus composed of a *burst generator* and a *cycle-timing generator,* which are driven by the pacemaker and which provide regular discharges to a *sensorimotor integrator.* Cycle timing and burst-pattern formation are distinct functions (Fig. 5-2); the timer does not affect the output of the burst-pattern generator, and inhibition is not necessary for cycle timing but can contribute to burst-pattern generation.[12] The sensorimotor integrator is composed of the dorsal and ventral respiratory groups and perhaps other specific respiratory premotor neurons; this integrator receives and processes afferent activity from peripheral and central chemoreceptors and from the mechanoreceptors. The mechano- and chemoreceptor afferents also provide neuronal input to the burst generator. The sensorimotor integrator then processes these discharges and commands the diaphragm, intercostal muscles, and upper airway respiratory muscles to contract. This model is consistent with recently available evidence.[12]

Undoubtedly, our understanding of how respiratory pattern generation can fail will be enhanced when the mechanisms of normal respiratory rhythmogenesis are elucidated.

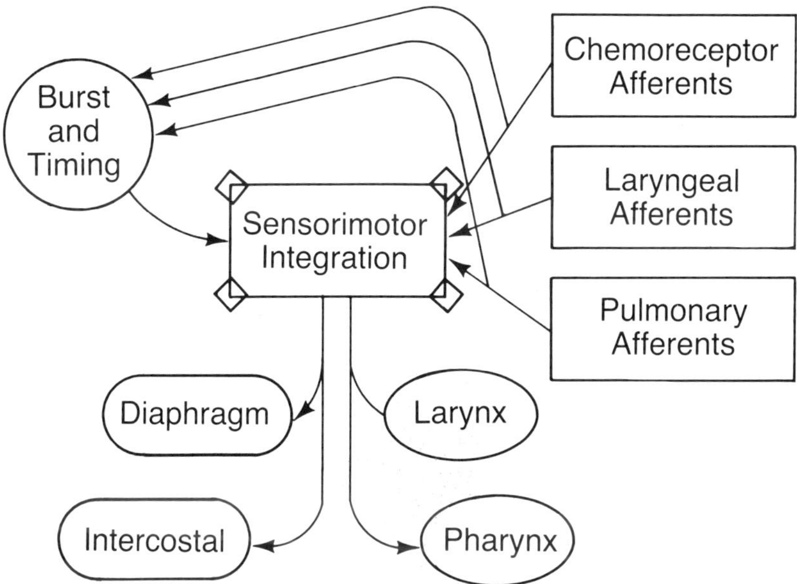

Fig. 5.2. Model of respiratory pattern generation as proposed by Feldman and colleagues (see text). (Feldman JL, Smith JC, McCrimmon DR, et al: Generation of respiratory pattern in mammals. In Cohen AH, Grillner S, Rossignol S (eds): The Neural Control of Rhythmic Movements in Vertebrates. J. Wiley & Sons, New York, In Press. Reprinted by permission of John Wiley & Sons, Inc.)

Brain Stem Immaturity in the Preterm Infant

Recent indirect evidence suggests that immaturity of the brain stem centers that regulate breathing may be a major factor in the pathogenesis of idiopathic AOP (Fig. 5-3). The proximity of the auditory pathways to the cardiorespiratory centers in the brain stem provides a method for examining the relationship between the stage of brain stem development and AOP. Henderson-Smart et al.[13] found that the conduction velocity of the auditory evoked response (wave V-I interval) through the brain stem is slower in preterm infants with apnea than in age-matched controls. Apneic episodes were found to resolve when conduction velocity returned to the levels observed in normal infants of the same postconceptual age. These clinical data provide indirect support of the hypothesis that brain stem immaturity adversely affects the rhythmic firing of brain stem respiratory neurons, resulting in apnea. Resolution of apnea may occur as the developing dendrites of respiratory neurons elongate to receive their mature synaptic connections.

There is clearly a need to examine the anatomy and physiology of the various groups of respiratory neurons over a developmental timespan in order to understand how the integration of respiratory rhythm is influenced by the evolving synaptic connectivity. The normal sequence of neuronal development must be understood before hypotheses can be generated as bases for testing potential sites of dysfunction. Only one study to date has examined the discharge characteristics

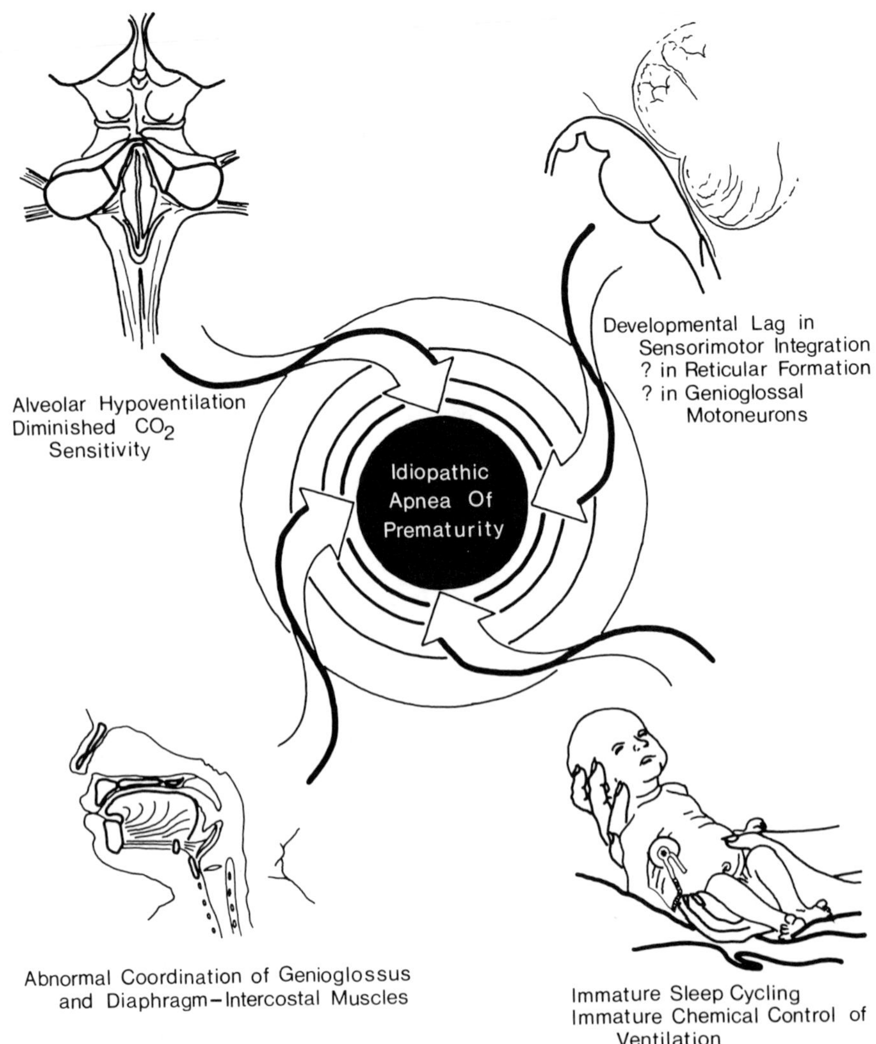

Fig. 5.3. Factors influencing the pathogenesis of idiopathic apnea of prematurity.

of a respiratory motoneuron population during normal development.[14] The investigators found a greater frequency of discharge (peak and mean) of individual phrenic motoneurons in the kitten as compared to the adult cat. They also found few "early recruited" phrenic motoneurons in animals less than 3 weeks of age. They concluded that the immaturity of phrenic motor output in the newborn was due either to a small number of active early bulbospinal neurons or to intrinsic electrical and morphologic properties of kitten phrenic motoneurons. More detailed studies of developmental changes in the electrophysiology and morphology of phrenic motoneurons are clearly needed.

The normal development of genioglossal motoneurons and their synaptic connections might also be important to the development of a regular, unobstructed breathing pattern. As discussed above, many of the apneic episodes in preterm infants are mixed or obstructive, and the upper airway (the region controlled by contraction of the genioglossus muscle) is the most likely site of obstruction.[8] It is also clear in adult animal models that genioglossal motoneurons provide synchronous inspiratory discharges to the muscle, which are important in the maintenance of upper airway patency during normal and stimulated breathing (see "Coordination of Respiratory Muscle Function," below). Moreover, the dendrites of the hypoglossal nucleus have been described as projecting to four distinct areas, among them the reticular formation and the nucleus and tractus solitarius.[15] Both brain stem areas are known to be important in respiratory control. Therefore, an understanding of the normal sequence of development in genioglossal motoneurons would provide data relevant to theories of the pathogenesis of AOP.

We have studied the anatomic maturation of the genioglossal motoneurons during development in a newborn animal model to identify changes in cell-body surface area, volume, and shape. Representative genioglossal motoneurons are shown in transverse section in Figure 5-4. Preliminary data indicate that the surface area of the cell body increases approximately 93 percent ($r = 0.96$; $P < 0.001$) over the first 2 months of postnatal life. Assuming a parallel growth in the dendrites, there would be a marked increase in the area available for synapse formation. Current studies in our laboratory are comparing the rate of development of the genioglossal motoneurons with that of the phrenic motoneurons (unpublished observations, Dr. William Cameron). Future studies will attempt to define the intricate interconnections of these respiratory premotor and motoneuron populations over the same developmental period.

Future investigations

A detailed analysis of brain stem respiratory nuclei in preterm infants with and without apnea, using rapid Golgi staining techniques, would be of interest. For example, a developmental delay in maturation of the reticular formation as judged by growth of dendrites could explain some of the pathophysiology of AOP. Known functions of the reticular formation include facilitation of respiration, maintenance of airway patency, induction of rapid eye movement (REM) sleep, and mediation of the arousal response.[16,17] Recently, St. John[18] has demonstrated that respiratory modulation of hypoglossal discharges is influenced by reticular mechanisms. Electrical stimulation and microinjection of glutamate into specific loci in the reticular formation increased hypoglossal activity more than phrenic activity; hypoglossal activity also normally preceded phrenic activity. A lag in the neuroanatomic or functional maturation of the pontine and medullary reticular formation may prove to be a critical link in the pathogenesis of AOP (Fig. 5-3). According to this hypothesis, specific neurons in the reticular formation would form a critical component of the sensorimotor integrator proposed by Feldman and colleagues,[11] and would therefore be necessary for generation of a regular, unobstructed pattern of respiration.

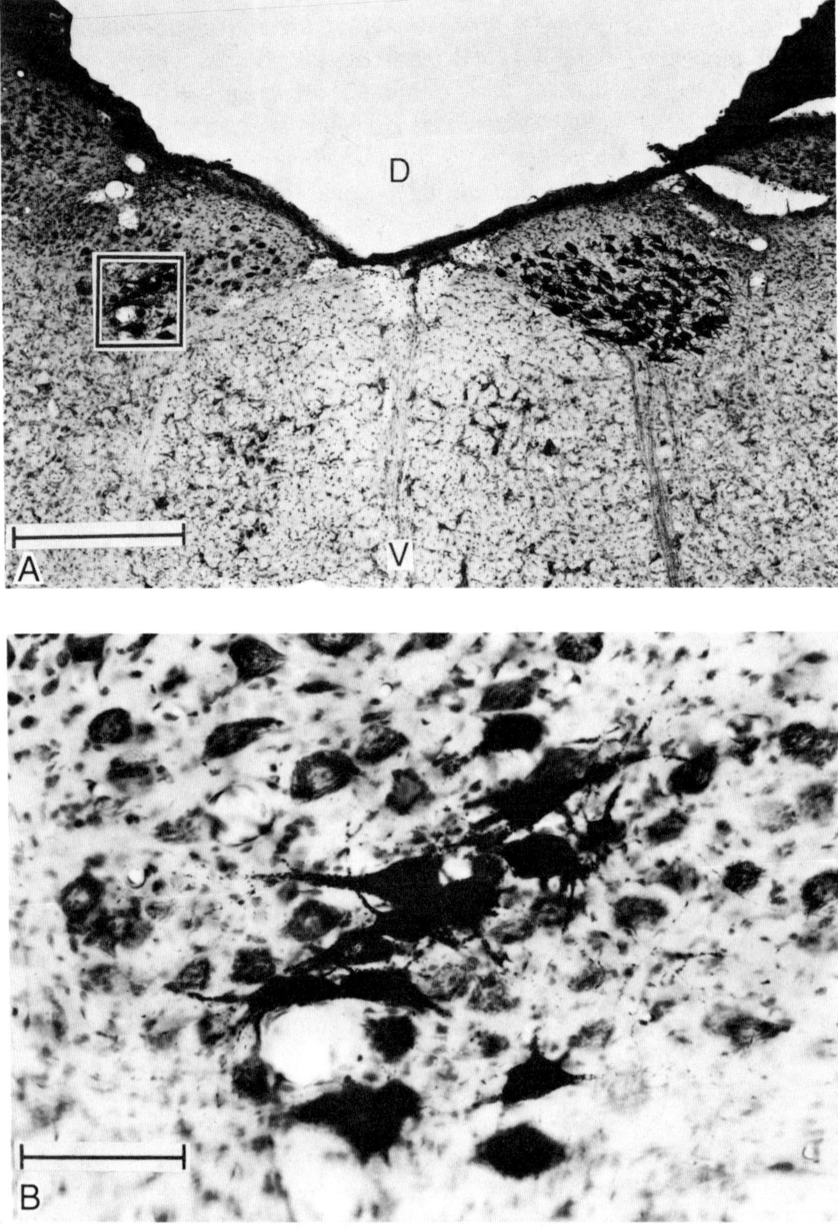

Fig. 5.4. (**A**) Lower power photomicrograph of a 50-μm-thick section of the brain stem of a 35-day-old kitten 1.1 mm rostral to the obex. The hypoglossal motor nucleus (right) was retrogradely labeled by soaking the nerve in a 40 percent solution of horseradish peroxidase (HRP). On the contralateral side, the genioglossal motoneurons (left) were labeled by injecting cholera-toxin-bound HRP into the genioglossus muscle. The sections were reacted with TMB and counterstained with neural red. Calibration bar = 500 μm; D = dorsal; V = ventral. (**B**) Higher power photomicrograph of the genioglossal motoneurons outlined in A (same orientation). Calibration bar = 100 μm. (Brozanski BS, Guthrie RD, Cameron WE: Morphology of genioglossal motoneurons in the developing kitten. Am Rev Respir Dis 135:A173, 1987 (Abstract).)

Development of Chemical Control of Respiration

Carbon dioxide

Major changes in the chemical control of respiration occur in neonates over the postnatal timespan when apneic episodes are frequent. The slope of the steady-state ventilatory response to carbon dioxide (here defined as CO_2 sensitivity—$\Delta \dot{V}_E / \Delta PaCO_2$) increases progressively from birth to 3 to 4 weeks postnatal age in premature infants and in premature primates[19–22] (Fig. 5-5). The mechanism of this change remains unknown. Developmental changes in respiratory mechanics, in the efficiency of respiratory muscle contraction, or in central chemosensitivity to H^+, CO_2, or both are theoretical possibilities. It is unlikely that an improvement in respiratory mechanics with age is responsible, and more research is necessary to clarify the mechanism.[20]

Sleep state does not influence CO_2 sensitivity in the immediate neonatal period. However, by 3 weeks of age in the premature primate, CO_2 sensitivity is decreased

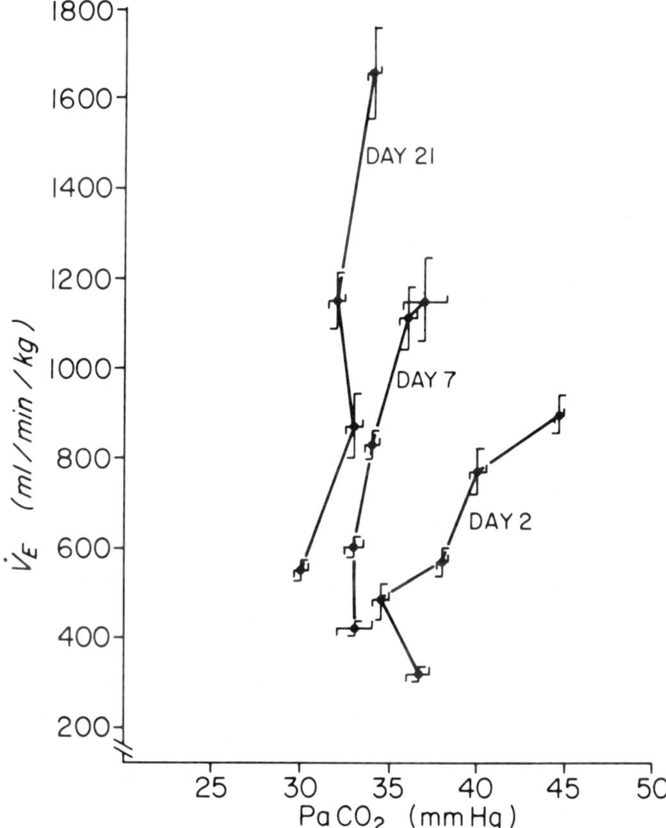

Fig. 5.5. Postnatal maturation of CO_2 sensitivity during NREM sleep in the premature primate. Note progressive shift to left and increase in slope of the hypercapnic ventilatory curve. $\dot{V}_E$, minute volume, $PaCO_2$, arterial CO_2 tension. (Guthrie RD, Standaert TA, Hodson WA, Woodrum DE: Development of CO_2 sensitivity: Effects of gestational age, postnatal age, and sleep state. J Appl Physiol 50:956, 1981).

in REM sleep as compared to non-rapid eye movement (NREM) sleep, as is classically reported in adult humans and animals.[23,24]

Hypoxia

The ventilatory response to acute hypoxia also differs between newborns and adults. Human preterm infants and infants of various animal species respond to an acute hypoxic stimulus with an immediate increase in minute ventilation ($\dot{V}_E$) followed by a return of $\dot{V}_E$ to or below baseline values by 5 to 7 minutes after the stimulus.[25,26] Indeed, some preterm infants actually become apneic.[27] This biphasic response may depend upon sleep state, although the evidence is contradictory.[20,26,28] In contrast, adult subjects given a hypoxic stimulus sustain hyperventilation as a normal defense mechanism for maintaining arterial oxygen saturation at as high a level as possible.[29] This unique biphasic ventilatory response to hypoxia in neonates normally converts to sustained hyperventilation by 3 to 4 weeks of age, and the maturation of the hypoxic ventilatory response must therefore be a normal developmental phenomenon.[25,26]

The precise mechanism of the biphasic response to hypoxia remains unknown. Peripheral chemoreceptor activity shows a sustained increase during hypoxia, and the response therefore does not appear to be secondary to a failure or diminution of chemoreception of the low PaO_2 at the carotid body.[30] Some investigators contend that central depression occurs (i.e., phrenic nerve output increases and then decreases to or below baseline values during hypoxia in the anesthetized, newborn animal).[31] In contrast, we have demonstrated during acute hypoxia in the unanesthetized premature primate that airway occlusion pressures ($P_{0.2}$—an indirect measure of central respiratory drive) and the moving average of crural diaphragmatic electromyograms (EMG_{di}) show a sustained increase above control values even though minute ventilation is decreasing below baseline values[32,33] (Fig. 5-6). After several minutes, in the late ventilatory response to hypoxia, EMG_{di} and $P_{0.2}$ decrease from the peak response at 1 to 2 minutes but remain above baseline values. In summary, the central depressant effects of hypoxia alone cannot explain the biphasic ventilatory phenomenon in the unanesthetized subject, since depression of measures of central respiratory drive below eupneic breathing values does not occur. Anesthesia appears to accentuate the depressant effects of hypoxia on central respiratory output.

Other mechanisms have been proposed to explain the biphasic nature of the ventilatory response to hypoxia. LaFramboise et al.[32] have documented a decrease in dynamic lung compliance and an increase in functional residual capacity during acute hypoxia. These data suggest that a decrease in dynamic lung compliance during acute hypoxia at least partly accounts for the biphasic ventilatory response. Diaphragmatic "fatigue," as reflected in shifts in the power spectra of the EMG_{di} or its centroid frequency (an index of the relative contribution of low- and high-frequency components in a given bandwidth), also does not occur during hypoxia in the neonate.[34] Alterations in certain putative neurotransmitters or neuromodulators such as serotonin, the endorphins, substance P, and glutamate have been proposed to explain the biphasic response.[35,36] Lawson has documented changes in serotonin concentration in selected brain stem respiratory nuclei during acute hypoxia, but it is not clear whether these changes induce the ventilatory response

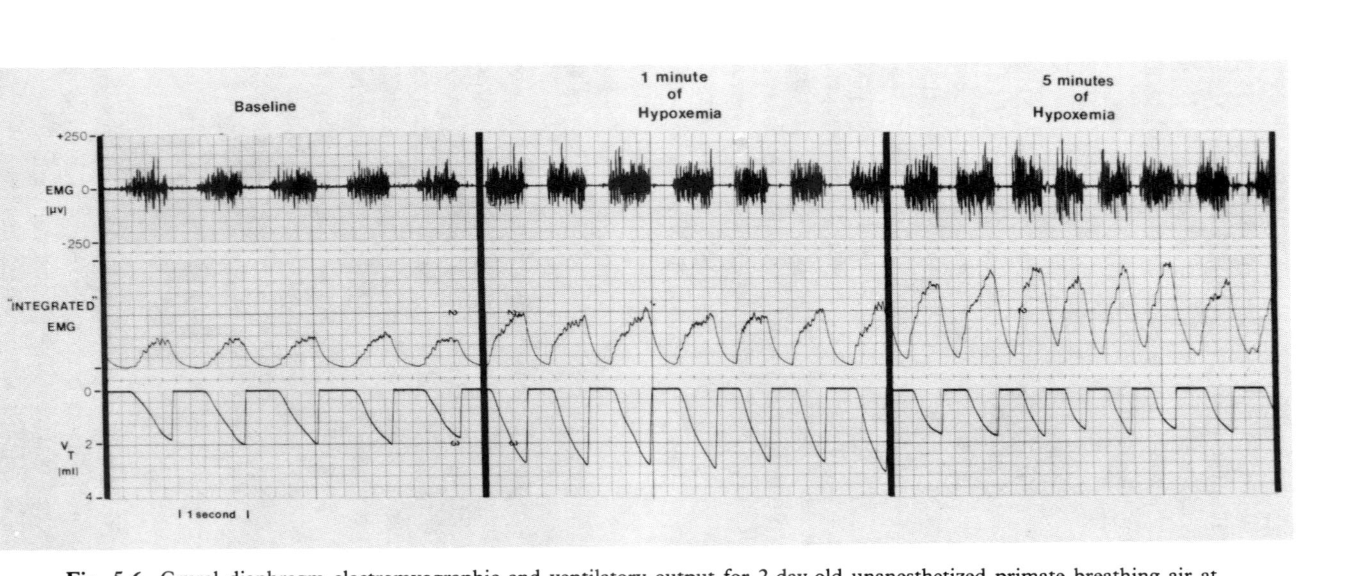

Fig. 5.6. Crural diaphragm electromyographic and ventilatory output for 2-day-old unanesthetized primate breathing air at baseline, followed by sampling of data at 1 and 5 minutes after being switched to inspiratory gas of 12 percent O_2–88 percent N_2 composition. Note sustained increase of raw and integrated (moving average) EMGs above baseline values as minute ventilation decreases below baseline values. V_T, tidal volume. (LaFramboise WA, Woodrum DE: Elevated diaphragm electromyogram during neonatal hypoxic ventilatory depression. J Appl Physiol 59:1040, 1985.)

or are secondary to it.[36] The potential role of neurotransmitters in explaining this phenomenon remains intriguing but very difficult to study using "physiologic" cellular levels of stimuli. Other mechanisms for the biphasic response that have not been excluded are a dynamic change in O_2 consumption in preterm subjects in a neutral thermal environment, and a hypoxia-induced increase in brain stem blood flow and subsequent washout of the CO_2/H^+ stimulus. Nevertheless, the end result remains the same: acute hypoxia can induce apnea in some preterm infants—by whatever mechanism—because the preterm infant lacks the normal defense of sustained hyperventilation in response to hypoxia.

O_2–CO_2 interaction

The ventilatory interaction between hypoxia and carbon dioxide sensitivity in the newborn is the opposite of the classic interaction seen in adults. In adult subjects, hypoxia enhances CO_2 sensitivity whereas hyperoxia reduces it. The inverse of this O_2–CO_2 interaction occurs in the newborn. Hypoxia depresses the slope of the CO_2 ventilatory response curve and hyperoxia increases it remarkably—to near infinity in some subjects.[37] The mechanism responsible for this inverse ventilatory interaction of O_2 and CO_2 in the newborn is unknown, but an exaggerated response to hypoxia-induced alterations of newborn brain stem blood flow (and subsequent washout of the H^+/CO_2 stimulus) seems most probable (see Ch. 6).

In summary, dramatic changes in the chemical control of respiration occur in the neonatal period, when apneic episodes are frequent. Premature infants with apnea demonstrate exaggerations of this normal developmental sequence, as discussed below.

Abnormalities of Chemical Control of Respiration in Apnea of Prematurity

CO_2 sensitivity

Several lines of evidence support the hypothesis that the chemical control of respiration in preterm infants with AOP differs from that of appropriately matched controls who do not manifest apnea. Durand and colleagues[38] have shown a decrease in $\dot{V}_E$ in preterms with apnea and, concomitantly, the end-tidal $PaCO_2$ in these infants is higher than in controls; thus, preterm infants with apnea also hypoventilate even when breathing regularly. These same investigators and others have also demonstrated a significant depression in CO_2 sensitivity and a shift of its intercept to the right in apneic preterm infants between 30 and 33 weeks gestational age.[38,39] However, these abnormalities are likely to be secondary to some other primary brain stem maturational abnormality which causes the apnea; depressed CO_2 sensitivity by itself is not sufficient to cause apnea.

Sleep state

Sleep (as compared to wakefulness) may be associated with the pathogenesis of AOP. Prolonged apneic episodes have been reported by Schulte et al.[40] to occur predominantly in REM sleep, whereas Krauss and colleagues[41] found the more prolonged apneic episodes in NREM sleep. These contradictions might be explained by the inherent difficulties in sleep-state determination in preterm infants, and perhaps sleep, in whatever state, is associated with apnea. Failure of normal arousal from sleep during hypoventilation may be an important factor in the pathogenesis of apnea. It is a common clinical observation that preterm infants fail to arouse in the face of arterial oxygen tensions below 50 mmHg and arterial carbon dioxide tensions greater than 65 mmHg. Also, arousal in newborn calves occurs at lower oxygen saturations in REM sleep than in NREM sleep.[42] Normal arousal mechanisms may not be fully developed in preterm infants, in association with their relative brain stem immaturity, and preterm infants with apnea may experience even greater delay in the development of normal arousal mechanisms.

As discussed earlier, hypoxia is followed by apnea in a small but significant percentage of preterm infants. The youngest neonate lacks a normal defense mechanism against hypoxia—that of sustained hyperventilation. Although hypoxemia does not precede the vast majority of episodes of idiopathic AOP, the breathing pause itself may lead to recurrent apnea, especially in REM sleep, due to decreased oxygen "stores." Metabolic O_2 consumption is two- to threefold greater in relation to the available O_2 in infants than in adults. In REM sleep, the further reduction in O_2 "stores" in the lung secondary to loss of intercostal muscle activity and a reduction in functional residual capacity might lead to an even more rapid drop in arterial oxygen saturation.[43] Therefore, it becomes prudent to aggressively treat apneic episodes that occur in clusters.

Neurotransmitters

Developmental changes in the function of brain stem neurotransmitters that influence respiratory control have not been well studied in apnea of prematurity for obvious technical reasons. Investigators have examined the urine of preterm infants for the presence of various biogenic amines which have been implicated as transmitter substances mediating sleep states within the central nervous system, and as controllers of peripheral chemoreceptor sensitivity. Levels of dopamine, epinephrine, and norepinephrine were all found to be lower in 15 infants with idiopathic apnea than in 7 controls.[44] However, urine levels would not be expected to reflect specific abnormalities in brain stem respiratory nuclei, and the significance of this finding is unclear. A delayed maturational change in neurotransmitter function in specific respiratory nuclei remains a tenable hypothesis for AOP; the investigation of this theory, however, awaits animal models of apnea and technical advances. Certainly the therapeutic success of methylxanthines in the treatment of AOP supports this hypothesis indirectly (see "Treatment," below).

Coordination of Respiratory Muscle Function

As previously noted, greater appreciation for the role of airway obstruction in idiopathic AOP has emerged in recent years, though its contribution to some apneic episodes in the newborn has long been recognized. Animal and adult human studies, and recent clinical investigations in the preterm infant, have documented a coordinated interaction among the major respiratory muscles (intercostals, diaphragm) and those of the upper airway (alae nasi, genioglossus, laryngeal abductors) that normally assures airway patency. Since other complex brain stem integrations (i.e., sucking and swallowing while synchronously breathing) are not developed completely in preterm infants, it seems reasonable to hypothesize that the integration among these muscles is also immature. Chemical stimulation (hypoxia, hypercapnia), mechanical loading (airway occlusion), sleep state, and numerous pharmacologic agents influence this sophisticated coordination as well.

Airway obstruction in AOP

Until recently, it was generally accepted that the site of obstruction in preterm infants was the larynx (glottis),[45,46] but further investigation has demonstrated conclusively that the level of obstruction is most commonly in the high pharyngeal region. In an elegant study, Mathew and co-workers[8] reported on the incidence and site of obstruction in nine preterm infants with the clinical diagnosis of apnea and bradycardia. Heart rate, abdominal respiratory excursion, and nasal/oral airflow were monitored. Additionally, a saline-filled catheter connected to a pressure transducer was inserted through the nostril and positioned with its tip in the pharynx. High pharyngeal obstruction was reflected in absence of airflow with characteristic negative pressure changes within the catheter, whereas obstruction below the level of the catheter tip (at the larynx) was recorded as absence of both airflow and pressure changes. Eight central, 27 obstructive, and 70 mixed apneic episodes were detected; of the 94 obstructive or mixed apneas subsequently analyzed for level of airway occlusion, 87 occurred in the high pharyngeal region.

Function of the genioglossus and other upper airway muscles in adults

Attention has increasingly focused upon the genioglossus as the primary obstructive element in AOP, given its relative mobility in the otherwise bony and cartilaginous upper pharynx. Though other muscles of the upper airway may contribute to the overall resistance to airflow, radiographic and endoscopic studies in older children and adults confirm the occlusive movement of the tongue.[47,48]

Continuing the pioneering work of Gastaut[49] and Sauerland,[50,51] Remmers et al.[52] in 1978 demonstrated the phasic activity of the genioglossal electromyogram (EMG) in 10 obese adult patients with daytime somnolence and obstructive apnea; they further observed that high negative pharyngeal pressure (as during inspiration) promoted pharyngeal closure, while preferential activation of the genioglossus terminated the obstruction. Subsequently, Brouillette and Thach[53] showed activation of the genioglossus to occur earlier in inspiration than that of the diaphragm in anesthetized rabbits, even during tidal breathing. These data extended earlier findings in animals of phasic inspiratory activity of the posterior cricoarytenoid (a laryngeal abductor)[54] and the geniohyoid[55] muscles. Similarly, upper airway muscle contraction, preceding or coincident with the onset of diaphragmatic contraction and airflow, was confirmed in the normal adult human for the alae nasi[56] and for the genioglossus under conditions of both hypercapnia[57] and isocapnic hypoxia.[58] Thus, a logical sequence of investigations in adult animals and humans has shown that inspiratory activity of several upper airway abductors occurs not only at the termination of obstructive apnea, but in synchrony with normal tidal respiration. These studies have also shown that the activity of these abductors can be recruited by both chemical stimulation[56–58] and inspiratory resistive loading.[59] Finally, the data suggest that the upper airway muscles and diaphragm share similar central control mechanisms in the adult.

Animal studies of respiratory muscle coordination in the newborn

Given that the usual site of airway obstruction in preterm infants is at the level of the genioglossus, and that a vital respiratory function of this muscle has been proven in adults, attention has recently focused on its physiology and that of other upper airway muscles in the newborn period.

In 1985, England et al.[60] expanding on preliminary studies by Harding[61] in fetal and neonatal lambs, developed a chronic preparation for the study of posterior cricoarytenoid (PCA), thyroarytenoid (TA), and diaphragm muscle activities. Utilizing chronically implanted electrodes in the puppy, the authors demonstrated prominent inspiratory PCA activity in all behavioral states; activity of the TA, a laryngeal adductor, was consistently high during expiration in quiet wakefulness and NREM sleep, but decreased dramatically in REM sleep. Additionally, Bruce and Hoh[62] have shown a rapid increase in activity of both the phrenic and hypoglossal nerves in anesthetized, paralyzed, and ventilated kittens in response to moderate hypoxia.

We have investigated the coordination of the genioglossus with the costal diaphragm, crural diaphragm, and external intercostal muscles in lightly anesthetized but spontaneously breathing 3- to 4-week-old kittens. Utilizing surgically implanted bipolar electrodes, we have recorded the EMG activities during eupneic respiration and in response to hyperoxic hypercapnia (8 percent CO_2) and isocapnic hypoxia (13 and 10 percent O_2). Preliminary data show little spontaneous phasic genioglossal activity during eupneic respiration (perhaps secondary to halothane anesthesia), but rapid recruitment upon presentation of a chemical stimulus. This response is distinctly transient during hypoxia in the youngest kittens (see Fig. 5-7), but is more sustained during hypercapnia at all ages. The inspiratory contraction of the genioglossus appears to occur in phase with other muscles of the respiratory system. Because phasic inspiratory activity always occurs during breathing stimulated by hypercapnia in 8-week-old, lightly anesthetized kittens (unpublished observations, Dr. Ryoichi Ochiai), we speculate that the sophisticated integration of genioglossal and diaphragmatic activities characteristic of adults is not completely developed in the immediate neonatal period.

Indeed, the progressive integration of upper airway muscle function with that of the diaphragm appears to begin in utero. Johnston and colleagues[63] have demonstrated phasic respiratory genioglossal and alae nasi activity in fetal sheep from 112 to 140 days gestation. Further, the activity varied markedly depending upon the pattern of electrocortical activity (sleep stage). The alae nasi rapidly developed an inspiratory rhythm during 5 percent CO_2 administration, though the genioglossus rarely showed inspiratory activity in synchrony with the diaphragm, even in response to 10 percent CO_2 stimulation. Hypoxia rapidly abolished the activity of both muscles.

In summary, investigations in newborn animals have demonstrated a functional but incomplete coordination of several upper airway muscles with the muscles of the "classic" respiratory pump. This integration is not completely developed in the fetal and early neonatal periods, and is not as responsive to chemical stimuli as is the sophisticated integration in adults. The immature response of the genioglossus to hypoxia and hypercapnia might predispose the newborn to obstructive or mixed apnea.

Comparisons among the few existing reports and, more importantly, their ap-

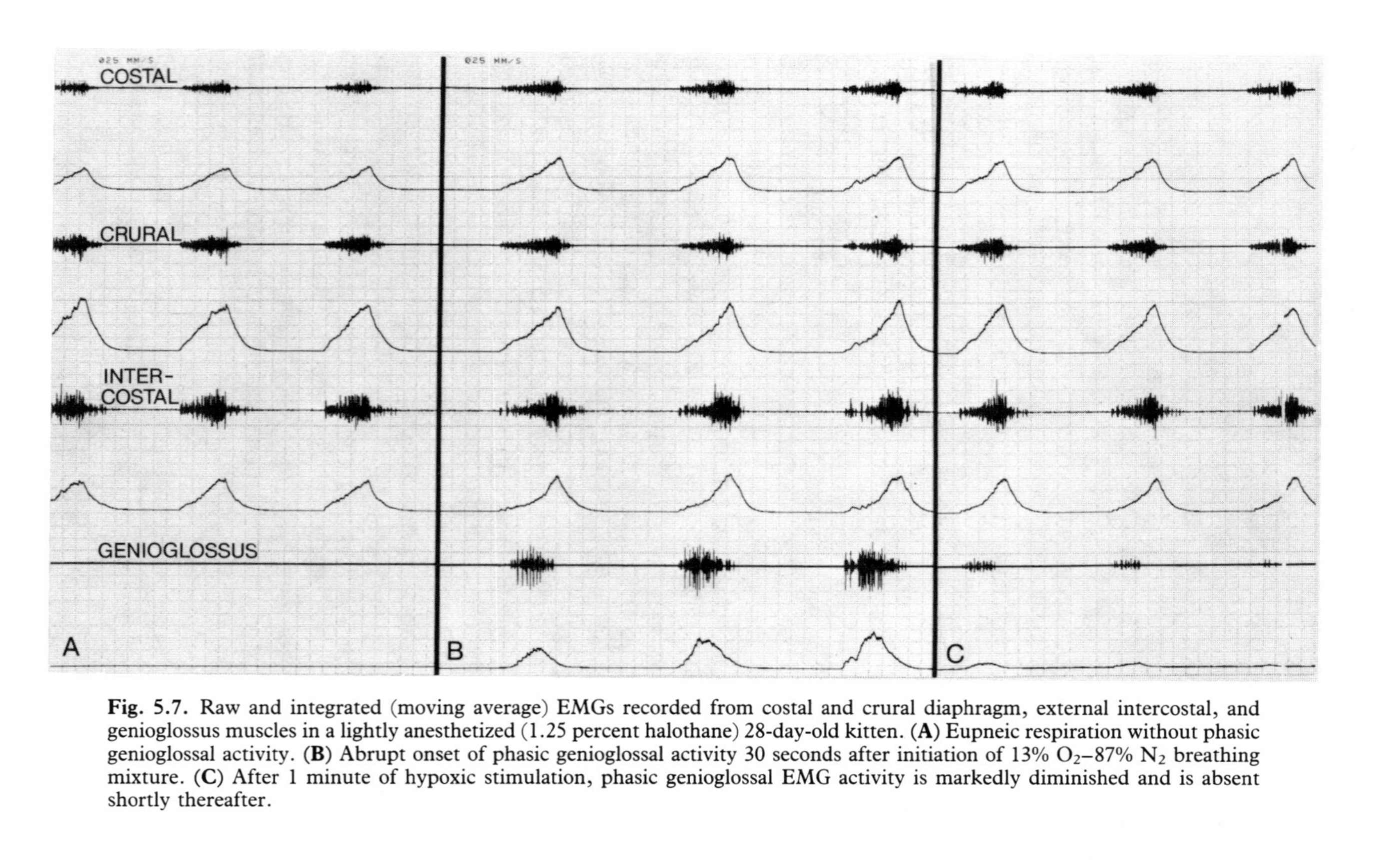

Fig. 5.7. Raw and integrated (moving average) EMGs recorded from costal and crural diaphragm, external intercostal, and genioglossus muscles in a lightly anesthetized (1.25 percent halothane) 28-day-old kitten. (**A**) Eupneic respiration without phasic genioglossal activity. (**B**) Abrupt onset of phasic genioglossal activity 30 seconds after initiation of 13% O_2–87% N_2 breathing mixture. (**C**) After 1 minute of hypoxic stimulation, phasic genioglossal EMG activity is markedly diminished and is absent shortly thereafter.

plicability to the human preterm neonate are confounded by species differences, degree of maturity, and effects of anesthesia. Nonetheless, they provide a basis for the pursuit of less invasive clinical studies of mixed and obstructive AOP.

Clinical studies of respiratory muscle coordination in the newborn

Surface electromyograms have been recorded from the alae nasi[64] and from the submental (genioglossal) area[65] in healthy preterm infants, and compared to diaphragmatic EMGs obtained with adhesive electrodes positioned at the right costal margin. Though electrical noise, ECG artifact, and EMG interference from adjacent muscles appeared more prominent in these recordings, they clearly showed inspiratory coordination of upper airway and chest wall muscles, both in time of onset of contraction and in time of peak activity. Onset of the alae nasi EMG preceded that of the diaphragmatic EMG by 41 ± 8 msec, and preceded inspiratory airflow by 114 ± 29 msec, a relationship not altered by inhalation of 4 percent CO_2. Such early contraction might serve to decrease upper airway resistance, facilitating airflow during inspiration and preventing the development of a large negative (collapsing) pharyngeal pressure during inspiration.[66] In contrast, with increasing chemical drive (2 to 4 percent CO_2), the peak diaphragm EMG activity and tidal volume progressively increased, while peak alae nasi EMG activity was consistently recruited only during 4 percent CO_2 inhalation. The authors concluded that the nonlinear alae nasi response to CO_2, in contrast to that seen in adults,[56] might be viewed as a developmental phenomenon that contributes to the high incidence of breathing disturbances in preterm infants. They also suggested, however, that the activity of the alae nasi may indeed be linear within a higher hypercapnic range, where a decrease in nasal resistance during high inspiratory airflow would be of most benefit.[64] In this regard, several investigators[67,70] have recently reported that as the duration of apnea increases, mixed rather than central apneas predominate, the actual obstructive component usually being manifest toward the end of the episode. A rapid increase in chemoreceptor drive during the initial central apneic component, followed by recruitment of diaphragm activity before that of the upper airway muscles (as evidenced above), would explain why the airway is often briefly obstructed as breathing efforts resume. It is important to recall, however, that the level of obstruction in AOP is high pharyngeal (not nasal). Studies should also be done on the chemical response of the genioglossus in preterm infants with and without apnea.

In response to end-expiratory airway (nasal) occlusion, a progressive increase in the peak amplitude of the submental EMG was shown in 10 sleeping preterm infants.[65] Though the diaphragmatic EMG increased significantly only by the third occluded effort, an increase in the submental EMG was seen even with the first occluded breath, thus invariably maintaining pharyngeal patency and, presumably, preventing the development of obstructive apnea. In four infants who experienced spontaneous obstructive apnea, a sharp burst of submental EMG activity was seen to coincide with a larger negative pressure swing in the esophageal catheter and a restitution of nasal airflow, indicating resolution of the obstruction as adhesive forces between the tongue and posterior pharyngeal wall were overcome. Multiple investigations lend support to this mechanism for the recovery of airway patency.[68–71]

Coordination of respiratory muscle function during sleep

In a recent review of the influence of sleep state on the coordination of upper airway muscles and the diaphragm, the authors concluded that the contribution of behavioral state to upper airway muscle activity in the newborn is important but poorly documented.[72] During the transition from quiet waking to NREM to REM sleep, the genioglossal EMG activity progressively declines in adult humans,[73] but results of the influence of sleep state in the newborn vary greatly, depending upon the species and the specific upper airway muscle studied. Carlo et al.[64] have shown augmentation of the alae nasi and diaphragmatic activities in REM sleep, when intercostal muscle activity decreases[74]; the authors speculate that the resulting increase in transdiaphragmatic pressure might predispose to higher negative pharyngeal pressures and pharyngeal collapse. An increase in alae nasi activity would serve to lower the resistance in the upper airway, preventing airway collapse and obstruction. In a recent study, Cohen and Henderson-Smart[68] examined the effect of manual end-expiratory airway occlusion on upper airway stability in 22 preterm infants, of whom 17 had clinical apnea. Airway collapse occurred in five infants, more commonly in NREM than in REM sleep. In addition, obstructive and mixed apneas were more common in those infants with airway collapse than in those without. These data support the concept that obstructive apnea in some preterm infants may be related to upper airway muscle dysfunction.

Drug effects on respiratory muscle coordination

Finally, numerous pharmacologic agents and anesthetics have been shown in adult animals and humans to have a profound effect on upper airway muscles. Ethanol[75] and diazepam[76] selectively depress activity of the genioglossus and PCA muscles in cats, possibly by a direct effect on the reticular formation, whereas protryptiline,[76] an antidepressant, selectively stimulates these muscles. By its action on peripheral chemoreceptors, dopamine[77] depresses activity of the hypoglossal nerve compared to that of the phrenic nerve, whereas isoproterenol,[77] lobeline,[77] and almitrine[78] selectively stimulate the hypoglossal nerve. Anesthetics including chloralose, pentobarbital, ketamine, and halothane[79] all selectively depress respiratory activity of the hypoglossal nerve, perhaps accounting for the high incidence of upper airway obstruction with the use of these agents. While the response of the preterm human newborn to these drugs has not been investigated, similar or exaggerated results might be expected. The ability, then, to selectively manipulate the respiratory activity of upper airway muscles raises exciting possibilities for the future therapy of mixed and obstructive AOP.

Airway Mechanoreceptors and Chest Wall Reflexes

While afferent input from airway stretch, irritant, and flow receptors, and from muscle-spindle reflexes affects respiratory timing in the newborn, their exact role in the normal cycle of breathing is unclear, and their contribution to AOP remains speculative.

Slowly adapting stretch receptors located within the trachea and large airways, and more widely scattered airway irritant receptors responding to stretch (rapidly adapting), mechanical, and chemical stimuli, have long been recognized. In 1868, Hering and Breuer[80] first noted effects of sustained lung inflation on prolonging the expiratory time (Te) of subsequent breaths and thus decreasing the respiratory rate. Mediated by vagal afferent feedback from the slowly adapting stretch receptors, this reflex is particularly strong in the preterm infant, but difficult to demonstrate in the adult.[81] Stimulation of irritant airway receptors by noxious stimuli, on the other hand, results in a decreased inspiratory time (Ti) and tidal volume (the vagally mediated deflation reflex), and may result in apnea.[82] These receptor activities are readily demonstrable in numerous species, and can be manipulated by a variety of experimental conditions (vagotomy, airway anesthesia). In the preterm human, their effects are several. Because of the highly compliant chest wall of the neonate, the resting lung volume (functional residual capacity) is low, and decreased stretch receptor activity may decrease Te and so attempt to maintain lung volume.[83] When stretch receptor activation is prevented by end-expiratory airway occlusion, inspiration is prolonged[84] and upper airway muscles are preferentially activated to dilate the upper airway and relieve the obstruction.[65]

Receptors that respond to changes in flow and pressure have been identified in the upper airways of newborn infants, though their contribution to respiratory control may be limited to the immediate neonatal period. Fisher and colleagues[85] have shown that both inspiratory and expiratory airflow and negative pressure applied to the isolated upper airway of young, anesthetized puppies caused either immediate prolongations of Ti and Te or apnea. These reflexes were abolished by section of the superior laryngeal nerves (part of the vagal system), and were inoperative by 1 month of age. In addition, stimulation of these receptors may contribute to the selective activation of upper-airway-dilating muscles.

The intercostal muscles are particularly rich in proprioceptive muscle spindles that also impact on respiratory timing. In the face of airway obstruction, the muscle spindles shorten more than the muscles themselves and, by way of sensory feedback, a more forceful, prolonged contraction of the intercostal muscles results.[86] Finally, an intercostal-phrenic reflex that inhibits inspiration when the lower rib-cage is distorted has been identified, and may be partially responsible for the erratic breathing pattern seen in REM sleep.[87]

Species differences and the confounding effects of anesthesia and various behavioral states make comparisons of the numerous mechanoreceptor studies hazardous. In any event, it appears that the relative contribution of these receptors to the central integrative process changes greatly with maturation.[88]

Summary of Pathogenesis of Idiopathic Apnea of Prematurity

The pathogenesis of idiopathic apnea of prematurity remains unknown. Any unifying theory must explain the observation that these episodes of apnea may be central, mixed, or obstructive. Reproducible evidence documents that preterm infants with apnea hypoventilate and have a diminished CO_2 sensitivity (Fig. 5-5). The chemical control of respiration, which normally provides a defense against apnea, is not yet fully developed in the preterm infant. Additionally, the mechanism of upper airway obstruction in many of the apneic events in premature infants has not been elucidated. A functional or anatomic lag in the development of coordination of upper airway muscles with the diaphragm and intercostal muscles seems a reasonable unifying hypothesis. A likely central locus for this developmental lag is the "sensorimotor integrator" suggested by Feldman and colleagues.[11] Chemical stimuli and mechanoreceptor afferent activity are integrated at this site in the maintenance of normal control of the respiratory pattern generator. Incomplete development of such a complex and sophisticated integrating mechanism would be a logical explanation for system failure. The reticular formation is anatomically and neurophysiologically central to the facilitation of respiration, coordination of upper airway muscles, control of sleep state, and regulation of the arousal response. A role for the reticular formation in the sensorimotor integration of respiration seems probable, particularly as a locus for the potential developmental lag. Definitive proof of this hypothesis will be challenging because of the obvious technical difficulties involved in studying this complex brain stem circuitry.

CLINICAL DIAGNOSIS

Differential Diagnosis

Apnea is a common nonspecific manifestation of underlying illness in the preterm infant, and may also result from any noxious stimulation of the patient (catheter suctioning, gavage feeding). Therefore, true AOP must first be distinguished from secondary apnea before appropriate therapy can be instituted. Apnea is seldom the sole manifestation of serious illness in the newborn; accompanying signs and symptoms will generally direct the clinician toward the appropriate diagnosis.

Respiratory disease and accompanying hypoxemia, intracranial hemorrhage, septicemia, patent ductus arteriosus, anemia, hypoglycemia, hyperthermia, gastroesophageal reflux, and depression by drugs (opiates, magnesium sulfate) have all been associated with secondary central and mixed apnea. Hypocalcemia has been implicated in neonatal apnea, but this cause is exceedingly rare in our experience; more likely, both the hypocalcemia and apnea are simply related to perinatal stress.[89] Seizures are often mentioned as a cause of apnea as well, but a recent review of prolonged EEG recordings in 37 neonates who experienced 153 apneic episodes unassociated with clinical seizures showed no detectable EEG seizure activity.[90] Conversely, since the establishment of regular EEG monitoring of infants at Magee-Womens Hospital in 1983, only 1 of 71 infants with documented electrocortical seizures experienced apnea as the sole clinical manifestation of this abnormality (personal communication, Dr. Mark Scher). Therefore, in the workup of episodic neonatal apnea, EEG monitoring appears of little value except in the term infant or in cases in which the apnea is not accompanied by bradycardia.[91]

Congenital malformations can cause upper airway obstruction and obstructive apnea, among them the Robin sequence and the Treacher Collins syndrome (both with mandibular hypoplasia), and the CHARGE association (choanal atresia). A recent study noted that among 28 preterm infants, purely obstructive apnea was the least common type and that, as a group, those infants with obstructive apnea of greater than 20 seconds duration had evidence of neurologic abnormality (generally intracranial hemorrhage).[67]

Apnea Detection

The use of transthoracic impedance monitoring (impedance pneumography) to detect apnea in the newborn has gained wide acceptance despite its limitations. This technique is based on the observation that the conduction of a small alternating electric current across the thorax fluctuates during breathing (the measured resistances are called impedances).[92] Apnea monitors register a breath above a predetermined level of transthoracic impedance and, failing to detect a change in impedance, will trigger an alarm after a given time interval. Since Daily's report[3] in 1969 on their clinical applicability, the use of such monitors in the nursery has superseded all other detection methods: the apnea mattress alarm system, esophageal and pharyngeal pressure manometers, and O_2/CO_2 transcutaneous electrodes. It has been long recognized, however, that body movement and heartbeat can register as changes in impedence during true central apnea,[93,94] a false-negative effect that may occur commonly.[95] More importantly, these monitors fail to detect the absence of airflow in obstructive apnea and in mixed apnea when obstruction precedes the central pause. That such episodes may be accompanied by hypoxemia without being detected[96] has spurred the development of new technologies for the specific detection of airflow. An excellent review of these methods has recently been published.[97] Current research methods for the quantitative measurement of respiratory airflow utilize a face-mask[98] or nasal[99] pneumotachygraph. More clinically useful qualitative detection techniques include acoustic recording of breath sounds,[100] measurement of exhaled carbon dioxide,[101] and monitoring the fluctuation of the air stream temperature between inspiration and expiration.[96,102] The capnograph and nasal thermistor share the distinct advantages of being nonrestrictive, generally reliable with minimal supervision, and commercially available. If these techniques were to be combined with the determination of heart rate by electrocardiography and with impedance pneumography, perhaps in conjunction with noninvasive measurement of oxygen saturation, the ideal, reliable monitor for AOP might be achieved. A statement urging the commercial development and standardization of such devices, for research, clinical, and home use, has recently been issued.[1]

TREATMENT

Numerous treatment protocols have been proposed for AOP, though the test of time has shown some methods to be clearly more beneficial than others. Recent advances in understanding the chemical control of ventilation, the potential role of newly discovered neurotransmitters, and drug effects on the integration of upper and lower airway muscles hold the promise of more effective pharmacotherapy for AOP in the future. In the interim, however, we continue to utilize many of the same techniques reviewed by Kattwinkel[103] a decade ago and summarized in Table 5-1.

When to Treat

The therapy of secondary apnea in the newborn infant must obviously be directed at the underlying illness (treatment of septicemia, etc.). With concurrent illness, idiopathic or primary AOP may still occur and may be impossible to distinguish from secondary apnea until the specific disorder has resolved. Idiopathic AOP can occur as early as the first or second day of life, especially in infants without respiratory disease, but its peak incidence has been shown to occur later in those with RDS, generally coincident with resolution of the lung disease.[104]

Table 5-1. Therapeutic Recommendations for Idiopathic Apnea of Prematurity

Intervention	Comment
Intermittent cutaneous stimulation	May be adequate for neonate approaching term
Positioning with mild extension of neck	Neck flexion associated with upper airway obstruction
Maintenance of thermoneutral environment	Central apnea exacerbated by iatrogenic overheating
25–30% FIO_2 delivered by head hood or nasal cannula	May be helpful for apneic episodes occurring frequently and accompanied by hypoxemia
Methylxanthines Caffeine 10.0 mg/kg IV or PO loading 2.5 mg/kg IV or PO q 24 hour maintenance Theophylline 5.0 mg/kg IV loading 2.0 mg/kg IV q 12 hour maintenance	Dose and interval vary depending upon specific salt form, route of administration, and postconceptional age (see text); therapeutic serum concentrations: Caffeine 5–25 μg/ml Theophylline 5–15 μg/ml
Nasal or nasopharyngeal CPAP of 3–6 cm H_2O	May be particularly effective for mixed and obstructive apnea
Doxapram: 0.5 mg/kg/hour continuous IV infusion, increasing by 0.5 mg/kg/hour increments to maximum of 2.5 mg/kg/hour	May be effective for central apnea refractory to methylxanthines, but pharmacokinetics in neonate poorly studied
Mechanical ventilation	Seldom necessary and use should prompt renewed search for underlying illness

A paucity of adequately controlled studies on the short- and long-term effects of untreated AOP, and the sure knowledge that no mode of therapy is entirely benign, make it difficult to define exactly when treatment is warranted. The threshold for intervention, therefore, varies widely among neonatologists. Nonetheless, somewhat arbitrary guidelines can be offered beyond using "good clinical judgment." If episodes of primary AOP consistently occur more frequently than two to three times per hour, or require more than moderate cutaneous stimulation, particularly if accompanied by a prolonged recovery time, we recommend the early use of methylxanthines. The rationale for this intervention is further explained below.

Sensory Stimulation

Simple tactile stimulation is frequently effective in aborting mild apneic spells by means of nonspecific afferent input to the respiratory control centers. Numerous other methods of sensory stimulation have been investigated, including mild electric shock, flashing lights, intermittent loud sounds, a cold airstream to the skin, and a rapidly inflating balloon beneath the infant.[105] Perhaps the only alternative that has gained a measure of acceptance is the oscillating water mattress, a device initially proposed by Millen[106] and Lee,[107] but introduced by Korner[7,108] as a means of simulating the vestibular-proprioceptive input normally experienced in utero. In both a pilot study[108] and in a later report on eight preterm infants who served as their own controls (crossover design),[7] Korner and co-workers demonstrated this method to be both safe and effective in reducing the incidence of severe apneic and bradycardic episodes. In a later report, however, the incidence of residual apnea in 17 theophylline-treated preterm infants was not reduced by the water mattress.[109] Most recently, in a randomized clinical trial with 1-year follow-up, an oscillating air mattress was shown to confer no benefit in reducing apnea or enhancing growth and neurobehavioral performance.[110] Additional, carefully designed studies of the efficacy of the oscillating mattress, perhaps used in conjunction with other sensory stimuli (i.e., auditory) are needed, but at present, the preponderance of evidence indicates that its clinical usefulness is limited.

Avoidance of noxious sensory stimuli and maintenance of a thermoneutral environment are, of course, basic to the prevention of AOP.

Oxygen

Mild hypoxemia clearly can result in increased periodic breathing and apnea in the preterm infant, and such patients often benefit from the use of 25 to 30 percent O_2 delivered by head hood or nasal cannula. However, several studies of preterm infants with apnea have failed to detect hypoxemia preceding the apneic episodes.[39] Furthermore, a study of matched preterm infants with and without apnea revealed comparable PaO_2 values between the two groups. Hypoxemia is more important as a result than as a cause of AOP.

Continuous Positive Airway Pressure (CPAP) and Mechanical Ventilation

Early observation of an increase in the frequency of apneic episodes upon discontinuation of CPAP in infants recovering from respiratory distress syndrome led clinicians to advocate its use for the treatment of AOP.[111,112] The mode of action of CPAP is still unclear, although current evidence suggests that it may splint the upper airway and thus relieve obstruction. In this regard, Miller and colleagues[113] have shown a decreased incidence of mixed and obstructive apnea, but no effect on central apnea, with the application of CPAP. If CPAP acts through the Hering-Breuer lung inflation reflex,[114] or even simply by means of improved oxygenation, the frequency of central apnea should also have diminished. In those infants in whom mixed and obstructive apnea predominate, CPAP may be shown to be the therapy of choice.

AOP is rarely so severe as to require mechanical ventilation, and in those infants in whom it is utilized, a vigorous effort should be made to rule out underlying illness.

Methylxanthines

The methylxanthines, including caffeine and theophylline, have become the mainstay of therapy for idiopathic AOP. Since the pioneering report of Kuzemko and Paala in 1973,[115] numerous investigations have decumented the efficacy and general safety of their use in the preterm neonate for reducing the incidence and severity of AOP.[116–120] Yet despite the plethora of studies, many questions remain about their metabolism at various gestational ages, their systemic effects, and their effectiveness in shortening the course of AOP. Though other medications have achieved a measure of clinical utility, such as doxapram for refractory apnea, the widespread preferential use of the methylxanthines is unlikely to diminish in the near future.

Pharmacology

The absorption, distribution, metabolism, and excretion of caffeine and theophylline have been extensively studied in the neonate, but the results are frequently conflicting because of differences in study design, patient population, clinical status of the patients, and analytical techniques used for the measurement of serum concentrations. Several excellent reviews of the basic and clinical pharmacology of the methylxanthines are available.[121–123]

Caffeine is a naturally occurring, lipid-soluble methylated xanthine that is widely distributed (mean volume of distribution 0.8 to 0.9 L/kg) and uniformly concentrated among various tissues in the neonate.[124] A cerebrospinal fluid (CSF) concentration almost equivalent to that in the plasma is achieved shortly after its administration.[125] It is rapidly and completely absorbed from the gastrointestinal tract.[126] Parenteral administration is generally limited to the intravenous route; intramuscular injection should be used with caution because of the acidity of aqueous preparations of caffeine. Approximately 25 percent of caffeine is bound to plasma protein.[127]

The liver microsomal cytochrome P450 system is responsible for the metabolism of caffeine, although during the first 3 months of life the drug is excreted in the urine largely in unchanged form. Thereafter, an increased capacity to produce demethylated metabolites causes the slow plasma clearance to approach adult rates.[128]

The drug theophylline differs from caffeine only by the presence of a methyl group at the number seven position of the xanthine ring. Its most common salt form, aminophylline, achieves greater water solubility through its ethylenediamine complex. Theophylline also is widely distributed in the body (0.7 to 0.9 L/kg), with its concentrations in blood and tissues being equal after prolonged therapy.[129] Its rate of gastrointestinal absorption is variable as a result of local irritation and interference by food.[130] The absorption of theophylline is erratic after rectal administration and, as with caffeine, intramuscular injection should be avoided. Approximately 36 percent of theophylline is protein bound.[131]

Theophylline is metabolized by a cytochrome P450 mixed-function oxidase. Additionally, a metabolic pathway unique to the neonate permits the methylation of theophylline, to yield caffeine. In neonates treated with theophylline, the mean plasma ratio of caffeine to theophylline is 0.3.[132,133] The age at which the methylation pathway becomes inactive is unclear, although children greater than 16 months of age show no metabolism to caffeine.[123] Pharmacokinetic studies show a direct correlation between postconceptional age and clearance of theophylline in infants.[134]

While the numerous pharmacologic effects of caffeine and theophylline are similar, the two drugs differ considerably in the intensity of these actions. Roberts[123] has recently provided a concise review of the comparative potencies and proposed mechanisms of action of theophylline and caffeine in affecting AOP. Methylxanthines act as potent general stimulants of the central nervous system, although their central respirogenic effect appears centered on the brain stem. Caffeine is relatively more potent in its stimulation of the medullary respiratory centers and reticular formation,[135] though the central mechanism of theophylline's action has been more extensively studied. At a cellular level, the actions of the methylxanthines are partially mediated by adenosine receptor blockade, resulting in release of excitatory neurotransmitters in the CNS and of norepinephrine from autonomic nerve endings.[136]

Other systemic effects

Though studies in the neonate are incomplete and often conflicting, the effects of therapeutic levels of methylxanthines on the cardiovascular system generally include an increase in heart rate and contractile force, peripheral vasodilation,[137] and constriction of cerebral blood vessels.[138] An increased capacity for skeletal muscle work, including contraction of the diaphragm, has been shown, particularly with caffeine use.[139,140] Theophylline is far more potent in its ability to relax bronchial smooth muscle and dilate pulmonary arterioles.[141] It also has a greater effect in increasing the glomerular filtration rate, although this diuretic action is mild and of little clinical utility.[142] Theophylline alters the sleep state in preterm infants,[143] and because the frequency and type of apnea may be related to sleep state, such alteration may serve as yet another mechanism for affecting AOP.

While theophylline can cause an acute increase in plasma glucose concentration, the effect of methylxanthines on plasma glucose levels during chronic therapy remains to be clarified.[144]

Clinical toxicity

Beyond mild tachycardia, adverse reactions to the methylxanthines are uncommon when levels of these drugs are carefully monitored and maintained within the therapeutic range. Despite a documented constriction of cerebral vessels and reduction of blood flow with caffeine treatment, no such effect on retinal blood vessels has been seen, and the incidence of retrolental fibroplasia is not increased in treated infants.[145] Early clinical reports suggesting an association of methylxanthine use and necrotizing enterocolitis[146] have not been substantiated by subsequent epidemiologic[147] and retrospective clinical studies.[148] Supraventricular tachycardia[149] and seizures[150] have been reported in the neonatal period at serum concentrations well above 20 mg/ml for theophylline. The potent effect of methylxanthines on lipid synthesis in cultured glial cells and in aggregating brain-cell cultures, two models of developing neural systems, has caused concern for the long term neurodevelopment of neonates undergoing prolonged treatment for apnea. Volpe[151] has further suggested that the effects of the drugs on brain structure and function may be subtle and difficult to define. However, limited neurologic follow-up studies to date suggest no adverse effects up to 4 years after treatment.[152]

Dosage schedules

The use of both caffeine and theophylline is widespread, and one or the other may be preferred solely on the basis of greater clinical familiarity with it. Proponents of caffeine, however, point to several advantages: greater specificity in its stimulation of the brain stem respiratory center (documented primarily in the adult literature), a higher therapeutic index, a once-daily dosing schedule, and lack of active metabolites. The relative efficacy of the two agents has not been thoroughly investigated.

Dosage recommendations and therapeutic serum levels are provided in Table 5-1 for the parent (base) compounds. It is imperative to recognize that maintenance schedules (dose and interval) for theophylline and caffeine will vary, depending upon postconceptional age and, for oral administration, on the specific salt form employed. Careful monitoring of serum concentrations is essential: within 48 hours of the loading dose, peak and trough theophylline levels should be obtained. After adjustment of the maintenance schedule based on the pharmacokinetics in a given infant, levels of the methylxanthines should be monitored. In the preterm infant, elimination of caffeine occurs very slowly, and a steady state may not be achieved for as long as 2 weeks after a change in the maintenance dose. It is the rare infant who, while failing to respond at normal therapeutic serum levels, experiences a reduction in the frequency or severity of apnea, or both at higher drug concentrations. Such an effect should not be anticipated.

Other medications

Doxapram is an analeptic agent and a respiratory stimulant that has been used extensively in adults for primary alveolar hypoventilation and in the treatment of respiratory insufficiency caused by obstructive lung disease, postanesthetic depression, and drug overdose. Reports about its safety and efficacy in the neonatal period are sparse. At low dosages, doxapram is thought to act by stimulating carotid-body chemoreceptors, accounting for its reported usefulness in the central congenital hypoventilation syndrome (Ondine's curse).[153] Larger doses appear to directly affect central respiratory neurons as well.[154] Preliminary reports on the effectiveness of doxapram as the primary treatment for apnea of prematurity or as an alternative agent in the treatment of refractory apnea have been encouraging.[155] Most recently, Eyal and colleagues[156] have shown that in 8 of 10 infants with apnea unresponsive to aminophylline therapy, the simultaneous use of doxapram resulted in complete cessation of apnea. Nine infants who received placebo in addition to aminophylline experienced no reduction in the frequency of their apneic episodes. At present, recommendations call for an initial continuous intravenous infusion of 0.5 mg/kg/hour, to be increased in increments of 0.5 mg/kg/hour every 24 hours to a maximum of 2.5 mg/kg/hour or until an adequate response has occurred.[156,157] The most common side effect of doxapram, hypertension, may be seen at doses greater than 1.5 mg/kg/hour.[157] Transient jitteriness has also been noted. The optimal dosage, therapeutic serum levels, and complete range of adverse side effects remain to be determined in the preterm neonate.

FUTURE DIRECTIONS

While our understanding of the pathogenesis of idiopathic apnea of prematurity is incomplete, and our therapy therefore imperfect, the goals of future investigations can now be more clearly defined. The preterm infant who "forgets to breathe" does so not of his own volition, but because of the apparent immaturity of those brain stem centers that generate the inspiratory rhythm and that integrate afferent feedback from central and peripheral receptors. The application of sophisticated neurophysiologic techniques, such as single-cell recording of electrical "pacemaker" activity, or the microinjection of neurotransmitters into specific medullary loci, may soon allow a more precise definition of the central respiratory pattern generator. Studies of the complex synaptic interconnections among the various brain stem motor nuclei, the reticular formation, and the receptor afferents will clarify how numerous sensory (i.e., sleep) and motor (i.e., upper airway muscle) influences develop into a mature, integrated system of respiratory control.

Of more immediate concern, the introduction of new clinical monitors capable of detecting respiratory airflow will certainly enhance the identification of airway obstruction. With this, therapy might be directed specifically at the predominant type of apnea in a given infant: central, obstructive, or mixed. Selective pharmacologic manipulation of the upper airway muscles, and in particular the genioglossus, has been demonstrated experimentally. The clinical utility and safety of the requisite pharmacologic agents, however, have not been investigated in the preterm infant. In the past, various methods of treatment have been introduced without a firm understanding of their modes of action. Given the rapid increase in our knowledge of the development of respiratory control, future therapy will probably be based more securely on the actual pathophysiology of AOP.

ACKNOWLEDGMENTS

We wish to express our sincere appreciation to Ms. Karen Brustle for her preparation of the manuscript, and to Mr. Terrence O'Day for the illustrations. This work was supported in part by grants from The Twenty-Five Club of Magee-Womens Hospital, the Richard King Mellon Foundation, the Magee-Womens Hospital Research Fund, and by a Training Fellowship Award (KWK) from the American Lung Association.

REFERENCES

1. Consensus Development Panel, Little GA, Chairman: Draft consensus statement on infantile apnea and home monitoring. National Institutes of Health Consensus Development Conference; 1986 September 29–October 1; Bethesda, MD. Available from: NICHHD Office of Research Reporting, Bethesda, MD.
2. Kelly DH, Shannon DC: Periodic breathing in infants with near-miss sudden infant death syndrome. Pediatrics 63:355, 1979
3. Daily WJR, Klaus M, Meyer HBP: Apnea in premature infants: Monitoring, incidence, heart rate changes, and an effect of environmental temperature. Pediatrics 43:510, 1969
4. Henderson-Smart DJ: The effect of gestational age on the incidence and duration of recurrent apnoea in newborn babies. Aust Paediatr J 17:273, 1981
5. Tudehope DI, Rogers Y: Clinical spectrum of neonatal apnoea in very low birthweight infants. Aust Paediatr J 20:131, 1984
6. Guilleminault C, Peraita R, Souquet M, et al: Apneas during sleep in infants: Possible relationship with sudden infant death syndrome. Science 190:677, 1975
7. Korner AF, Guilleminault C, Hoed J Van den, Baldwin RB: Reduction of sleep apnea and bradycardia in preterm infants on oscillating water beds: A controlled polygraphic study. Pediatrics 61:528, 1978
8. Mathew OP, Roberts JL, Thach BT: Pharyngeal airway obstruction in preterm infants during mixed and obstructive apnea. J Pediatr 100:964, 1982
9. Dransfield DA, Spitzer AR, Fox WW: Episodic airway obstruction in premature infants. Am J Dis Child 137:441, 1983
10. Euler, C von: On the central pattern generator for the basic breathing rhythmicity. J Appl Physiol 55:1647, 1983
11. Feldman JL, Smith JC, McCrimmon DR, et al: Generation of respiratory pattern in mammals. In Cohen AH, Grillner S, Rossignol S (eds): The Neural Control of Rhythmic Movements Vertebrates. John Wiley and Sons, New York, In press
12. Smith JC, Feldman JL: Role of chloride-dependent synaptic inhibition in respiratory pattern generation. Studies in an in vitro mammalian brainstem-spinal cord preparation. Fed Proc 45:518, 1986, (Abstract)
13. Henderson-Smart DJ, Pettigrew AG, Campbell DJ: Clinical apnea and brain-stem neural function in preterm infants. N Engl J Med 308:353, 1983

14. Marlot D, Duron B: Postnatal development of the discharge pattern of phrenic motor units in the kitten. Respir Physiol 46:125, 1981
15. Wan XST, Trojanowski JQ, Gonates JO, Liu CN: Cytoarchitecture of extranuclear and commissural dendrites of hypoglossal neurons as revealed by conjugates of HRP with cholera toxin. Exp Neurol 78:167, 1982
16. Takashima S, Becker LE: Prenatal and postnatal maturation of medullary "respiratory centers." Dev Brain Res 26:173, 1986
17. McGinty DJ, Hoppenbrouwers T: The reticular formation, breathing disorders during sleep, and SIDS. p. 375. In Tilden J, Roeder LM, Steinschneider A (eds): Sudden Infant Death Syndrome. Academic Press, New York, 1983
18. St. John WM, Bledsoe TA: Comparison of respiratory-related trigeminal, hypoglossal and phrenic activities. Respir Physiol 62:61, 1985
19. Rigatto H, Brady JP, de la Torre Verduzco R: Chemoreceptor reflexes in preterm infants: II. The effect of gestational age and postnatal age on the ventilatory response to inhaled carbon dioxide. Pediatrics 55:614, 1975
20. Rigatto H: Control of ventilation in the newborn. Annu Rev Physiol 46:661, 1984
21. Guthrie RD, Standaert TA, Hodson WA, Woodrum DE: Sleep and maturation of eucapnic ventilation and CO_2 sensitivity in the premature primate. J Appl Physiol 48:347, 1980
22. Frantz ID, Adler SM, Thach BT, et al: Maturational effects on respiratory responses to carbon dioxide in premature infants. J Appl Physiol 41:41, 1976
23. Guthrie RD, Standaert TA, Hodson WA, Woodrum DE: Development of CO_2 sensitivity: Effects of gestational age, postnatal age and sleep state. J Appl Physiol 50:956, 1981
24. Phillipson EA: Control of breathing during sleep. Am Rev Respir Dis 118:909, 1978
25. Rigatto H, Brady JP, de la Torre Verduzco R: Chemoreceptor reflexes in preterm infants: I. The effect of gestational age and postnatal age on the ventilatory response to inhalation of 100% and 15% oxygen. Pediatrics 55:604, 1975
26. LaFramboise WA, Standaert TA, Woodrum DE, Guthrie RD: Occlusion pressures during the ventilatory response to hypoxemia in the newborn monkey. J Appl Physiol 51:1169, 1981
27. Rigatto H, Brady JP: Periodic breathing and apnea in preterm infants. II. Hypoxia as a primary event. Pediatrics 50:219, 1972
28. Haddad GG, Gandhi MR, Mellins RB: Maturation of ventilatory response to hypoxia in puppies during sleep. J Appl Physiol 52:309, 1982
29. Sankaran K, Wiebe H, Seshia MMK, et al: Immediate and late ventilatory response to high and low O_2 in preterm infants and adult subjects. Pediatr Res 13:875, 1979
30. Blanco CE, Hanson MA, Johnson P, Rigatto H: Breathing pattern of kittens during hypoxia. J Appl Physiol 56:12, 1984
31. Lawson EE, Long WA: Central origin of biphasic breathing pattern during hypoxia in newborns. J Appl Physiol 55:483, 1983
32. LaFramboise WA, Guthrie RD, Standaert TA, Woodrum DE: Pulmonary mechanics during the ventilatory response to hypoxemia in the newborn monkey. J Appl Physiol 55:1008, 1983
33. LaFramboise WA, Woodrum DE: Elevated diaphragm electromyogram during neonatal hypoxic ventilatory depression. J Appl Physiol 59:1040, 1985
34. Watchko JF, LaFramboise WA, Mayock DE et al: Spectral analysis of diaphragmatic EMG during the neonatal biphasic hypoxic ventilatory response. Am Rev Respir Dis 133:A104, 1986, (Abstract)
35. Eldridge FL, Millhorn DE: Central regulation of respiration by endogenous neurotransmitters and neuromodulators. Annu Rev Physiol 43:121, 1981
36. Lawson EE, Long WA, Gingras-Leatherman J, McNamara MC: Hypoxia and endogenous neurotransmitters in newborns. p. 422. In Bianchi AL, Denavit-Saubie M (eds): Neurogenesis of Central Respiratory Rhythm. MTP Press Limited, Lancaster, England, 1985
37. Guthrie RD, LaFramboise WA, Standaert TA, et al: Ventilatory interaction between oxygen and carbon dioxide in the preterm primate. Pediatr Res 19:528, 1985
38. Durand M, Georgie S, Barberis C, et al: Ventilatory response to CO_2 in preterm infants with idiopathic apnoea. p. 211. In Jones CT, Nathanielsz PW (eds): The Physiological Development of the Fetus and Newborn. Academic Press, London, 1985
39. Gerhardt T, Bancalari E: Apnea of prematurity: I. Lung function and regulation of breathing. Pediatrics 74:58, 1984
40. Schulte FJ: Apnea. Clin Perinatol 4:65, 1977
41. Krauss AN, Solomon GE, Auld PAM: Sleep state, apnea and bradycardia in preterm infants. Dev Med Child Neurol 19:160, 1977
42. Jeffery HE, Read DJC: Ventilatory responses of newborn calves to progressive hypoxia in quiet and active sleep. J Appl Physiol 48:892, 1980

43. Henderson-Smart DJ, Read DJC: Ventilatory responses to hypoxemia during sleep in the newborn. J Dev Physiol 1:195, 1979
44. Kattwinkel J, Mars H, Fanaroff AA, et al: Urinary biogenic amines in idiopathic apnea of prematurity. J Pediatr 88:1003, 1976
45. Stark AR, Thach BT: Mechanisms of airway obstruction leading to apnea in newborn infants. J Pediatr 89:982, 1976
46. Milner AD, Boon AW, Saunders RA, Hopkin IE: Upper airways obstruction and apnoea in preterm babies. Arch Dis Child 55:22, 1980
47. Brouillette RT, Hunt CE: Obstructive sleep apnea in infants and children. Pediatr Res 15:715, 1981
48. Walsh RE, Michaelson ED, Harkleroad LE, et al: Upper airway obstruction in obese patients with sleep disturbance and somnolence. Ann Intern Med 76:185, 1972
49. Gastaut H, Tassinari CA, Duron B: Polygraphic study of the episodic diurnal and nocturnal (hypnic and respiratory) manifestations of the Pickwick syndrome. Brain Res 1:167, 1966
50. Sauerland EK, Harper RM: The human tongue during sleep: electromyographic activity of the genioglossus muscle. Exp Neurol 51:160, 1976
51. Sauerland EK, Mitchell SP: Electromyographic activity of intrinsic and extrinsic muscles of the human tongue. Tex Rep Biol Med 33:445, 1975
52. Remmers JE, DeGroot WJ, Sauerland EK, Anch AM: Pathogenesis of upper airway occlusion during sleep. J Appl Physiol 44:931, 1978
53. Brouillette RT, Thach BT: Control of genioglossus muscle inspiratory activity. J Appl Physiol 49:801, 1980
54. Bartlett D, Remmers JE, Gautier H: Laryngeal regulation of respiratory airflow. Respir Physiol 18:194, 1973
55. Brouillette RT, Thach BT: A neuromuscular mechanism maintaining extrathoracic airway patency. J Appl Physiol 46:772, 1979
56. Strohl KP, Hensley MJ, Hallett M, et al: Activation of upper airway muscles before onset of inspiration in normal humans. J Appl Physiol 49:638, 1980
57. Onal E, Lopata M, O'Connor TD: Diaphragmatic and genioglossal electromyogram responses to CO_2 rebreathing in humans. J Appl Physiol 50:1052, 1981
58. Onal E, Lopata M, O'Connor TD: Diaphragmatic and genioglossal electromyogram responses to isocapnic hypoxia in humans. Am Rev Respir Dis 124:215, 1981
59. Patrick GB, Strohl KP, Rubin SB, Altose MD: Upper airway and diaphragm muscle responses to chemical stimulation and load. J Appl Physiol 53:1133, 1982
60. England SJ, Kent G, Stogryn HAF: Laryngeal muscle and diaphragmatic activities in conscious dog pups. Respir Physiol 60:95, 1985
61. Harding R, Johnson R, McClelland ME: Respiratory function of the larynx in developing sheep and the influence of sleep state. Respir Physiol 40:165, 1980
62. Bruce EN, Hoh C: Phrenic and hypoglossal nerve responses to hypoxia in anesthetized kittens. Fed Proc 42:742, 1983, (Abstract)
63. Johnston BM, Gunn TR, Gluckman PD: Genioglossus and alae nasi activity in fetal sheep. J Dev Physiol 8:323, 1986
64. Carlo WA, Martin RJ, Abboud EF, et al: Effect of sleep state and hypercapnia on alae nasi and diaphragm EMGs in preterm infants. J Appl Physiol 54:1590, 1983
65. Carlo WA, Miller MJ, Martin RJ: Differential response of respiratory muscles to airway occlusion in infants. J Appl Physiol 59:847, 1985
66. Carlo WA, Martin RJ, Bruce EN, et al: Ala nasi activation (nasal flaring) decreases nasal resistance in preterm infants. Pediatrics 72:338, 1983
67. Butcher-Puech MC, Henderson-Smart DJ, Holley D, et al: Relation between apnoea duration and type and neurological status of preterm infants. Arch Dis Child 60:953, 1985
68. Cohen G, Henderson-Smart DJ: Upper airway stability and apnea during nasal occlusion in newborn infants. J Appl Physiol 60:1511, 1986
69. Wilson SL, Thach BT, Brouillette RT, Abu-Osba YK: Upper airway patency in the human infant: influence of airway pressure and posture. J Appl Physiol 48:500, 1980
70. Stark AR, Thach BT: Recovery of airway patency after obstruction in normal infants. Am Rev Respir Dis 123:691, 1981
71. Roberts JL, Reed WR, Mathew OP, Thach BT: Control of respiratory activity of the genioglossus muscle in micrognathic infants. J Appl Physiol 61:1523, 1986
72. Read DJC, Henderson-Smart DJ: Regulation of breathing in the newborn during different behavioral states. Annu Rev Physiol 46:675, 1984
73. Sauerland EK, Orr WC, Hairston LE: EMG patterns of oropharyngeal muscles during respiration in wakefulness and sleep. Electromyogr Clin Neurophysiol 21:307, 1981

74. Prechtl HFR, Eykern LA van, O'Brien MJ: Respiratory muscle EMG in newborns: A nonintrusive method. Early Human Dev 1:265, 1977
75. Bonora M, Shields GI, Knuth SL, et al: Selective depression by ethanol of upper airway respiratory motor activity in cats. Am Rev Respir Dis 130:156, 1984
76. Bonora M, St. John WM, Bledsoe TA: Differential elevation by protryptiline and depression by diazepam of upper airway respiratory motor activity. Am Rev Respir Dis 131:41, 1985
77. Lunteren E van, Haxhiu MA, Mitra J, Cherniack NS: Effects of dopamine, isoproterenol, and lobeline on cranial and phrenic motoneurons. J Appl Physiol 56:737, 1984
78. Weese-Mayer DE, Brouillette RT, Klemka L, Hunt CE: Effects of almitrine on hypoglossal and phrenic electroneurograms. J Appl Physiol 59:105, 1985
79. Hwang JC, St. John WM, Bartlett D, Jr.: Respiratory-related hypoglossal nerve activity: Influence of anesthetics. J Appl Physiol 55:785, 1983
80. Hering E, Breuer J: Die selbsteurung der athmung durch den nervus vagus. Sitzberg Akad Wiss wein 57(II):672, 1868
81. Kirkpatrick SML, Olinsky A, Bryan MH, Bryan AC: Effect of premature delivery on the maturation of the Hering-Breuer inspiratory inhibitory reflex in human infants. J Pediatr 88:1010, 1976
82. Fleming PJ, Bryan AC, Bryan MH: Functional immaturity of pulmonary irritant receptors and apnea in newborn preterm infants. Pediatrics 61:515, 1978
83. Kosch PC, Stark AR: Dynamic maintenance of end-expiratory lung volume in full-term infants. J Appl Physiol 57:1126, 1984
84. Olinsky A, Bryan MH, Bryan AC: Influence of lung inflation on respiratory control in neonates. J Appl Physiol 36:426, 1974
85. Fisher JT, Mathew OP, Sant'Ambrogio FB, Sant'Ambrogio G: Reflex effects and receptor responses to upper airway pressure and flow stimuli in developing puppies. J Appl Physiol 58:258, 1985
86. Henderson-Smart DJ, Read DJC: Depression of respiratory muscles and defective responses to nasal obstruction during active sleep in the newborn. Aust Paediatr J 12:261, 1976
87. Knill R, Bryan AC: An intercostal-phrenic inhibitory reflex in human newborn infants. J Appl Physiol 40:352, 1976
88. Haddad GG, Mellins RB: The role of airway receptors in the control of respiration in infants: A review. J Pediatr 91:281, 1977
89. Gershanik JJ, Levkoff AH, Duncan R: The association of hypocalcemia and recurrent apnea in premature infants. Am J Obstet Gynecol 113:646, 1972
90. Bridgers SL, Ment LR, Ebersole JS, Ehrenkranz RA: Cassette electroencephalographic recording of neonates with apneic episodes. Pediatr Neurol 1:219, 1985
91. Fenichel GM, Olson BJ, Fitzpatrick JE: Heart rate changes in convulsive and nonconvulsive neonatal apnea. Ann Neurol 7:577, 1980
92. Ollson T, Daily W, Victorin L: Transthoracic impedance: I. Theoretical considerations and technical approach. Acta Pediatr Scand Suppl 207:15, 1970
93. Lucey JF: False alarms in the nursery. (Editorial). Pediatrics 61:665, 1978
94. Warburton D, Stark AR, Taeusch HW: Apnea monitor failure in infants with upper airway obstruction. Pediatrics 60:742, 1977
95. Southall DP, Levitt GA, Richards JM, et al: Undetected episodes of prolonged apnea and severe bradycardia in preterm infants. Pediatrics 72:541, 1983
96. Peabody JL, Gregory GA, Willis MM, et al: Failure of conventional monitoring to detect apnea resulting in hypoxemia. p. 275. In Huch A, Huch R, Lucey JF (eds): Continuous Transcutaneous Blood Gas Monitoring. Birth Defects: Original Article Series, Vol XV, Alan R. Liss, Inc., New York, 1979
97. Dransfield DA, Philip AGS: Respiratory airflow measurement in the neonate. Clin Perinatol 12:21, 1985
98. Gregory GA, Kitterman JA: Pneumotachygraph for use with infants during spontaneous or assisted ventilation. J Appl Physiol 31:766, 1971
99. Brouillette RT, Thach BT: A self-retaining nasal flowmeter for preterm infants. J Appl Physiol 48:569, 1980
100. Werthammer J, Krasner J, DiBenedetto J, Stark AR: Apnea monitoring by acoustic detection in airflow. Pediatrics 71:53, 1983
101. Thach BT, Stark AR: Spontaneous neck flexion and airway obstruction during apneic spells in preterm infants. J Pediatr 94:275, 1979
102. Dransfield DA, Fow WW: A noninvasive method for recording central and obstructive apnea with bradycardia in infants. Crit Care Med 8:663, 1980
103. Kattwinkel J: Neonatal apnea: Pathogenesis and therapy. J Pediatr 90:342, 1977

104. Carlo WA, Martin RJ, Versteegh FGA: The effect of respiratory distress syndrome on chest wall movements and respiratory pauses in preterm infants. Am Rev Respir Dis 126:103, 1982
105. Frank UA, Bordiuk JM, Borromeo-McGrail V, et al: Treatment of apnea in neonates with an automated monitor-actuated apnea arrestor. Pediatrics 51:878, 1973
106. Millen RS, Davies J: See-saw resuscitator for the treatment of asphyxia. Am J Obstet Gynecol 52:508, 1946
107. Lee HF: A rocking bed respirator for use with premature infants in incubators. J Pediatr 44:570, 1954
108. Korner AF, Kraemer HC, Haffner ME, Cosper LM: Effects of waterbed flotation on premature infants: A pilot study. Pediatrics 56:361, 1975
109. Korner AF, Ruppel EM, Rho JM: Effects of water beds on the sleep and motility of theophylline-treated preterm infants. Pediatrics 70:864, 1982
110. Saigal S, Watts J, Campbell D: Randomized clinical trial of an oscillating air mattress in preterm infants: effect on apnea, growth and development. J Pediatr 109:857, 1986
111. Kattwinkel J, Nearman HS, Fanaroff AA, et al: Apnea of prematurity: comparative therapeutic effects of cutaneous stimulation and nasal continuous positive airway pressure. J Pediatr 86:588, 1975
112. Speidel BD, Dunn PM: Use of nasal continuous positive airway pressure to treat severe recurrent apnoea in very preterm infants. Lancet 2:658, 1976
113. Miller MJ, Carlo WA, Martin RJ: Continuous positive airway pressure selectively reduces obstructive apnea in preterm infants. J Pediatr 106:91, 1985
114. Martin RJ, Nearman HS, Katona PG, Klaus MH: The effect of a low continuous positive airway pressure on the reflex control of respiration in the preterm infant. J Pediatr 90:976, 1977
115. Kuzemko JA, Paala J: Apnoeic attacks in the newborn treated with aminophylline. Arch Dis Child 48:404, 1973
116. Shannon DC, Gotay F, Stein IM, et al: Prevention of apnea and bradycardia in low-birthweight infants. Pediatrics 55:589, 1975
117. Bednarek FJ, Roloff DW: Treatment of apnea of prematurity with aminophylline. Pediatrics 58:335, 1976
118. Aranda JV, Gorman W, Bergsteinsson H, Gunn T: Efficacy of caffeine in treatment of apnea in the low-birth-weight infant. J Pediatr 90:467, 1977
119. Meyers TF, Milsap RL, Krauss AN, et al: Low-dose theophylline therapy in idiopathic apnea of prematurity. J Pediatr 96:99, 1980
120. Brouard C, Moriette G, Murat I, et al: Comparative efficacy of theophylline and caffeine in the treatment of idiopathic apnea in premature infants. Am J Dis Child 139:698, 1985
121. Aranda JV, Turmen T: Methylxanthines in apnea of prematurity. Clin Perinatol 6:87, 1979
122. Soyka LF: Developmental pharmacology of the methylxanthines. Semin Perinatol 5(4), 1981
123. Roberts RJ (ed): Methylxanthine therapy: Caffeine and theophylline. p. 119. In Roberts RJ (ed): Drug Therapy in Infants: Pharmacologic Principles and Clinical Experience. W.B. Saunders, Philadelphia, 1984
124. Warszawski D, Gorodischer R: Tissue distribution of caffeine in premature infants and in newborn and adult dogs. Pediatr Pharmacol 1:341, 1981
125. Turmen T, Louridas TA, Aranda JV: Relationship of plasma and CSF concentrations of caffeine in neonates with apnea. J Pediatr 95:644, 1979
126. Aranda JV, Cook CE, Gorman W, et al: Pharmacokinetic profile of caffeine in the premature newborn infant with apnea. J Pediatr 94:663, 1979
127. Tyrala EE, Dodson WE: Caffeine secretion into breast milk. Arch Dis Child 54:787, 1979
128. Aranda JV, Collinge JM, Zinman R, Watters G: Maturation of caffeine elimination in infancy. Arch Dis Child 54:946, 1979
129. Bonati M, Latini R, Marra G, et al: Theophylline distribution in the premature neonate. Dev Pharmacol Ther 3:65, 1981
130. Heimann G, Murgescu J, Bergt U: Influence of food intake on bioavailability of theophylline in premature infants. Eur J Clin Pharmacol 22:171, 1982
131. Aranda JV, Sitar DS, Parsons WD, et al: Pharmacokinetic aspects of theophylline in premature newborns. N Engl J Med 295:413, 1976
132. Bory C, Baltassat P, Porthault M, et al: Metabolism of theophylline to caffeine in premature newborn infants. J Pediatr 94:988, 1979
133. Brazier JL, Salle B, Ribon B, et al: In vivo N7 methylation of theophylline to caffeine in premature infants. Dev Pharmacol Ther 2:137, 1981
134. Tserng K-Y, King KC, Takieddine FN: Theophylline metabolism in premature infants. Clin Pharmacol Ther 29:594, 1981
135. Foote WE, Holmes P, Pritchard A, et al: Neurophysiological and pharmacodynamic studies on

caffeine and on interactions between caffeine and nicotinic acid in the rat. Neuropharmacology 17:7, 1978

136. Rall TW: Central nervous system stimulants in the methylxanthines. p. 589. In Gilman AG, Goodman LS, Rall TW, Murad F (eds): The Pharmacological Basis of Therapeutics, 7th Ed. Macmillan, New York, 1985
137. Howell J, Clozel M, Aranda JV: Adverse effects of caffeine and theophylline in the newborn infant. Semin Perinatol 5:359, 1981
138. Rosenkrantz TS, Oh W: Reduction of cerebral blood flow (CBF) in low birth weight (LBW) infants after aminophylline administration. Pediatr Res 16:306A, 1982, (Abstract)
139. Supinski GS, Deal EC, Jr, Kelsen SG: The effects of caffeine and theophylline on diaphragm contractility. Am Rev Respir Dis 130:429, 1984
140. Murciano D, Aubier M, Lecocguic Y, Pariente R: Effects of theophylline on diaphragmatic strength and fatigue in patients with chronic obstructive pulmonary disease. N Engl J Med 311:349, 1984
141. Trippenbach T: Effects of drugs on the respiratory control system in the perinatal period and during postnatal development. Pharmacol Ther 20:307, 1983
142. Zakauddin S, Leake RD, Trygstad CW: Theophylline increases glomerular filtration rate in preterm infants. Dev Pharmacol Ther 1:333, 1980
143. Dietrich J, Krauss AN, Reidenberg M, et al: Alterations in state in apneic pre-term infants receiving theophylline. Clin Pharmacol Ther 24:474, 1978
144. Srinivasan G, Pildes RS, Jaspan JB, et al: Metabolic effects of theophylline in preterm infants. J Pediatr 98:815, 1981
145. Gunn TR, Metrakos K, Riley P, et al: Sequelae of caffeine treatment in preterm infants with apnea. J Pediatr 94:106, 1979
146. Robinson MJ, Clayden GS, Smith MF: Xanthines and necrotising enterocolitis. (Letter). Arch Dis Child 55:494, 1980
147. Kliegman RM, Hack M, Jones P, Fanaroff AA: Epidemiologic study of necrotizing enterocolitis among low birth weight infants: absence of identifiable risk factors. J Pediatr 100:440, 1982
148. Davis JM, Abbasi S, Spitzer AR, Johnson L: Role of theophylline in pathogenesis of necrotizing enterocolitis. J Pediatr 109:344, 1986
149. Loughnan PM, McNamara JM: Paroxysmal supraventricular tachycardia during theophylline therapy in a premature infant. J Pediatr 92:1016, 1978
150. Simons FER, Friesen FR, Simons KJ: Theophylline toxicity in term infants. Am J Dis Child 134:39, 1980
151. Volpe JJ: Effects of methylxanthines on lipid synthesis in developing neural systems. Semin Perinatol 5:395, 1981
152. Nelson RM, Jr., Resnick MB: Long-term outcome of premature infants treated with theophylline. Semin Perinatol 5:370, 1981
153. Hunt CE, Inwood RJ, Shannon DC: Respiratory and nonrespiratory effects of doxapram in congenital central hypoventilation syndrome. Am Rev Respir Dis 119:263, 1979
154. Franz DN: Central nervous system stimulants: strychnine, picrotoxin, pentylenetetrazol, and miscellaneous agents (doxapram, nikethamide, methlyphenidate). p. 582. In Gilman AG, Goodman LS, Rall TW, Murad F (eds): The Pharmacological Basis of Therapeutics, 7th Ed. Macmillan, New York, 1985
155. Burnard ED, Moore RG, Nichol H: A trial of doxapram in the recurrent apnea of prematurity. p. 143. In Stern L, Oh W, Friis-Hansen B (eds): Intensive Care in the Newborn. II. Masson, New York, 1978
156. Eyal F, Alpan G, Sagi E, et al: Aminophylline versus doxapram in idiopathic apnea of prematurity: A double-blind controlled study. Pediatrics 75:709, 1985
157. Barrington K, Torok-Both G, Finer N, Jamali F: Dose-response relationship of doxapram in refractory idiopathic apnea of prematurity. Am Rev Respir Dis 133:A105, 1986 (Abstract)

6
Regulation of Cerebral Blood Flow in the Fetus, Newborn, and Adult

M. Douglas Jones, Jr.
Raymond C. Koehler
Richard J. Traystman

The importance of the cerebral circulation to the survival of the newborn animal after an asphyxial episode was recognized over 150 years ago by Le Galois (cited by Dawes[1]), but quantitative data defining the tolerable limits of the balance between cerebral blood flow (CBF) and the developing brain's needs for oxygen and metabolic substrate are only now becoming available. A growing literature is in the process of answering such questions as: What are the criteria by which CBF should be judged sufficient or insufficient? Does the definition of sufficiency change during brain development? Do the mechanisms that regulate the cerebrovascular bed differ among fetuses, newborns, and adults? What are the implications of any such differences for the pathophysiology of neurologic disorders in the developing brain? This review will summarize recent information relating to each of these questions, but will concentrate on mechanisms of CBF regulation and how they pertain to the developing brain's need to maintain an adequate oxygen supply.

BLOOD FLOW AND METABOLISM

The longstanding controversy over whether cardiac output was determined centrally, by the heart itself, or peripherally, by the individual organs, was not finally settled until Guyton and others demonstrated definitively that cardiac output should be considered as the sum of individual organ blood flows, with each organ regulating flow according to its own needs.[2] Organ blood flow thus became more than simply an entity delivered by a remote heart operating in isolation; rather, flow was locally tailored to the needs of the organ, and the heart was expected to make the best of the situation.

In that context, a description of organ blood flow as high or low gives rise immediately to the question: "High or low relative to what?" For instance, the oxygen needs of the brain represent an important determinant of its need for flow. Thus, in order to judge the adequacy of a given level of CBF, one must have a reliable measurement of the cerebral metabolic rate for oxygen ($CMRO_2$).[3] In comparing resting and exercising muscle, a change in metabolic requirements is obvious, and it is clear that this has to be considered before a particular value for blood flow can be evaluated. The analogy to resting and exercising muscle may seem inappropriate for the brain, since overall brain metabolism is not measurably changed by mental activity[4]; however, in a number of circumstances (e.g., after asphyxia or trauma, or in seizures) cerebral metabolism varies considerably.[3–6] In fact, it is no less important to relate blood flow to simultaneous measurements of metabolic rate for the brain than it is for any other organ.[3]

It is especially difficult to interpret changes in CBF alone under circumstances in which $CMRO_2$ and oxygen availability change simultaneously. In those situations, the responses of the cerebrovascular bed are more easily described with variables that link CBF to its physiologic purpose.[7,8] We will define these variables now, since they appear repeatedly in the subsequent discussion.

One such variable is cerebral oxygen delivery, or perhaps more accurately, cerebral oxygen transport. The latter designation is preferable because "oxygen delivery" implies to some investigators the delivery of molecular oxygen to the mitochondrial electron transport chain. Cerebral oxygen transport (OT) refers only to the convective transport of oxygen to the vascular exchange site, and is defined by the equation:

$$OT = CBF \times CaO_2, \tag{1}$$

where CaO_2 is the arterial oxygen content in milliliters of oxygen per 100 ml of blood (vol%). Thus, OT represents the total amount of oxygen presented to the brain. The determinants of CaO_2 are the blood oxygen carrying capacity and arterial PO_2. The oxygen carrying capacity depends in turn on the hemoglobin concentration, number of hemoglobin binding sites for oxygen, and oxygen affinity of each site, as defined by the oxyhemoglobin dissociation curve.

The relationship between OT and $CMRO_2$ can be summarized by using the ratio: $CMRO_2/OT$. Since both $CMRO_2$ and OT are measured in milliliters of oxygen per 100 g of brain per minute, the ratio is dimensionless. It expresses cerebral oxygen consumption as a fraction of the total amount of oxygen transported to the brain, and is variously referred to as cerebral fractional O_2 extraction (E) or, when multiplied by 100, as percentage oxygen extraction. This review will express the ratio as a decimal fraction:

$$E = CMRO_2/OT. \tag{2}$$

To date, E has not been commonly used because it requires measurement of the oxygen content (see Eq. 6), until recently a tedious and time-consuming procedure. But new technology has simplified the measurement of oxygen content,[8] and the introduction of positron emission tomography (PET) as a clinical and research tool has made it possible to measure E directly.[3,9] The PET literature employs the designation oxygen extraction ratio (OER)[3] or oxygen extraction fraction (OEF)[9] for E. Comparisons among species[7] and, using PET techniques, among regions of the individual brain[10] show that E is relatively tightly controlled between 0.30 and 0.50. This compares with values of fractional extraction for the kidney of approximately 0.10 and for the heart of 0.70.[11]

In situations in which CaO_2 is constant, one may correct for variations in $CMRO_2$ by using the ratio $CBF/CMRO_2$. This corrects blood flow for variations in metabolism, and at the same time reduces to an expression that does not require the direct measurement of flow at all. Since, according to the Fick principle:

$$CMRO_2 = CBF\,(CaO_2 - CvO_2), \tag{3}$$

in which CvO_2 represents the oxygen content in cerebral venous blood, CBF/$CMRO_2$ reduces to:

$$CBF/CMRO_2 = 1/(CaO_2 - CvO_2), \tag{4}$$

which is the reciprocal of the arteriovenous difference of oxygen content across the brain. As long as the uptake and metabolism of oxygen are in a steady state, the requirements of the Fick principle are satisfied,[12] and CBF/$CMRO_2$ is a valid and useful variable. The same requirement for a steady state applies to the measurement of E, which also reduces to a simple expression:

$$E = CBF(CaO_2 - CvO_2)/CBF(CaO_2) \tag{5}$$

$$E = 1 - (CvO_2/CaO_2) \tag{6}$$

HYPOXIA, ISCHEMIA AND TISSUE OXYGEN INSUFFICIENCY

The brain compensates for decreases in CaO_2 or PO_2 by increasing CBF (Fig. 6-1).[8] When the capacity of that mechanism is overwhelmed, E rises until eventually, $CMRO_2$ can no longer be sustained and oxygen insufficiency results in tissue injury. In the case of ischemia, where the decrease in CBF is the primary abnormality, an increase in E is the only mechanism by which $CMRO_2$ can be sustained.[3] This

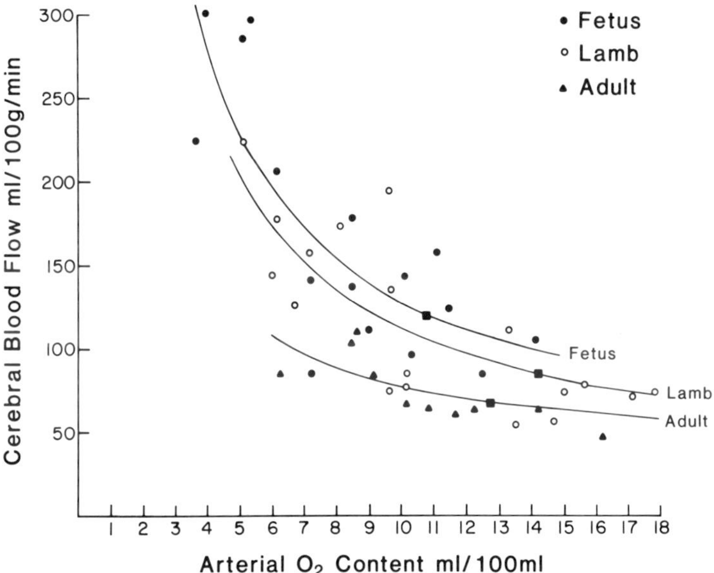

Fig. 6-1. The relationship of cerebral blood flow to arterial O_2 content during acute isocapnic hypoxic hypoxia in fetal, newborn, and adult sheep. The square symbol along each line identifies approximate normal values.

section will review the brain's responses to hypoxia and ischemia, and will attempt to arrive at a physiologic definition of insufficient CBF.

Hypoxic Hypoxia

A fall in arterial PO_2 results in hypoxic hypoxia. As mentioned above, $CMRO_2$ is essentially constant despite wide variations in arterial PO_2 (see Jones and Traystman[8]). The cerebral fractional oxygen extraction (E) is constant over most of the PO_2 range because the increase in CBF maintains OT,[7] but during severe hypoxic hypoxia OT cannot be sustained[13] and E rises. If the PO_2 is lower still, the capacity of the brain to extract oxygen is exceeded and $CMRO_2$ falls.[14] The ability to extract oxygen is presumably limited by the PO_2 in cerebral venous (and therefore end-capillary) blood. Even though the PO_2 necessary to support ATP generation by the mitochondrion is extraordinarily low, the gradient between intravascular and mitochondrial PO_2 must be sufficient to sustain diffusion.[15]

The increase in CBF during hypoxic hypoxia may be conveniently indexed by calculating the resulting OT. As mentioned above, this is accomplished by multiplying CBF by CaO_2 (Eq. 1). Examination of the behavior of OT during hypoxic hypoxia discloses the interesting property just mentioned: If arterial PCO_2 is unchanged (isocapnic hypoxic hypoxia), OT is virtually constant as CaO_2 changes (Fig. 6-2).[7,8]

Maintenance of OT during acute isocapnic hypoxic hypoxia is characteristic of a wide variety of experimental situations in humans and other species.[7] (Chronic isocapnic, or for that matter hypocapnic, hypoxia is a different and less well-studied phenomenon.[16]) As can be deduced from a re-examination of Equation 1, OT will

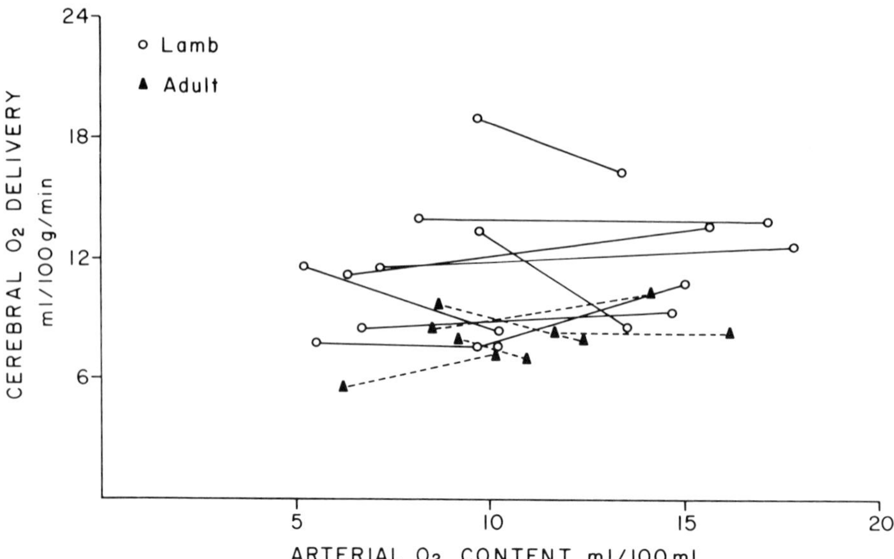

Fig. 6-2. The relationship between cerebral O_2 delivery and arterial O_2 content in newborn and adult sheep, using data from Figure 6-1. No systematic relationship is evident.

be maintained only if the decrease in CaO_2 is accompanied by a proportional rise in CBF:

$$CBF \times CaO_2 = OT = \text{a constant} \quad (1a)$$

The mechanism by which the brain achieves this rather precise regulation of OT is not clear. One possibility is that it senses changes in CaO_2 directly. At least one CaO_2 receptor exists in the body. Even though the carotid chemoreceptor is affected only by changes in arterial PO_2, the aortic chemoreceptors can respond to changes in CaO_2 in the absence of a change in arterial PO_2.[17] There is no evidence, however, that aortic chemoreceptors influence the CBF response to hypoxic hypoxia.[18] It is conceivable that an area in the brain operating according to the same principle as the aortic chemoreceptor might sense changes in CaO_2, but there is at present no evidence to support this hypothesis either. A more likely explanation is that CaO_2 is not in fact sensed directly. This possibility will be discussed at the end of the section.

CBF Response to Hypoxic Hypoxia: A Threshold Effect?

Before considering mechanisms by which hypoxic hypoxia causes cerebral vasodilation, it is important to be as precise as possible about how CBF behaves when oxygen availability falls. Careful measurements disclose that CBF increases even with decreases in CaO_2 or arterial PO_2 within the "normoxic" range.[7,19] This conflicts with an early view of the hypoxic response as a threshold phenomenon, in the sense that CBF will not increase until a "critical" PO_2 is reached.[20–22] At present there is little reason to think that a "critical" PO_2 does exist, first because of the experimental results mentioned above and others, involving changes in oxyhemoglobin affinity, to be discussed later, and second because of a better understanding of how oxygen effects cellular metabolism in intact biologic systems.[22,23] The situation may be summarized as follows: A threshold response to a decrease in arterial PO_2 appears to be present because either the PO_2 in the arteriolar network as a whole or the parenchymal PO_2, most probably the latter,[24] is the major determinant of CBF. Furthermore, because of loss of oxygen from larger arterioles[25] and the sigmoid shape of the oxyhemoglobin dissociation curve (Fig. 6-3), large changes in arterial PO_2 will result in comparatively small changes in PO_2 in small arterioles and tissues. Moreover, any changes in CBF that occur at high levels of arterial PO_2 will be on the relatively flat portion of the hyperbolic response curve[8] (see Fig. 6-1) and will be difficult to measure. The CBF response to hypoxic hypoxia is best thought of as a continuous hyperbolic function that applies over a wide range of PO_2 values. Experiments in which oxyhemoglobin affinity is altered (see below) provide additional evidence for this description.

Mechanisms of OT Maintenance in Hypoxic Hypoxia

With the above in mind we can reconsider the remarkably tight link between CBF and CaO_2. Although the existence of a central (cerebral) chemoreceptor that senses CaO_2 needs to be explored, it is equally likely that the important relationship is not between CaO_2 and CBF, but rather between microvascular or tissue PO_2 and CBF. How then is OT, which reflects CaO_2, so well maintained when PO_2 is the controlling variable? Again, the important consideration may be the shape of the

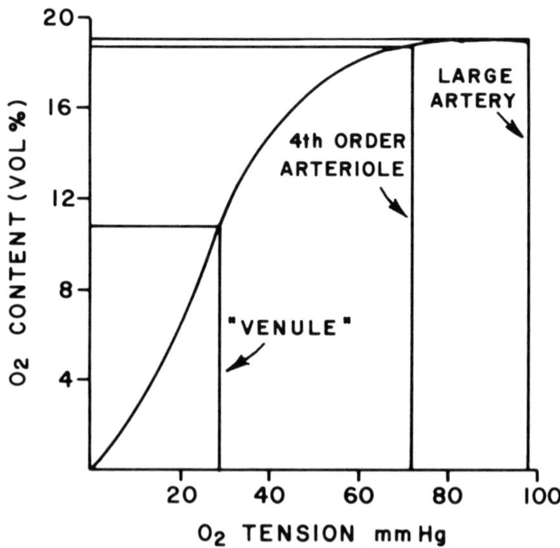

Fig. 6-3. The relationship between O_2 tension and content in large arteries, in fourth-order pial arterioles, and in cerebral "venules" plotted on the human oxyhemoglobin dissociation curve. These relationships are approximate. The arteriolar value is taken from the work of Duling and co-workers in pial vessels in cats,[25] and the "venular" value is not measured directly, but rather calculated from the oxygen extraction fraction measured with positron emission tomography (PET).[10] The resulting "venular" PO_2 is approximately 5 mmHg lower than that measured in jugular venous blood (see Paulson et al.[46] and Cohen et al.,[129] below). Venular PO_2 would have been slightly higher if we had corrected for the Bohr effect; the remaining difference could reflect extracerebral contamination of jugular venous blood or a methodologic error in the PET estimate.

oxyhemoglobin dissociation curve. Although the overall relationship between oxygen content and PO_2 is sigmoid (see Fig. 6-3), it is approximately linear along the steep portion of the curve, over the range of CaO_2 and PO_2 values that are characteristic of moderate to severe hypoxic hypoxia. Moreover, arterial, venous, and tissue PO_2 values are relatively close to one another during hypoxic hypoxia, because all lie on the steep portion of the oxyhemoglobin dissociation curve. Thus, CaO_2 is not a bad "assay" for tissue PO_2 during hypoxic hypoxia in the sense that: (1) the two are linearly related, and (2) CaO_2 can be measured with a high degree of accuracy. Consideration of the connection between CaO_2 and CBF as an indirect one in no way diminishes the importance of the maintenance of OT. It simply makes all the more interesting the mechanism by which this is accomplished.

The Oxyhemoglobin Dissociation Curve and CBF

In the preceding discussion, reference was made to the importance of the sigmoid shape of the oxyhemoglobin dissociation curve in an understanding of the effects of hypoxic hypoxia. We will now consider the effects of changes in oxyhemoglobin affinity on CBF. These studies are particularly pertinent to an understanding of perinatal changes in CBF because of the marked change in oxyhemoglobin affinity that occurs just after birth in humans and other mammals.[26,27] Moreover, studies of the effects of shifts in the oxyhemoglobin dissociation curve provide convincing evidence of the importance of cerebral tissue PO_2 to the regulation of CBF under both normoxic and hypoxic conditions.

Changing the position of the oxyhemoglobin dissociation curve for cerebral blood has been shown to alter CBF in fetal, newborn, and adult animals,[28–31] and in adult humans.[32] Wade et al. measured unexpectedly high CBF values in adult men with a high-affinity hemoglobin variant.[32] The mean P_{50} (the PO_2 at which oxyhemoglobin is 50 percent saturated with oxygen) in the study group was 13 mmHg, as compared with 28 mmHg in normal controls, and their CBF was almost twice the control value. The higher CBF could be tentatively interpreted as compensation for decreased oxygen availability. This interpretation is confirmed by experiments in a perfused brain preparation in which CBF was held constant as P_{50} was decreased from 30 to 18 mmHg.[33] The EEG deteriorated within 60 seconds of introducing high-affinity blood, and the $CMRO_2$ fell by 25 percent. The latter study documents a decrease in oxygen availability within the brain, and by implication demonstrates the importance of the increase in CBF.

The human newborn has, in a manner of speaking, a high-affinity hemoglobin variant. The majority of its hemoglobin is still fetal hemoglobin.[26] A prime determinant of oxygen affinity in the adult red cell is the concentration of 2,3-diphosphoglycerate (2,3-DPG),[34] but fetal hemoglobin is relatively unaffected by 2,3-DPG, and since 2,3-DPG lowers oxygen affinity, the affinity of fetal hemoglobin for oxygen is increased.[27] As a result, P_{50} changes from 19 mmHg on the first day of life, when fetal hemoglobin levels are high, to 27 mmHg at 3 months of age, when fetal hemoglobin is virtually absent.[26]

We have studied the effects of alterations in oxyhemoglobin affinity using two models: fetal and newborn sheep transfused with adult sheep red cells,[28–30] and both adult and newborn sheep exposed to carbon monoxide.[28,35] The fetal sheep near term has a P_{50} of approximately 18 mmHg.[36] The adult animal with type B hemoglobin has a P_{50} over 40 mmHg.[37] The large difference between fetus and adult make the sheep an ideal model for these studies.

P_{50} Alterations by Exchange Transfusion

Changes in oxyhemoglobin affinity have marked effects in fetal sheep. Under ordinary circumstances, fetal CBF is much higher than in adult sheep at the same CaO_2.[38] Indeed, OT in the fetus exceeds that in the adult by over 60 percent. The increase in OT is not due to a high fetal $CMRO_2$. In fact, fetal and adult $CMRO_2$ values are approximately equivalent.[38] Thus, E in fetal sheep ranges from 0.30 to 0.40, whereas adult values are between 0.50 and 0.60. When we increased the P_{50} from 17 to 30 mmHg in fetal sheep by performing an in utero exchange transfusion with adult blood, E rose from 0.30 to 0.50 (Fig. 6-4).[38] There was no alteration in $CMRO_2$; the rise in E was due to a 45 percent fall in OT.

This study demonstrates that (1) The high CBF in fetuses is not the result of a unique cerebrovascular physiology. If oxyhemoglobin affinity is the same in fetus and adult, they will have similar relationships among CaO_2, CBF, and $CMRO_2$, as indicated by the finding that fetal values of E after exchange transfusion were similar to the adult. (2) A shift of oxyhemoglobin affinity over the range occurring normally in humans has pronounced effects on the oxygen economy of the brain.

These experiments are interesting not only because of their implications for

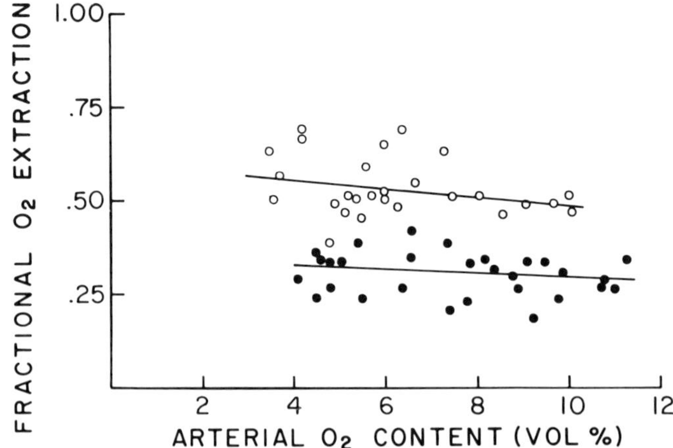

Fig. 6-4. The effect of increasing the P_{50} on cerebral fractional oxygen extraction during acute hypoxic hypoxia in fetal sheep. The increased P_{50} is accompanied by a parallel downward shift in the response. ● = low P_{50}; ○ = high P_{50}. (Data from Rosenberg AA, Harris AP, Koehler RC, et al: Role of O_2-hemoglobin affinity in the regulation of cerebral blood flow in fetal sheep. Am J Physiol 251 [Heart Circ Physiol 25]: HSG, 1986.)

understanding developmental differences in CBF. The effect of shifts in oxyhemoglobin affinity offers an interesting perspective on the mechanisms by which changes in oxygenation regulate the cerebral circulation. Specifically, a shift in the dissociation curve does not alter arterial PO_2 in well-oxygenated subjects, but as blood enters arterioles and oxygen is removed from hemoglobin, the PO_2 within the vessel is changed in proportion to the shift in the P_{50}. Thus, as blood moves from large arteries into the arterioles and capillaries, the PO_2 at the more distal sites will depend on the P_{50} (see below). Alterations in oxyhemoglobin affinity therefore provide a means of separating the effects on CBF of arterial from arteriolar and (or) "tissue" PO_2. Studies in the fetus are not completely successful in this regard because, due to the properties of the placental circulation, fetal arterial PO_2 and P_{50} vary directly.[29] As a result, fetal arterial PO_2 was somewhat higher after the exchange transfusion. Studies in lambs, on the other hand, show unequivocally that a decrease in oxyhemoglobin affinity can alter CBF in the absence of any alteration in arterial PO_2. When well-oxygenated lambs are exchange-transfused with adult blood such that their P_{50} is increased from 26 to 37 mmHg, their CBF falls by 22 percent.[30] As a result, their OT falls by a similar amount. Since, once again, $CMRO_2$ is unaltered, E increases proportionally.

These experiments have a number of implications for our understanding of the effects of oxygen on CBF, but first we should reconsider in more detail the influence of a shift in P_{50} on the tissue PO_2. At saturations between 20 and 80 percent, the oxyhemoglobin dissociation curve is accurately described by the Hill equation[39]:

$$PO_2 = P_{50} [SO_2/(100 - SO_2)] \exp 1/n,$$

in which SO_2 is oxyhemoglobin saturation and n is a constant. This equation quantifies the relationship between PO_2 and P_{50} for oxyhemoglobin saturations from 20 to 80 percent, coincidentally over the range of moderate to severe hypoxic hypoxia. It is apparent by inspection that PO_2 will be altered in direct proportion to any alteration in P_{50}. This means that as the intravascular oxyhemoglobin saturation falls below 80 percent, PO_2 will be changed in the same proportion as P_{50}. Cerebral venous PO_2, which presumably reflects the lowest microvascular PO_2 the brain parenchyma sees, will change in the same proportion as the higher PO_2 values in arterioles and capillaries as long as all oxyhemoglobin saturations lie between 20 and 80 percent. With this in mind, we will discuss the implications of the exchange-transfusion experiments for our understanding of CBF responses to hypoxic hypoxia.

First of all, the decrease in CBF in normoxic lambs demonstrates that oxygen exerts a tonic effect on cerebrovascular resistance even when arterial PO_2 is in the normal range. This is compelling evidence against the existence of an oxygen "threshold" (see above).[28]

Second, the magnitude of the fall in CBF shows something of the brain's strategy in coping with changing oxygen availability. The cerebrovascular bed might respond to the increased P_{50} in one of two ways. It might not respond at all, in the sense that CBF could remain constant. In that case, tissue PO_2 would rise in exactly the same proportion as the P_{50}. Alternatively it might decrease CBF to the point at which tissue PO_2 would remain constant. In that case CBF would have to decrease dramatically in experiments such as these in which P_{50} is altered by 40 percent. In fact, the brain selects the middle ground, in the sense that tissue PO_2 (at least to the extent that it is reflected by cerebral venous PO_2) rises, and CBF falls. To be more precise, because of the fall in CBF, the cerebral venous PO_2 in our study rose by just half the amount predicted by the increase in P_{50} (Fig. 6-5).

Third, this particular study showed not only that CBF was changed during normoxia, but that it was also altered during hypoxic hypoxia. Moreover, CBF during hypoxic hypoxia was lowered in exact proportion to the fall in normoxia. Proportionate alterations in CBF all along the hypoxic response curve mean a similarly proportionate change in the slope of that curve (i.e., in the hypoxic response itself). This result is interesting because the hypoxic response could easily be regarded as a fixed property of the cerebral vessels; however, the hypoxic response can apparently quickly adapt to a new baseline state of oxygen availability.

Fourth, and a corollary to the above, a proportional change in the hypoxic response means that OT is equally well maintained at each P_{50}. The fall in CBF after exchange transfusion means an equal fall in OT. However, the new, lower OT was maintained as well as the original OT. In regard to this last point, we have recently shown that this change in cerebrovascular responsivity is not simply the result of the change in CBF itself. In separate experiments, we raised CBF and OT with hypercapnia until both were twice the control values. However, the hypoxic response was not proportionally increased, as one would expect if the baseline CBF value itself determined hypoxic responsivity. It was in fact identical to the control value.[40]

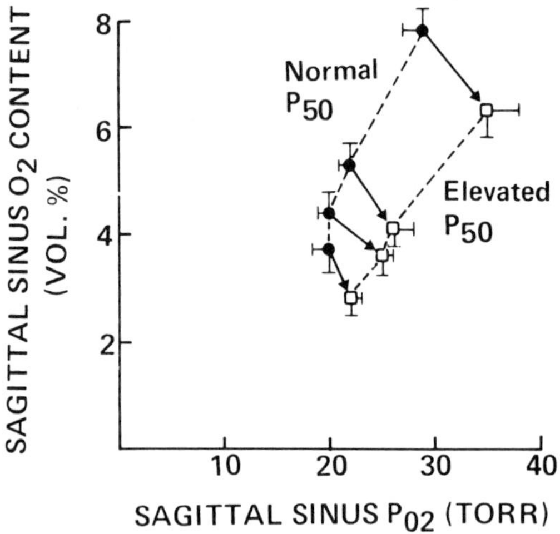

Fig. 6-5. Paired values for O_2 content and PO_2 in sagittal sinus blood during hypoxic hypoxia in lambs. The arrows connect points that share the same arterial O_2 contents before and after an increase in P_{50}. If CBF had remained constant, the arrow would have been horizontal, since the arteriovenous difference of O_2 content would not have changed; if the venous PO_2 had been constant, the arrow would have been vertical. The observed response includes both and increase in venous PO_2 and a fall in CBF, the latter causing a fall in venous O_2 content. (Koehler RC, Traystman RJ, Jones MD Jr: Influence of reduced oxyhemoglobin affinity on cerebrovascular response to hypoxic hypoxia. Am J Physiol 251 [Heart Circ Physiol 20]: H756, 1986.)

P_{50} Alterations by Carbon Monoxide

Whereas exchange transfusion experiments shift the oxyhemoglobin dissociation curve to the right and therefore decrease oxyhemoglobin affinity, carbon monoxide exposure causes a leftward shift and increased affinity. An increase in affinity with carbon monoxide occurs because as each of the four oxygen binding sites on hemoglobin are occupied by a molecule of carbon monoxide, the affinity of the remaining sites for oxygen increases.[41] Thus, as Haldane pointed out 75 years ago, carbon monoxide has a dual effect on oxygen availability: it decreases CaO_2 and decreases P_{50}.[42]

By comparing the CBF with and without carbon monoxide exposure at the same CaO_2, the effect of the change in P_{50} can be identified. We have completed such experiments in both lambs and adult sheep.[35] They show that CBF at the same CaO_2 is increased in direct proportion to the decrease in P_{50}. Moderate levels of carbon monoxide have no effect on $CMRO_2$; thus, E falls as the carboxyhemoglobin level rises. The experiments in adult sheep gave identical results. We used a combined approach to show that the increased OT is due primarily to the influence of a change in oxyhemoglobin affinity.[28] We measured CBF and $CMRO_2$ in lambs before and after an exchange transfusion with adult blood. The P_{50} was increased by 10 mmHg after the transfusion and, as expected, CBF fell and E rose. We then exposed the animals to carbon monoxide to the extent that P_{50} fell to the original control value. We found that OT and E also returned to their original value. These experiments show that the difference between hypoxic and carbon monoxide hypoxia may be attributed to the difference in oxyhemoglobin affinity.

P_{50} Alterations: A Synthesis

As a final note, it is of interest to compare the effects of increasing P_{50} by exchange transfusion in fetuses and lambs with the effects of decreasing P_{50} with carbon monoxide. Although precise quantitative comparisons are not justified, the effects are qualitatively the same[30]: When CaO_2 and $CMRO_2$ are held constant, an increase in P_{50} decreases CBF, while a decrease in P_{50} has the opposite effect.

The data also show that for the same alteration in cerebral venous PO_2, the consequences of a shift in P_{50} are the same as the consequences of hypoxic hypoxia.[30] In other words, an alteration in cerebral venous PO_2 after the exchange transfusion has the same effect on CBF/$CMRO_2$ as an equivalent change produced by a fall in arterial PO_2 (Fig. 6-6). Under these circumstances, arterial PO_2 itself is clearly irrelevant to the control of CBF. The data further imply that the so-called mean tissue PO_2 is probably not the PO_2 that controls cerebrovascular resistance. Since arterial PO_2 is normal in carbon monoxide hypoxia, the mean tissue PO_2 should be considerably higher than with hypoxic hypoxia. Yet CBF is higher, not lower, in CO hypoxia. Similarly, the effect of a given change in cerebral venous PO_2 secondary to altering P_{50} is indistinguishable from the effect of the same change in venous PO_2 secondary to altering arterial PO_2, yet the mean tissue PO_2 values in these two situations should be different: the cerebral venous PO_2 values are the same at very different levels of arterial PO_2. Taken together, these data imply that cerebrovascular resistance is regulated by the minimum rather than the mean tissue PO_2.

The basic similarity of the response of the cerebrovascular beds in fetal, newborn, and adult sheep to hypoxic hypoxia can be seen by plotting CBF/$CMRO_2$ for all three groups on the same axis. A plot of CBF/$CMRO_2$ against CaO_2 in fetal,

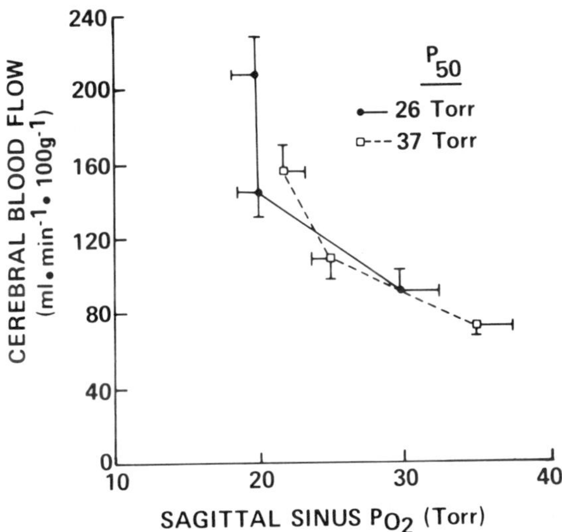

Fig. 6-6. The relationship between sagittal sinus PO_2 and cerebral blood flow in lambs during acute hypoxic hypoxia studied at low and high P_{50}. The change induced by hypoxic hypoxia is equivalent to that induced by the shift in P_{50}. (Koehler RC, Traystman RJ, Jones MD Jr: Influence of reduced oxyhemoglobin affinity on cerebrovascular response to hypoxic hypoxia. Am J Physiol 251 [Heart Circ Physiol 20]: H75, 1986.)

newborn, and adult sheep describes roughly a single function (Fig. 6-7A), but with a lot of variability.[29,30] If the same animals are studied after exchange transfusion has brought the fetal and lamb P_{50} closer to adults, the correlation is vastly improved (Fig. 6-7B).

Anemic Hypoxia

This section is entitled "anemic hypoxia," with the *caveat* that the response of CBF to changes in hemotocrit, like the response to changes in PO_2, should be considered as a continuous function, beginning at high hematocrits and extending down over a wide range of values. If the response is thought of in this way, the designation "anemic hypoxia" is somewhat arbitrary. However, since the literature typically divides aberrations of hemoglobin and hematocrit into either anemia or polycythemia, we will follow that convention.

The remarkable thing about the curve describing the response of CBF to changes in CaO_2 during anemic hypoxia is that it is superimposable on the curve during hypoxic hypoxia.[7] This is not surprising if one postulates a chemoreceptor that senses changes in CaO_2, but as was just discussed, the evidence for such a receptor (except, one might say, for the striking correspondence between these two response curves) is lacking. Since the response curves to anemic and hypoxic hypoxia are identical, the properties of the responses, insofar as maintenance of OT and E, are also the same. That these properties extend into the polycythemic range has been demonstrated in both humans and animals.[43–45] This is the reason for the above statement that the CBF response to a change in hematocrit should be considered as a single function extending over a wide range of values.

There are obviously limits to the brain's ability to maintain OT when hemotocrit changes. If anemia is severe enough, OT will fall[45] just as it does during hypoxic hypoxia. There are insufficient data to determine whether this happens at roughly comparable levels of CaO_2. If polycythemia is severe enough, OT will also fall.[45] In the latter instance, the most likely reason for the fall, although other factors may contribute to it, is increased blood viscosity.

The similarity in the CBF response to anemic and hypoxic hypoxia is intriguing. Just what the correspondence means is not clear, but it does not imply an equivalent degree of tissue hypoxia as measured by either cerebral venous PO_2 or tissue levels of lactate and high energy phosphates. Studies of anemia have been unable to correlate the rise in CBF with a fall in cerebral venous PO_2.[46,47] This is in contrast to well-documented decreases in PO_2 in subcutaneous tissue and in the peritoneum in anemia,[48,49] and it is worth considering how tissue hypoxia might contribute to the increase in spite of a normal venous PO_2.

One explanation is that cerebral venous PO_2 is an ambiguous indicator of cerebral oxygenation.[50] It is possible that anemia alters the microvascular distribution of red cells in a way that causes patchy tissue hypoxia. This would not necessarily be reflected in mixed cerebral venous blood because mixed venous blood would represent the hypoxic areas along with areas that receive a relative excess of red cells. In support of possible maldistribution of red cells during anemia are in vitro studies showing that red cells are not always distributed equally at microvascular bifurcations.[51] Specifically, the red cell flux to a daughter branch is not linearly dependent on the flow into that branch. The result is that the red cell fraction

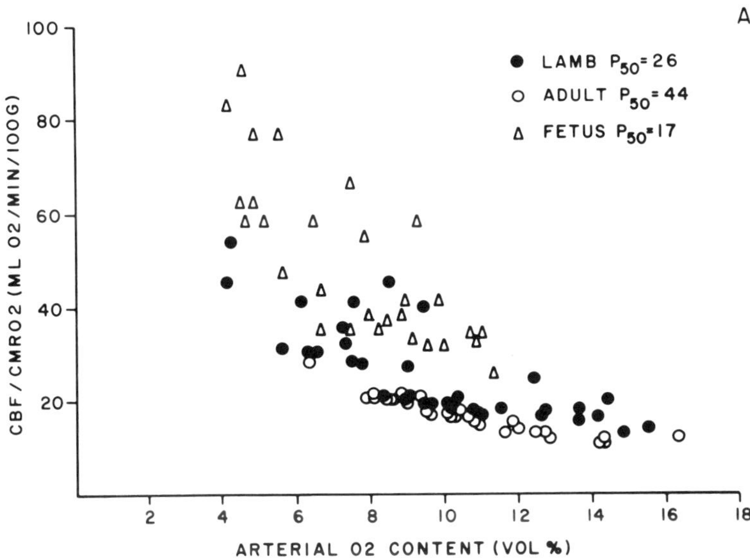

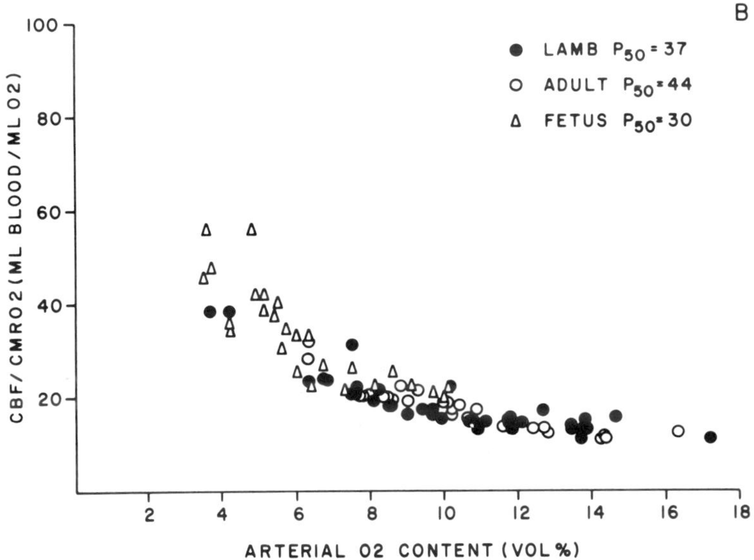

Fig. 6-7. Relationship between arterial O_2 content and $CBF/CMRO_2$ in fetal, newborn, and adult sheep studied during acute hypoxic hypoxia. The data represent pooled data from the studies of Rosenberg et al.[29] in fetal sheep before (**A**) and after (**B**) exchange transfusion with adult blood, from Koehler et al.[30] in lambs treated in the same manner (**A** and **B**, respectively), and from Koehler and co-workers[35] in adult sheep. The data in **B** approximate a single function because all subjects are studied at approximately the same P_{50}.

falls more rapidly than the flow fraction; at low flow rates the flow to a daughter branch may be made up of plasma alone. This represents a variety of "plasma skimming," and would tend to distribute red cells away from lower flow bifurcations and lead to an overall picture of uneven oxygen availability.[52] This tendency is markedly accentuated as the hematocrit falls.[51] It is also important to mention that increased heterogeneity of red cell distribution during anemia has not been documented in vivo.

Against the hypothesis that tissue oxygen availability plays a role, at least over much of the hematocrit range, are the findings of Johannsson and Siesjo.[53] An analysis of cerebral tissue metabolites showed no evidence of hypoxia unless hematocrit values were on the order of 10 percent. Enormous changes in CBF thus occurred without biochemical evidence of tissue hypoxia. It is possible that, because of a patchy nature of tissue hypoxia in anemia, metabolites in whole brain will give the appearance of normality when some microregions are actually hypoxic. This is highly speculative, however, and at this point it must be admitted that except during severe anemia, any influence of hematocrit on tissue oxygenation is hypothetical.

Viscosity and CBF

The arterial oxygen content, CaO_2, is of course only one of the variables that change with hematocrit. The other is blood viscosity. Studies in which the influence of viscosity has been measured directly are few, and the results are conflicting. There is general agreement that alterations in plasma viscosity, unless extreme, have little influence on CBF.[54–56] However, it is difficult to know what this means for changes in hematocrit. Although plasma viscosity is a component of whole-blood viscosity, it is by no means clear that for the same change in whole-blood viscosity, changes in plasma and red cell viscosity have equivalent physiologic consequences. Few studies have directly measured the effect of an isolated increase in red cell viscosity. One study concluded that red cell viscosity has no influence on CBF during polycythemia.[57] The investigators dissociated CaO_2 from hematocrit by using an infusion of sodium nitrite to convert oxyhemoglobin to methemoglobin. This lowers CaO_2 by rendering useless a portion of the hemoglobin binding sites for oxygen[39] while leaving the hematocrit unchanged. The relationship between CaO_2 and CBF was unaffected by this procedure, and the investigators inferred that red cell viscosity made no independent contribution to the decrease in CBF. However, their conclusion must be regarded as tentative, because methemoglobin produced in this manner is associated with increased oxyhemoglobin affinity.[39] The mechanism of the increase is presumably analogous to that occurring with carbon monoxide exposure. Thus, while the investigators were looking for a depressive effect of blood viscosity, the CBF was probably being simultaneously elevated by increased oxyhemoglobin affinity.

Methemoglobin can be produced in vitro in a way that inactivates all hemoglobin-oxygen binding sites with no alteration in oxygen affinity.[58] Using this approach, Hudak et al.[59] and Massik et al.[44] dissociated the effects of hematocrit and CaO_2 over the hematocrit ranges of 20 to 40 percent and 32 to 55 percent, respectively. In both instances, approximately half of the change in blood flow could be attributed to the change in hematocrit alone (Fig. 6-8).

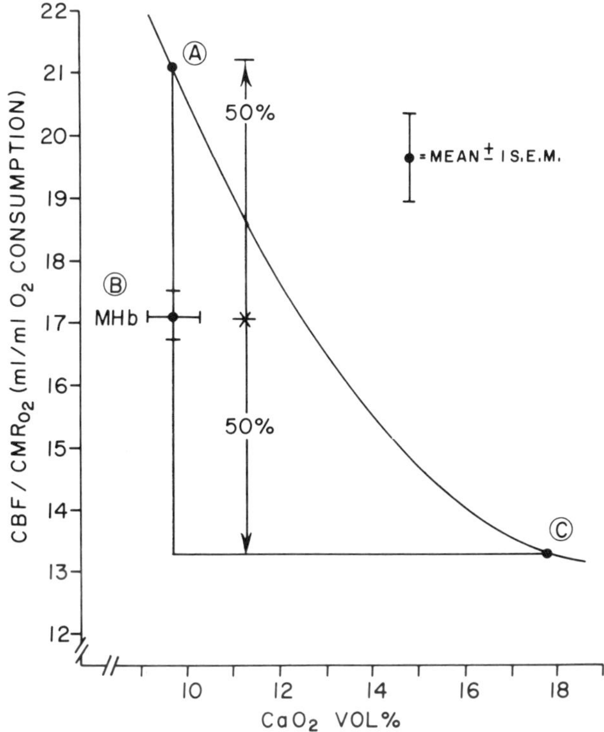

Fig. 6-8. The effect on cerebral blood flow corrected for O_2 consumption ($CBF/CMRO_2$) of increasing hematocrit without increasing arterial O_2 content (CaO_2) in lambs. The vertical distance between A and C represents the fall in $CBF/CMRO_2$ caused by a combined increase in hematocrit and CaO_2. The distance A–B represents the fall induced by increasing the hematocrit at constant CaO_2 using methemoglobin-containing red blood cells; it represents approximately 50 percent of the total.

In summary, when hematocrit changes, CBF is inversely related to CaO_2 by a function that is virtually identical to the one that applies when PO_2 changes. Changes in red cell viscosity account for a portion of the change in CBF. Mechanisms responsible for the remainder are obscure, and the reasons, if any, for the striking homology between the CBF responses to anemic and hypoxic hypoxia are unknown.

Blood Pressure and the Cerebral Circulation

The response of the cerebral circulation to changes in blood pressure will be discussed at this point because there is good evidence that one of the mechanisms that regulates cerebral vascular resistance when the blood pressure changes is very similar, if not identical, to the mechanism that regulates cerebral oxygen delivery during hypoxic hypoxia.[24] Before proceeding, it should be mentioned that the discussion applies generally to changes in perfusion pressure. An increase in intracranial pressure or cerebral venous pressure has the same physical effect on CBF as lowering the blood-pressure, and appears to provoke generally the same response from cerebral vessels.[60,61]

The term used to describe the tendency of cerebral blood flow to remain constant despite changes in cerebral perfusion pressure is "autoregulation."[62] This refers to reciprocal changes in cerebral vascular resistance that accompany changes in perfusion pressure and have the result of maintaining constant flow within an "autoregulatory range." The autoregulatory range is limited at both its low[63,64] and high[65,66] extremes; beyond these limits, CBF is the passive result of changes in perfusion pressure.

As mentioned, autoregulatory changes in vascular resistance appear to arise in part from the tissue hypoxia (or hyperoxia) that accompanies an initial, uncompensated change in perfusion pressure.[24] This has been referred to as the metabolic mechanism of autoregulation, because the elaboration of a hypothetical vasoactive compound would depend on the relation between oxygen supply and tissue metabolism. Other mechanisms that may be important are "myogenic" changes in vascular tone[62] and, perhaps, a local reflex arc that responds to local mechanoreceptors.[67]

Of the latter two, the myogenic mechanism is by far the best studied. In vitro, vascular tone changes in response to alterations in transmural pressure.[68] Since this property necessarily resides in the vessel itself, it has been called a myogenic response. From an overall perspective, myogenic changes in arteriolar tone may be seen as one mechanism maintaining constant capillary pressure and thus constant tissue fluid volume.[68] When increases in venous pressure increase the transmural pressure of the capillaries and small arterioles, the arterioles constrict in order to avoid a potentially massive capillary filtration of fluid. The opposite effect would apply when venous pressure falls. Moreover, a myogenic response in pre-capillary vessels would prevent the transmission of potentially damaging surges of pressure to capillaries and venules, and at the same time protect the tissue from ischemia if the perfusion pressure suddenly falls. Although myogenic responses are well documented in vessels from a variety of sites in vitro and in skeletal muscle vessels in vivo,[68] their importance in the brain is not clear.[62,64,69–71] The most attractive hypothesis is that both myogenic and metabolic mechanisms operate, but that their relative importance changes with the situation.[71] This parallels the situation in skeletal muscle, as described by Morff and Granger.[72] These investigators used elevation of venous pressure as a convenient way to separate metabolic and myogenic regulation of vascular resistance. Elevation of venous pressure will decrease blood flow. If a metabolic mechanism predominates, arterioles will dilate; if a myogenic mechanism prevails, the increased transmural pressure will cause arteriolar constriction. Morff and Granger found that elevation of venous pressure provoked myogenic constriction, but that the intensity varied with the state of tissue oxygenation. It was most apparent when tissue oxygenation was excellent (i.e., when any metabolic mechanism was suppressed). The brain extracts approximately 50 percent of the oxygen available to it, and by comparison to many other tissues is relatively poorly oxygenated.[11] Wei and Kontos found that under ordinary circumstances, increases in venous pressure provoked dilation of pial arterioles, demonstrating a predominantly metabolic mechanism[69]; but when the brain was locally hyperoxygenated by superfusion with an oxygen-saturated fluorocarbon solution, they were able to identify myogenic arteriolar constriction.[71]

Autoregulation is obviously a fundamentally important mechanism, and it is somewhat surprising that it is rather easily disturbed. For instance, relatively mild trauma[73] or relatively brief asphyxial episodes[74] may attenuate or even abolish autoregulation. This will be discussed in detail in connection with data on fetal and newborn subjects.

Sufficiency of CBF: A Definition

Since the above discussion of cerebrovascular responses makes repeated references to tissue oxygen sufficiency as a regulator of CBF, it should be clear, as was said at the beginning of the foregoing section, that a particular level of CBF can be evaluated only in relation to the oxygen status of the brain. A principal determinant of oxygen status is the rate at which oxygen is consumed. A good example is the subject in which $CMRO_2$ is suppressed by pentobarbital coma.[75] The CBF is approximately half that in awake subjects, yet, since $CMRO_2$ is also depressed by half, E is unchanged. Similarly, although the hypoxic and autoregulatory responses are half those found in awake animals when considered in absolute terms, they are appropriate to the new $CMRO_2$. The hypoxic response still maintains OT, albeit at the lower level typical of coma, and autoregulation, defined as the maintenance of the lower baseline CBF, is no less effective than when the animal is awake.

The best index of impending insufficiency of CBF is a rise in E.[3]

ACID–BASE DISORDERS: CARBON DIOXIDE AND CBF

In this section we will discuss the effect of changes in acid-base balance on CBF. The consequences of a change in arterial PCO_2 will be discussed at the same time, since CO_2 acts on cerebral arterioles by changing perivascular pH.

Carbon dioxide is a particularly potent regulator of CBF in well-oxygenated subjects whose blood pressure is within the autoregulatory range and whose hematocrit is normal[62,76] (i.e., in normal subjects at sea level). The mechanism by which CO_2 dilates cerebral vessels is, by comparison to the mechanisms of hypoxia and autoregulation, well understood. Cerebral arteries and arterioles are quite sensitive to changes in the pH of interstitial fluid,[77] and since changes in PCO_2 result in prompt changes in interstitial fluid pH, PCO_2 is an important determinant of cerebral vascular tone. Several groups have shown that the important element in governing this tone is the alteration in pH and not the change in PCO_2 itself.[77–79]

It should be emphasized that cerebral blood vessels are sensitive to periarteriolar pH, but not to blood pH except as it effects the pH of interstitial fluid. For example, acute metabolic acidosis or alkalosis have little effect on CBF because, unlike CO_2, bicarbonate equilibrates only slowly across the blood-brain barrier.[80,81] Therefore, CBF is altered only if the disorder is prolonged enough to produce a change in CSF pH,[82] or if respiratory compensation results in a change in arterial PCO_2. Small changes in CBF during metabolic acid-base disorders are probably the result of changes in oxyhemoglobin affinity mediated by the Bohr effect.[39] For example, an increased CBF when metabolic alkalosis is superimposed on already severe respiratory alkalosis[83] has been attributed to the increase in oxyhemoglobin affinity.[84] Because of its particular importance to clinical management, we should mention one other situation in which an acute alteration in extracellular pH can alter CBF. Arvidsson and co-workers found that the administration of large amounts of sodium bicarbonate to hypercapneic animals was associated with an acute decrease in CBF. They hypothesized that hypercapnia and the hyperosmolality of the bicarbonate solution disrupted the blood-brain barrier and exposed cerebral resistance vessels directly to the alkaline intravascular pH.[85]

The consequences of chronic disorders of acid-base balance are considerably more complicated, but will be mentioned because of their importance for patient management. There is no question that the pH of CSF varies much less than the systemic pH in chronic metabolic acidosis and alkalosis (see Siesjo[86]). The mechanism for the compensation is not clear,[86–88] but whatever the mechanism, changes in the CSF bicarbonate content minimize alterations in CSF pH.[87] This means that therapeutic intervention to "normalize" the PCO_2 may have undesirable consequences for CBF. Oliva described a patient with severe chronic metabolic acidosis that was partially compensated by carbon dioxide retention (arterial pH = 7.50; arterial PCO_2 = 75 mmHg).[89] The patient developed seizures when voluntary hyperventilation reduced the arterial PCO_2 to 28 mmHg. Despite a markedly elevated PCO_2, this patient very probably had a normal CBF associated with a baseline CSF pH that was measured at 7.41. Hyperventilation lowered the CBF enough to result in tissue hypoxia and seizures, a situation that may have been aggravated by a Bohr shift-mediated increase in oxyhemoglobin affinity. Although patients with especially severe hypercapnia on the basis of severe chronic lung disease may have persistently low CSF pH values, possibly because coexisting tissue hypoxia and impaired myocardial function increase hydrogen ion production by brain tissue,[86,87] the CSF pH and CBF in patients with less severe lung disease (PCO_2 below 55 to 60 mmHg) are in the normal range,[90,91] and forced ventilation to a "normal" PCO_2 will result in a pronounced decline in CBF[91] and deterioration in mental status (see below).

For completeness, two other influences on the responsivity of cerebral vessels to CO_2 should be mentioned. The first, $CMRO_2$, is well documented.[92,93] Grubb and colleagues have summarized data showing that carbon dioxide responsivity is a simple linear function of $CMRO_2$, at least when variations in $CMRO_2$ are the result of differences among species or depression by anesthetic agents.[93] Clearly, one must consider $CMRO_2$ before carbon dioxide responsivity can be evaluated.

The other influence is more controversial, and its overall importance remains to be established. It will be mentioned both because it was recently received a good deal of attention, and because it involves a drug that is frequently used in neonatal intensive care, albeit at lower doses than employed experimentally. A number of investigators have shown a dramatic reduction of CO_2 responsivity after pretreatment with indomethacin (see Busija and Heistad[94]). The effect of indomethacin is well established,[94–97] but the implications of this for the participation of prostaglandins in the carbon dioxide response are not. One reason is that the effect is not demonstrable in all species.[98,99] Another is that it is not seen with all inhibitors of prostaglandin synthetase.[100] This suggests that attenuation of the CO_2 response is due to properties of indomethacin other than its inhibition of prostaglandin synthesis.

CARBON DIOXIDE: INTERACTIONS WITH HYPOXIA AND AUTOREGULATION

The effects of simultaneous hypercapnia and hypoxia have not been studied in detail, but the data on both phenomena point to additive rather than interactive effects. In other words, hypercapnia does not appear to enhance the response to hypoxic hypoxia.[40,101] An additive effect is odd in the context of a mechanism of hypoxic vasodilation that depends on a vasoactive compound whose concentration is proportional to tissue oxygenation (see above). One would expect, since hypercapnia elevates tissue PO_2,[50] that the hypoxic response would be diminished; conversely, hypocapnia should enhance the response. Yet neither appears to occur.[40,102] Indeed, hypocapnia hastens the onset of EEG changes and neurologic symptoms with hypoxic hypoxia.[103] Moreover, it has been clear for many years that autoregulatory vasodilation is not maximal even at the lower limit of the autoregulatory range, when CBF begins to fall[104,105]; a further decrease in vascular resistance can be achieved by elevating the PCO_2.[105] The level of PCO_2 appears to delimit the decrease in vascular tone in a way that the vessels are powerless to overcome. An explanation of this paradox would undoubtedly throw considerable light on the mechanisms of hypoxic and autoregulatory vasodilation.

Hypocapnic Hypoxic Hypoxia

The combination of hypocapnia and hypoxia requires special attention because of its relevance to the use of sustained hyperventilation in the management of infants with persistent pulmonary hypertension.[106] Evidence for tissue hypoxia based on the direct measurement of brain metabolites in hypocapnic animals is necessarily somewhat equivocal, because of the direct effects of carbon dioxide on cellular carbohydrate metabolism (see Siesjo[87]). Hypocapnia stimulates and hypercapnia inhibits the production of lactate. Since lactate accumulation is a sign of tissue hypoxia, it cannot be absolutely clear whether increased brain lactate during hypocapnia is the result of a direct metabolic effect or of tissue hypoxia. However, in addition to the increase in tissue lactate, extreme hyperventilation (PCO_2 = 10 mmHg) causes subtle deterioration of the cellular energy state.[107] The combination of hypoxic hypoxia (PO_2 = 30 mmHg) and less severe hypocapnia (PCO_2 = 18 mmHg) does the same.[108] The significance of these rather minor changes is unclear, and it is still true, as it was in 1974, that the interpretation of the metabolic data "in terms of tissue survival must await direct functional and histological assessment."[108] A recent study of the effects of hyperventilation in puppies[109] has not further clarified this problem.

Although these metabolic data during hypocapnic hypoxia are somewhat reassuring in that severe derangements in high energy phosphates were not found, the possibility of damage from combined hypoxia and hypocapnic cannot be dismissed. One reason for not dismissing the possibility of damage is that if anemic hypoxia is severe enough (hematocrit approximately 15), extreme hyperventilation (PCO_2 = 10 mmHg) causes a decline in $CMRO_2$,[110] although it must be admitted that any long term consequences of this are unknown. Second, as already mentioned, modest reductions in arterial PCO_2 in adults with chronic carbon dioxide retention can cause seizures and coma, and can be fatal if hyperventilation continues.[111,112] It is by no means clear whether one should compare mild hypocapnia in chronically hypercapneic patients with severe hypocapnia in normocapneic subjects, but the grim outcome in the former is sobering.

NEURAL INFLUENCES ON CBF

The overall importance of peripheral and central neurogenic mechanisms in the control of CBF has been vigorously debated for a number of years.[94,113] The circumstances under which neural influences assume importance in adult animals is only now becoming clear, and experiments that contrast adult with newborn or fetal animals are few. This important area will therefore not be covered at this time. We refer the reader to the excellent review of Busija and Heistad,[94] and to recent articles by Busija et al.[114] and Wagerle[115,116] and his co-workers.

CONTROL OF CBF IN THE FETUS AND NEWBORN

Studies in the fetus and newborn have been mentioned in the preceding sections, where they illustrate general principles of CBF regulation. In the following section we will review work that is of interest to those interested particularly in fetal and newborn subjects.

The Fetus and Newborn: $CMRO_2$, Hypoxia, and CBF

CBF and $CMRO_2$

In comparing different species, one is struck by the lack of correlation between brain development and the time of birth.[117] Some species, like rats, are extremely immature, whereas others, like ruminants, are capable of sophisticated CNS function within the first few hours of postnatal life. With this as a background, it is easy to see that it is difficult to differentiate between CNS characteristics that are simply manifestations of immaturity and those that are adaptations to the fetal environment. One question serves to illustrate this point: Does the apparent resistance of the newborn brain to hypoxic damage depend altogether on immaturity, or is it in part the result of persistent, although presumably disappearing, adaptations to the relative hypoxia of fetal life? There is at present no answer to this question. It is an important question, however, because until we understand the difference between immaturity and fetal adaptations, it will be difficult to understand the pathophysiology of perinatal brain damage.

Kennedy and co-workers were the first to make careful measurements of CBF using the same technique at different stages of brain development within the same species.[118] Their results in dogs correspond in a general way to early measurements of in vitro glucose utilization by the immature brain of the rat.[119,120] Two trends were evident in the dog: (1) There is a general increase in CBF over the first few weeks of life that peaks, depending on the specific brain region, between 20 and 60 days. After this, CBF declines toward adult values. Blood flow increases and peaks first in the brain stem and last in the cortex. Kennedy et al. speculate that the increased flow reflects increased metabolic activity, possibly associated with myelination. Part of the increase is due to the physiologic decrease in hemoglobin that occurs in the puppy, but anemia can account for only a portion of the overall increase, and can account not at all for temporal differences among regions. (2) Simultaneously, a relatively homogeneous regional flow pattern at birth progresses to the highly differentiated pattern of the adult. At birth the values in grey and white matter overlap. In the mature brain, blood flow is distinctly lower in white matter.

Differences in technique and experimental circumstances preclude detailed comparisons among studies, but data in humans and other species are consistent with the pattern established in the dog. Several groups have shown that values for CBF and $CMRO_2$ in normal children are higher than in adult humans,[121,122] and results in premature and full-term human infants and experimental animals are generally indicative of values lower than in adults.[123–128]

Hypoxic and anemic hypoxia

Maintenance of OT during hypoxic hypoxia is a property common to fetal sheep, and to newborns and adults of a variety of species including adult humans (see Jones and Traystman[8]).[129,130] Data in human newborns show that there is a qualitative decrease in CBF when the inspired oxygen content is raised.[131] Quantitative measurements of CBF in human newborns are not possible with most techniques currently available.[132] Anemic hypoxia has not been as well studied, but it appears that OT is maintained over a wide range of hematocrits in fetal sheep,[133] newborn sheep,[44,59] and adult humans.[8,134] Preliminary data in chronically anemic human newborns suggest that the CBF response may be only about half that necessary to sustain OT.[135]

The response to hypoxic hypoxia varies among regions of the fetal and newborn brain, with the brainstem showing the greatest increment in flow and white matter showing the least.[35,136–138] Response patterns have been compared directly in newborn and adult sheep.[139] In adult sheep the response to hypoxic hypoxia is equivalent in the forebrain, midbrain, and brainstem, but the newborn, like the fetus, shows a greater response in the brainstem than in the forebrain. The radioactive microsphere technique used in the sheep does not permit the degree of spatial resolution of the antipyrine technique,[118] but the pattern parallels that found with antipyrine in the puppy.[138]

The reason for regional differences in hypoxic responsivity of the brain is unclear. One possibility is that it reflects similar regional differences in baseline $CMRO_2$. This concept is supported by data in fetal sheep[137] showing that while the absolute responses are higher in brain stem than in cortical structures, the percentage increases are the same. This is what one would expect if OT in both regions were maintained at the level set by the regional $CMRO_2$. However, this does not hold for the puppy; in this animal the percentage brain stem response is threefold that in the cortex.[138] Moreover, areas in which the flow response was "excessive" in these latter studies were not those showing an increase in regional cerebral glucose uptake. Indeed, the overall correlation between increases in regional glucose uptake and blood flow was negative, with several white-matter areas showing fourfold increases in glucose uptake and little change in flow. A negative correlation between activation of glucose uptake and the percentage increase in blood flow raises the possibility, to which we will return later, of an anaerobic activation of glycolysis by insufficient oxygen availability. The increased response in the brain stem does not necessarily represent a hypoxic activation of brain stem respiratory centers, because regional differences in blood flow persist with carbon monoxide hypoxia,[35] and carbon monoxide hypoxia does not stimulate respiration.[139] On the other hand, the exaggerated response seen in caudal structures in the chronically hypoxic adult sheep is abolished by sinoaortic denervation.[16] Neubauer and Edelman reduced the relatively larger response in the medulla-pons of the adult cat by superior cervical ganglionectomy,[140] implying modulation by sympathetic tone. Lou et al. have recently raised the interesting possibility that opiate receptors mediate the increased brain stem response. In five anesthetized lambs they were able to abolish regional differences with naloxone.[141] As can be seen, the reason(s) for the caudal-to-rostral progression in the hypoxic response is unclear.

The Fetus and Newborn: Acid–Base and Carbon Dioxide Effects

Cerebral vascular responsivity to CO_2 is less in fetal and newborn animals than in adults.[127,142–144] In the puppy this has been attributed to its relatively low $CMRO_2$.[143] Studies by Rosenberg and co-workers, comparing fetal, newborn, and adult sheep, suggest that there is also be a real decrease in the sensitivity of immature cerebral vessels to CO_2. They found that the difference between fetal and newborn animals on the one hand and adults on the other persisted despite correction for variations in $CMRO_2$ (Fig. 6-9).[127] One study failed to find a significant effect of CO_2 in fetal sheep that were simultaneously severely hypoxic, some to the point of marked acidosis.[145] Although this may represent a true depression of CO_2 sensitivity, it more likely reflects the difficulty in identifying CO_2 effects in the face of enormous variability in CBF measurements along the steep portion of the hyperbolic hypoxic response curve.

It is interesting that regional differences in the response to CO_2 parallel those in hypoxic hypoxia. The adult may differ from the fetus and newborn in this regard.[127] In the fetal and newborn sheep the brain stem is more responsive to CO_2 than the forebrain as a whole,[127,146] whereas in the adult brain stem response is indistinguishable from that of the forebrain.[127] In one of these studies,[127] the white matter in both adult and newborn sheep was found to be less responsive than the caudate nucleus, the only pure grey matter structure measured in that particular study. Studying puppies, Shapiro et al. were able to achieve better spatial resolution with the antipyrine technique, and also found that white matter was less responsive than a number of grey matter structures, including the caudate.[144] Brain stem CO_2 responses have also been documented to be significantly higher than those of the forebrain in the piglet.[147]

There is no persuasive evidence that acute metabolic alkalosis or acidosis alters cerebral blood flow in newborn animals.[148,149] In two studies in which there was an acute change in CBF in the direction expected for a change in interstitial pH, it was difficult to be certain of the status of the blood-brain barrier. In one study, the subjects had been subjected to severe hypoxia,[150] and in the other, asphyxiated newborn infants were given a hyperosmolar injection of sodium bicarbonate.[151] The consequences of the latter in experimental animals[85] have been mentioned.

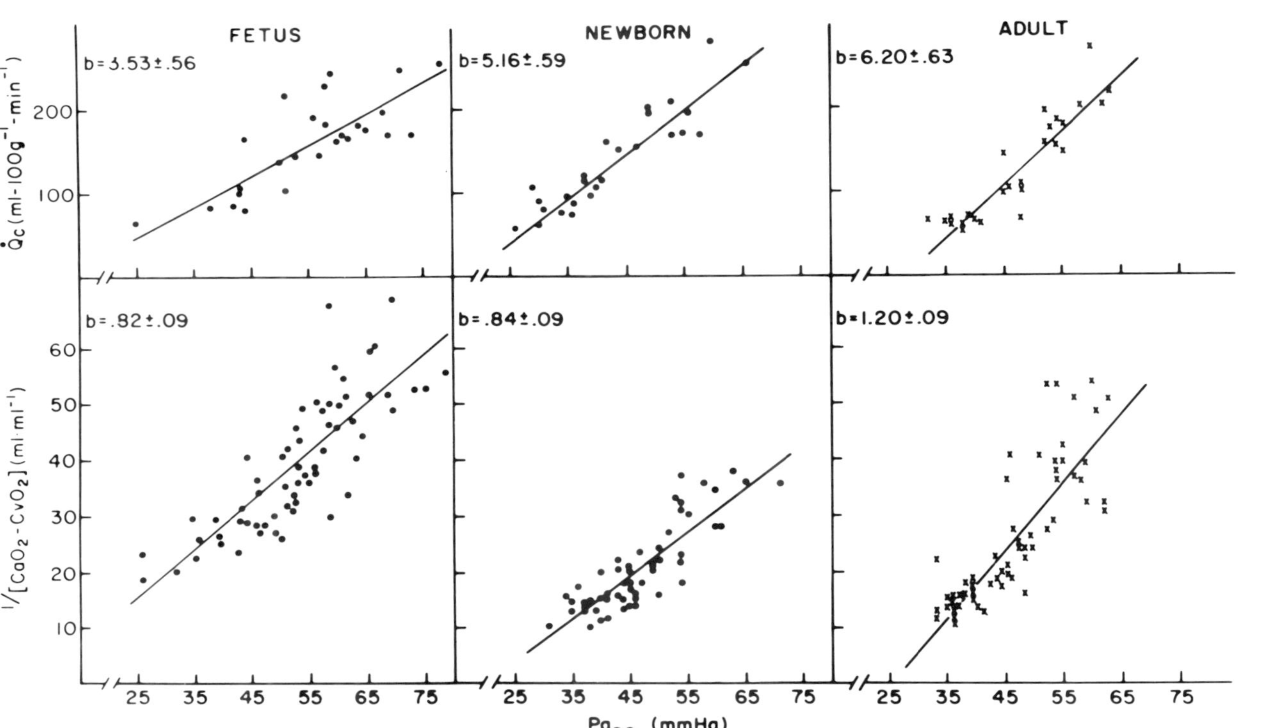

Fig. 6-9. The effect of varying arterial PCO_2 on cerebral blood flow (Q_C) and cerebral blood flow corrected for O_2 consumption ($1/[CaO_2 - CvO_2]$) in unanesthetized fetal, newborn, and adult sheep. b = regression coefficient. The difference between fetus and adult is significant ($P < 0.05$) even after correction for oxygen consumption. (Rosenberg AA, Jones MD Jr, Traystman J, et al: Response of cerebral blood flow to changes in PCO_2 in fetal, newborn, and adult sheep. Am J Physiol 242 [Heart Circ Physiol 11]: H862, 1982.)

The Fetus and Newborn: Autoregulation, Ischemia, and Intraventricular Hemorrhage

Autoregulation was first documented in fetal and newborn sheep by Purves and James.[152] It has since been confirmed in puppies,[130,148,153] in fetal sheep,[146,154–156] piglets,[157] and lambs.[75,158] The limits of autoregulation in immature animals differ from those in the adult in that both the high and lower limits of autoregulation are at lower pressures.[153,156] This is consistent with immature animals' lower baseline blood pressures.

There are important regional differences in the effectiveness of hypotensive autoregulation. Studying severely hypotensive piglets, Laptook et al. found that brain stem blood flow was better preserved than that in the forebrain.[157] Young and coworkers showed that white matter in puppies is particularly likely to exhibit a decrease in blood flow.[159] This confirms earlier preliminary work from the same group.[160] Ment et al. also showed that white matter was at particular risk in the hypotensive puppy,[161] and demonstrated increased glucose uptake in white matter, implying stimulation of glycolysis by tissue hypoxia. In view of the relatively great susceptibility of white matter to damage in the immature brain,[162] these data and those mentioned above, showing activation of glycolysis in white matter during pure hypoxic hypoxia,[138] are of particular interest.

As mentioned above, autoregulation may be disturbed with relative ease.[74] It is not surprising that severe hypercapnia (PCO_2 = 75 mmHg) impairs autoregulation,[63,64,163] or that the same occurs during severe hypoxic hypoxia (less than 40 percent arterial oxygen saturation)[105,163] or after profound asphyxia.[164] However, in lambs autoregulation is also transiently impaired by just 20 minutes of moderately severe normotensive hypoxia (arterial PO_2 = 30 mmHg).[74] It may also be impaired in newborn infants witth mild birth asphyxia.[125] Impairment of normal autoregulatory responses put the newborn infant at increased risk of ischemic injury, and perhaps of intraventricular hemorrhage as well.[165,166]

The Fetus and Newborn: Drugs and CBF

We have already mentioned sodium bicarbonate and its lack of effect in moderate doses on CBF. One other drug will be discussed briefly. The effects of indomethacin on resting CBF and the CO_2 response[94] have already been mentioned. Decreases in baseline CBF have been documented in fetal sheep[167] and newborn piglets given this drug.[168] Evidence of a similar phenomenon has recently been reported in human newborns receiving indomethacin to close a patent ductus arteriosus.[169] An effect in the CO_2 response has not been tested in newborn animals, but Leffler and colleagues documented that 5 mg/kg of intravenously administered indomethacin decreased CBF hyperemia during combined hypoxia and hypercapnia in the piglet.[168] They did not measure $CMRO_2$, however, and the meaning of the attenuated flow response is not clear.

SUMMARY

We have reviewed the regulation of cerebral blood flow in fetal, newborn, and adult animals. The fundamental principles that govern the cerebrovascular response to hypoxia, hyper- and hypocapnia, and changes in blood pressure do not appear to differ among the three populations, although differences in physiologic circumstances sometimes give that appearance. For instance, the fetus may appear to be exceptionally sensitive to hypoxic hypoxia. However, the response curve to hypoxia is not substantially different from that in adults. The difference is that normal fetal PO_2 values are on the steep portion of the hyperbolic response curve, whereas the adult values are on the flat portion of the same curve. Developmental differences in the importance of neural input to the control of cerebral circulation are more likely, but these have not as yet been systematically studied. The reasons for the apparent resistance of immature brain to anoxic damage are still not clear, but appear not to involve differences in the response of cerebral blood flow to changes in oxygen availability or blood pressure.

ACKNOWLEDGEMENT

Supported in part by the Hospital for Consumptives of Maryland (Eudowood) and by NIH Grant NS-20020.

REFERENCES

1. Dawes GS: Foetal and Neonatal Physiology. Year Book Medical Publishers, Chicago, 1969
2. Guyton AC, Jones CE, Coleman, TG: Circulatory Physiology: Cardiac Output and Its Regulation, 2nd Ed. W. B. Saunders, Philadelphia, 1973
3. Frackowiak RSJ: The pathophysiology of human cerebral ischaemia: A new perspective obtained with positron tomography. Q J Med 57:713, 1985
4. Sokoloff L: Relation between physiological function and energy metabolism in the central nervous system. J Neurochem 29:13, 1977
5. Frewen TC, Sumabat WO, Del Maestro RF: Cerebral blood flow, metabolic rate, and cross-brain oxygen consumption in brain injury. J Pediatr 107:510, 1985
6. Beckstead JE, Tweed WA, Lee J, et al: Cerebral blood flow and metabolism in man following cardiac arrest. Stroke 9:569, 1978
7. Jones MD, Jr, Traystman RJ, Simmons MA, et al: Effects of changes in arterial O_2 content on cerebral blood flow in the lamb. Am J Physiol 240 (Heart Circ Physiol 9):H209, 1981
8. Jones MD, Jr, Traystman RJ: Cerebral oxygenation of the fetus, newborn, and adult. Semin Perinatol 8:205, 1984
9. Phelps ME, Mazziotta JC, Huang S-C: Study of cerebral function with positron computed tomography. J Cereb Blood Flow Metab 2:113, 1982
10. Lebrun-Grandie P, Baron J-C, Soussaline F, et al: Coupling between regional blood flow and oxygen utilization in the normal human brain. Arch Neurol 40:230, 1983
11. Dejours P: Principles of Comparative Respiratory Physiology. 2nd Ed. Elsevier/North-Holland Biomedical Press, Amsterdam, 1981
12. Zierler KL: Theory of the use of arteriovenous concentration differences for measuring metabolism in steady and non-steady states. J Clin Invest 40:2111, 1961
13. Jones MD, Jr, Sheldon RE, Peeters LL, et al: Regulation of cerebral blood flow in the ovine fetus. Am J Physiol (Heart Circ Physiol 4): H162, 1978
14. McPherson RW, Zeger S, Traystman RJ: Relationship of somatosensory evoked potentials and cerebral oxygen consumption during hypoxic hypoxia in dogs. Stroke 17:30, 1986
15. Jones DP, Kennedy FG: Intracellular oxygen supply during hypoxia. Am J Physiol 243 (Cell Physiol 12):C247, 1982
16. Krasney JA, Miki K, McAndrews K, et al: Peripheral circulatory responses to 96 h of hypoxia in conscious sinoaortic-denervated sheep. Am J Physiol 250 (Regulatory Integrative Comp Physiol 19):R868, 1986
17. Lahiri S: Role of arterial O_2 flow in peripheral chemoreceptor excitation. Fed Proc 39:2648, 1980
18. Traystman RJ, Fitzgerald RS: Cerebrovascular response to hypoxia in baroreceptor- and chemoreceptor-denervated dogs. Am J Physiol 241 (Heart Circ Physiol 10):H724, 1981
19. Borgström L, Johannsson H, Siesjo BK: The relationship between arterial PO_2 and cerebral blood flow in hypoxic hypoxia. Acta Physiol Scand 93:423, 1975
20. McDowall DG: Interrelationships between blood oxygen tensions and cerebral blood flow. p.

205. In Payne JP, Hill DW, (eds): A Symposium on Oxygen Measurements in Blood and Tissues and their Significance. Churchill. London, 1966
21. Kogure K, Scheinberg P, Reinmuth OM, et al: Mechanisms of cerebral vasodilatation in hypoxia. J Appl Physiol 29:223, 1970.
22. Rosenthal M, Lamanna JC, Jobsis FF, et al: Effects of respiratory gases on cytochrome A in intact cerebral cortex: is there a critical PO_2? Brain Res 108:143, 1976
23. Wilson DF, Erecińska M, Drown C, et al: The oxygen dependence of cellular metabolism. Arch Biochem Biophys 195:485, 1979
24. Kontos HA, Wei EP, Raper AJ, et al: Role of tissue hypoxia in local regulation of cerebral microcirculation. Am J Physiol 234:H582, 1978
25. Duling BR, Kuschinsky W, Wahl M: Measurements of the perivascular PO_2 in the vicinity of the pial vessels of the cat. Pflugers Arch 383:29, 1979
26. Delivoria-Papadopoulos M, Roncevic NP, Oski FA: Postnatal changes in oxygen transport of term, premature, and sick infants: The role of red cell 2,3-diphosphoglycerate and adult hemoglobin. Pediatr Res 5:235, 1971
27. Novy MJ: Alterations in blood oxygen affinity during fetal and neonatal life. p. 696. In Rorth M, Astrup P (eds): Oxygen Affinity of Hemoglobin and Red Cell Acid Base Status. Academic Press, New York, 1972
28. Koehler RC, Traystman RJ, Rosenberg AA, et al: Role of O_2-hemoglobin affinity on cerebrovascular response to carbon monoxide hypoxia. Am J Physiol 245 (Heart Circ Physiol 14): H1019, 1983
29. Rosenberg AA, Harris AP, Keohler RC, et al: Role of O_2-hemoglobin affinity in the regulation of cerebral blood flow in fetal sheep. Am J Physiol 251 (Heart Circ Physiol 20):H56, 1986
30. Koehler RC, Traystman RJ, Jones MD Jr: Influence of reduced oxyhemoglobin affinity on cerebrovascular response to hypoxic hypoxia. Am J Physiol 251 (Heart Circ Physiol 20):H756, 1986
31. Woodson RD, Auerbach S: Effect of increased oxygen affinity and anemia on cardiac output and its distribution. J Appl Physiol: Respirat Environ Exercise Physiol 53:1299, 1982
32. Wade JPH, du Boulay GH, Marshall J, et al: Cerebral blood flow, haematocrit and viscosity in subjects with a high oxygen affinity haemoglobin variant. Acta Neurol Scand 61:210, 1980
33. Woodson RD, Fitzpatrick JH, Jr, Costello DJ, et al: Increased blood oxygen affinity decreases canine brain oxygen consumption. J Lab Clin Med 100:411, 1982
34. Benesch R, Benesch RE, Yu CI: Reciprocal binding of oxygen and diphosphoglycerate by human hemoglobin. Proc Natl Acad Sci USA 59:526, 1968
35. Koehler RC, Traystman RJ, Zeger S, et al: Comparison of cerebrovascular response to hypoxic and carbon monoxide hypoxia in newborn and adult sheep. J Cereb Blood Flow Metab 4:115, 1984
36. Bard H, Fouron J-C, Robillard JE, et al: Red cell oxygen affinity in fetal sheep: role of 2,3-DPG and adult hemoglobin. J Appl Physiol: Respirat Environ Exercise Physiol 45:7, 1978
37. Maginniss LA, Olszowka AJ, Reeves RB: Oxygen equilibrium curve shape in allohemoglobin interaction in sheep whole blood. Am J Physiol 250 (Regulatory Integrative Comp Physiol 19): R298, 1986
38. Jones MD Jr, Rosenberg AA, Simmons MA, et al: Oxygen delivery to the brain before and after birth. Science 216:324, 1982
39. Roughton FJW: Transport of oxygen and carbon dioxide. p. 767. In Fenn WO, Rahn H (eds): Handbook of Physiology, Sec. 3. Respiration, Vol. 1, American Physiological Society, Bethesda 1964
40. Massik J, Tang Y-L, Hudak ML, et al: Hypercapnia and the response of cerebral blood flow to hypoxia. Am J Physiol. Submitted for publication.
41. Zwart A, Kwant G, Oeseburg B, et al: Human whole-blood oxygen affinity: effect of carbon monoxide. J Appl Physiol: Respir Environ Exercise Physiol 57:14, 1984
42. Roughton FJW, Darling RC: The effect of carbon monoxide on the oxyhemoglobin dissociation curve. Am J Physiol 141:17, 1944
43. Brown MM, Wade JPH, Marshall J: Fundamental importance of arterial oxygen content in the regulation of cerebral blood flow in man. Brain 108:81, 1985
44. Massik J, Tang Y-L, Hudak ML, et al: The effect of hematocrit on cerebral blood flow in newborn lambs with induced polycythemia. J Appl Physiol. 62:1090, 1987
45. Fan F-C, Chen RYZ, Schuessler GB, et al: Effects of hematocrit variations on regional hemodynamics and oxygen transport in the dog. Am J Physiol 238 (Heart Circ Physiol 7):H545, 1980
46. Paulson OB, Parvin H-H, Olesen J, et al: Influence of carbon monoxide and of hemodilution on cerebral blood flow and blood gases in man. J Appl Physiol 35:111, 1973
47. Borgström L, Jóhannsson H, Siesjö BK: The influence of acute normovolemic anemia on cerebral blood flow and oxygen consumption of anesthetized rats. Acta Physiol Scand 93:505, 1975

48. Thorling EB, Erslev AJ: The "tissue" tension of oxygen and its relation to hematocrit and erythropoiesis. Blood 31:332, 1968
49. Bartlett D Jr, Tenney SM: Tissue gas tensions in experimental anemia. J Appl Physiol 18:734, 1963
50. Eklöf B, MacMillan BV, Siesjö BK: The effect of hypercapnic acidosis upon the energy metabolism of the brain in arterial hypotension caused by bleeding. Acta Physiol Scand 87:1, 1973
51. Fenton BM, Carr RT, Cokelet GR: Nonuniform red call distribution in 20 to 100 μm bifurcations. Microvasc Res 29:103, 1985
52. Schmid-Schonbein GW, Skalak R, Usami S, et al: Cell distribution in capillary networks. Microvasc Res 19:18, 1980
53. Jóhannson H, Seisjö BK: Brain energy metabolism in anesthetized rats in acute anemia. Acta Physiol Scand 93:515, 1975
54. Häggendal E, Norbäck B: Effect of viscosity on cerebral blood flow. Acta Chir Scand 132, suppl. 364:13–22, 1966
55. Brown MM, Marshall J: Effect of plasma exchange on blood viscosity and cerebral blood flow. Br Med J 284:1733, 1982
56. Brown MM, Marshall J: Regulation of cerebral blood flow in response to changes in blood viscosity. Lancet 1:604, 1985
57. Rosenkrantz TS, Stonestreet BS, Hansen NB, et al: Cerebral blood flow in the newborn lamb with polycythemia and hyperviscosity. J Pediatr 104:276, 1984
58. Murray JF, Escobar E: Circulatory effects of blood viscosity: Comparison of methemoglobinemia and anemia. J Appl Physiol 25:594, 1968
59. Hudak ML, Koehler RC, Rosenberg AA, et al: Effect of hematocrit on cerebral blood flow. Am J Physiol 251 (Heart Circ Physiol 20):H63, 1986
60. Wagner EM, Traystman RJ: Cerebral venous outflow and arterial microsphere flow with elevated venous pressure. Am J Physiol 244 (Heart Circ Physiol 13):H505, 1983
61. Häggendal E, Löfgren J, Nilsson NJ, et al: Effects of varied cerebrospinal fluid pressure on cerebral blood flow in dogs. Acta Physiol Scand 79:262, 1970
62. Lassen NA: Cerebral blood flow and oxygen consumption in man. Physiol Rev 39:183, 1959
63. Rapela CE, Green HD: Autoregulation of canine cerebral blood flow. Circ Res 24, 25, suppl. 1:I205–I211, 1964
64. Harper AM: Autoregulation of cerebral blood flow: influence of the arterial blood pressure on the blood flow through the cerebral cortex. J Neurol Neurosurg Psychiatry 29:398, 1966
65. Ekström-Jodal B, Häggendal E, Linder L-E, et al: Cerebral blood flow autoregulation at high arterial pressures and different levels of carbon dioxide tension in dogs. Eur Neurol 6, 1971/72
66. Strandgaard S, MacKenzie ET, Sengupta D, et al: Upper limit of autoregulation of cerebral blood flow in the baboon. Circ Res 34:435, 1974
67. Mchedlishvili GI, Nikolaishvili LS, Antia RV: Are the pial arterial responses dependent on the direct effect of intravascular pressure and extravascular and intravascular PO_2, PCO_2, and pH? Microvasc Res 10:298, 1976
68. Johnson PC: The myogenic response. p. 409. In Bohr DF, Somlyo AP, Sparks HV, Jr (eds): Handbook of Physiology. Section 2: The Cardiovascular System, Vol 2. American Physiological Society, Bethesda, MD, 1980
69. Wei EP, Kontos HA: Responses of cerebral arterioles to increased venous pressure. Am J Physiol 243 (Heart Circ Physiol 12):H442, 1982
70. Bohlen HG, Harper SL: Evidence of myogenic vascular control in the rat cerebral cortex. Circ Res 55:554, 1984
71. Wei EP, Kontos HA: Increased venous pressure causes myogenic constriction of cerebral arterioles during local hyperoxia. Circ Res 55:249, 1984
72. Morff RJ, Granger HJ: Autoregulation of blood flow within individual arterioles in the rat cremaster muscle. Circ Res 51:43, 1982
73. Lewelt W, Jenkins LW, Miller JD: Autoregulation of cerebral blood flow after experimental fluid percussion injury of the brain. J Neurosurg 53:500, 1980
74. Tweed A, Cote J, Lou H, et al: Impairment of cerebral blood flow autoregulation in the newborn lamb by hypoxia. Pediatr Res 20:516, 1986
75. Donegan JH, Traystman RJ, Koehler RC, et al: Cerebrovascular hypoxic and autoregulatory responses during reduced brain metabolism. Am J Physiol (Heart Circ Physiol 18): H421, 1985
76. Reivich M: Arterial PCO_2 and cerebral hemodynamics. Am J Physiol 206:25, 1964
77. Kontos HA, Raper AJ, Patterson JL Jr: Analysis of vasoactivity of local pH, PCO_2 and bicarbonate on pial vessels. Stroke 8:358, 1977
78. Levasseur JE, Wei EP, Kontos HA, et al: Responses of pial arterioles after prolonged hypercapnia and hypoxia in the awake rabbit. J Appl Physiol: Respir Environ Exercise Physiol 46:89, 1979

79. Koehler RC, Traystman RJ: Bicarbonate ion modulation of cerebral blood flow during hypoxia and hypercapnia. Am J Physiol 243 (Heart Circ Physiol 12):H33, 1982
80. Lambertsen CJ, Semple SJG, Smyth MG, et al: H^+ and pCO_2 as chemical factors in respiratory and cerebral circulatory control. J Appl Physiol 16:473, 1961
81. Harper AM, Bell RA: The effect of metabolic acidosis and alkalosis on the blood flow through the cerebral cortex. J Neurol Neurosurg Psychiatry 26:341, 1963
82. Pannier JL, Demeester G, Leusen I: The influence of nonrespiratory alkalosis on cerebral blood flow in cats. Stroke 5:324, 1974
83. Wollman H, Smith TC, Stephen GW, et al: Effects of extremes of respiratory and metabolic alkalosis on cerebral blood flow in man. J Appl Physiol 24:60, 1968
84. Alexander SC, Smith TC, Strobel G, et al: Cerebral carbohydrate metabolism of man during respiratory and metabolic alkalosis. J Appl Physiol 24:66, 1968
85. Arvidsson S, Häggendal E, Winsö I: Influence on cerebral blood flow of infusion of sodium bicarbonate during respiratory acidosis and alkalosis in the dog. Acta Anaesth Scand 25:146, 1981
86. Siesjö BK: The regulation of cerebrospinal fluid pH. Kidney Int 1:360, 1972
87. Siesjö BK: Brain Energy Metabolism. John Wiley & Sons, Chichester, England, 1978
88. Arieff AI, Kerian A, Massry SG, et al: Intracellular pH of brain: Alterations in acute respiratory acidosis and alkalosis. Am J Physiol 230:804, 1976
89. Oliva PB: Severe alveolar hypoventilation in a patient with metabolic acidosis. Am J Med 52:817, 1972
90. Huang CT, Lyons HA: The maintenance of acid-base balance between cerebrospinal fluid and arterial blood in patients with chronic respiratory disorders. Clin Sci 31:273, 1966
91. Skinhøj E: CBF adaption in man to chronic hypo- and hypercapnia and its relation to CSF pH. Scand J Lab & Clin Invest 22, Suppl. 102:VII:A, 1968
92. Fujishima M, Scheinberg P, Busto R, et al: The relation between cerebral oxygen consumption and cerebral vascular reactivity to carbon dioxide. Stroke 2:251, 1971
93. Grubb RL Jr, Raichle ME, Eichling JO, et al: The effects of changes in $PaCO_2$ on cerebral blood volume, blood flow, and vascular mean transit time. Stroke 5:630, 1974
94. Busija DW, Heistad DO: Factors involved in the physiological regulation of the cerebral circulation. Rev Physiol Biochem Pharmacol 101:161, 1984
95. Pickard JD, MacKenzie ET: Inhibition of prostaglandin synthesis and the response of baboon cerebral circulation to carbon dioxide. Nature 245:187, 1973
96. Dahlgren N, Nilsson B, Sakabe T, et al: The effect of indomethacin on cerebral blood flow and oxygen consumption in the rat at normal and increased carbon dioxide tensions. Acta Physiol Scand 111:475, 1981
97. Eriksson S, Hagenfeldt L, Law D, et al: Effect of prostaglandin synthesis inhibitors on basal and carbon dioxide stimulated cerebral blood flow in man. Acta Phys Scand 117:203, 1983
98. Busija DW, Heistad DD: Effects of indomethacin on cerebral blood flow during hypercapnia in cats. Am J Physiol 244 (Heart Circ Physiol 13):H519, 1983
99. Wei EP, Ellis EF, Kontos HA: Role of prostaglandins in pial arteriolar response to CO_2 and hypoxia. Am J Physiol 238 (Heart Circ Physiol 7):H226, 1980
100. Pickard JD, Rose JE, Shaw MDM, et al: The effect of sodium salicylate on cerebral blood flow and metabolism. Br J Pharmacol 68:407, 1980
101. Shapiro W, Wasserman AJ, Patterson JL, Jr: Human cerebrovascular response to combined hypoxia and hypercapnia. Circ Res 19:903, 1966
102. Häggendal E, Winsö I: The influence of arterial carbon dioxide tension on the cerebrovascular response to arterial hypoxia and to haemodilution. Acta Anesth Scand 19:134, 1975
103. Rebuck AS, Davis C, Longmire D, et al: Arterial oxygenation and carbon dioxide tensions in the production of hypoxic electroencephalographic changes in man. Clin Sci Mol Med 50:301, 1976
104. Stone HH, Mackrell TN, Brandstater BJ, et al: The effect of induced hemorrhagic shock on the cerebral circulation and metabolism of man. Surg Forum 5:789, 1954
105. Ekström-Jodal, B: On the relation between blood pressure and blood flow in the cerebral cortex of dogs. Acta Physiol Scand 80, Suppl. 350:29–42, 1970
106. Fox WW, Duara S: Persistent pulmonary hypertension in the neonate: Diagnosis and management. J Pediatr 103:505, 1983
107. MacMillan V, Siesjö BK: The influence of hypocapnia upon intracellular pH and upon some carbohydrate substrates, amino acids and organic phosphates in the brain. J Neurochem 21:1283, 1973
108. MacMillan V: The effect of combined hypocapnia and hypoxemia upon the energy metabolism of the brain. Can J Physiol Pharmacol 52:1136, 1974

109. Young RSK, Yagel SK: Cerebral physiological and metabolic effects of hyperventilation in the neonatal dog. Ann Neurol 16:337, 1984
110. Michenfelder JD, Theye RA: The effects of profound hypocapnia and dilutional anemia on canine cerebral metabolism and blood flow. Anesthesiology 31:449, 1969
111. Hamilton JD, Gross NJ: Unusual neurological and cardiovascular complications of respiratory failure. Br Med J 2:1092, 1963
112. Kilburn KH: Shock, seizures and coma with alkalosis during mechanical ventilation. Ann Intern Med 65:977, 1966
113. Heistad DD, Marcus ML: Evidence that neural mechanisms do not have important effects on cerebral blood flow. Circ Res 42:295, 1978
114. Busija DW, Leffler CW, Wagerle LC: Responses of newborn pig pial arteries to sympathetic nervous stimulation and exogenous norepinephrine. Pediatr Res 19:1210, 1985
115. Wagerle LC, Heffernan TM, Sacks LM, et al: Sympathetic effect on cerebral blood flow regulation in hypoxic newborn lambs. Am J Physiol 245 (Heart Circ Physiol 14):H487, 1983
116. Wagerle LC, Kumar SP, Delivoria-Papadopoulos M: Effect of sympathetic nerve stimulation on cerebral blood flow in newborn piglets. Pediatr Res 20:131, 1986
117. Jones MD Jr: Energy metabolism in the developing brain. Semin Perinatol 3:121, 1979
118. Kennedy C, Grave GD, Jehle JW, et al: Changes in blood flow in the component structures of the dog brain during postnatal maturation. J Neurochem 19:2423, 1972
119. Tyler DB, van Harreveld A: The respiration of the developing brain. Am J Physiol 136:600, 1942
120. Chesler A, Himwich HE: Comparative studies of the rates of oxidation and glycolysis in the cerebral cortex and brain stem of the rat. Am J Physiol 141:513, 1944
121. Kennedy C, Sokoloff L: An adaptation of the nitrous oxide method to the study of the cerebral circulation in children; normal values for cerebral blood flow and cerebral metabolic rate in childhood. J Clin Invest 36:1130, 1957
122. Mehta S, Kalsi HK, Nain CK, et al: Energy metabolism of brain in human protein-calorie malnutrition. Pediatr Res 11:290, 1977
123. Younkin DP, Reivich M, Jaggi J, et al: Noninvasive method of estimating human newborn regional cerebral blood flow. J Cereb Blood Flow Metab 2:415, 1982
124. Greisen G: Cerebral blood flow in preterm infants during the first week of life. Acta Paediatr Scand 75:43, 1986
125. Lou HL, Lassen NA, Friis-Hansen B: Impaired autoregulation of cerebral blood flow in the distressed newborn infant. J Pediatr 94:118, 1979
126. Kennedy C, Sakurada O, Shinohara M, et al: Local cerebral glucose utilization in the newborn macaque monkey. Ann Neurol 12:333, 1982
127. Rosenberg AA, Jones MD, Jr, Traystman J, et al: Response of cerebral blood flow to changes in PCO_2 in fetal, newborn, and adult sheep. Am J Physiol 242 (Heart Circ Physiol 11):H862, 1982
128. Abrams RM, Ito M, Frisinger JE, et al: Local cerebral glucose utilization in fetal and neonatal sheep. Am J Physiol 246 (Regulatory Integrative Comp Physiol 15): R608, 1984
129. Cohen PJ, Alexander SC, Smith TC, et al: Effects of hypoxia and normocarbia on cerebral blood flow and metabolism in conscious man. J Appl Physiol 23:183, 1967
130. Camp D, Kotagal UR, Kleinman LI: Preservation of cerebral autoregulation in the unanesthetized hypoxemic newborn dog. Brain Res 241:207, 1982
131. Rahilly PM: Effects of 2% carbon dioxide, 0.5% carbon dioxide, and 100% oxygen on cranial blood flow of the human neonate. Pediatrics 66:685, 1980
132. Kirsch JR, Traystman RJ, Rogers MC: Cerebral blood flow measurement techniques in infants and children. Pediatrics 75:887, 1985
133. Fumia FD, Edelstone DI, Holzman IR: Blood flow and oxygen delivery to fetal organs as functions of fetal hematocrit. Am J Obstet Gynecol 150:274, 1984
134. Heyman A, Patterson JL, Jr, Duke TW: Cerebral circulation and metabolism in sickle cell and other chronic anemias, with observations on the effects of oxygen inhalation. J Clin Invest 31:824, 1952
135. Younkin DP, Reivich M, Obrist WD, et al: Physiologic responses of neonatal CBF. J Cereb Blood Flow Metabol 1, Suppl. S273–S274, 1981
136. Johnson GN, Palahniuk RJ, Tweed WA, et al: Regional cerebral blood flow changes during severe fetal asphyxia produced by slow partial umbilical cord compression. Am J Obstet Gynecol 135:48, 1979
137. Ashwall S, Majcher JS, Vain N, et al: Patterns of fetal lamb regional cerebral blood flow during and after prolonged hypoxia. Pediatr Res 14:1104, 1980
138. Cavazzuti M, Duffy TE: Regulation of local cerebral blood flow in normal and hypoxic newborn dogs. Ann Neurol 11:247, 1982

139. Comroe JH: Physiology of Respiration. 2nd Ed. Year Book Medical Publishers, Chicago, 1977
140. Neubauer JA, Edelman NH: Nonuniform brain blood flow response to hypoxia. J Appl Physiol: Respirat Environ Exercise Physiol 57:1803, 1984
141. Lou HC, Tweed WA, Davies JM: Preferential blood flow increase to the brain stem in moderate neonatal hypoxia: Reversal by naloxone. Eur J Pediatr 144:225, 1985
142. Reivich M, Brann AW Jr, Shapiro H, et al: Reactivity of cerebral vessels to CO_2 in the newborn rhesus monkey. Eur Neurol 6:132, 1971/72
143. Hernandez MJ, Brennan RW, Vannucci RC, et al: Cerebral blood flow and oxygen consumption in the newborn dog. Am J Physiol 234 (Regulatory Integrative Comp Physiol 3):R209, 1978
144. Shapiro HM, Greenberg JH, Naughton KVH, et al: Heterogeneity of local cerebral blood flow-$PaCO_2$ sensitivity in neonatal dogs. J Appl Physiol: Respirat Environ Exercise Physiol 49:113, 1980
145. Kiellmer I, Karlsson K, Olsson T, et al: Cerebral reactions during intrauterine asphyxia in the sheep. I. Circulation and oxygen consumption in the fetal brain. Pediatr Res 8:50, 1974
146. Ashwal S, Dale PS, Longo LD: Regional cerebral blood flow: Studies in the fetal lamb during hypoxia, hypercapnia, acidosis, and hypotension. Pediatr Res 18:1309, 1984
147. Hansen NB, Brubakk A-M, Bratlid D, et al: The effects of variations in $PaCO_2$ on the brain blood flow and cardiac output in the newborn piglet. Pediatr Res 18:1132, 1984
148. Hermansen MC, Kotagal UR, Kleinman LI: The effect of metabolic acidosis upon autoregulation of cerebral blood flow in newborn dogs. Brain Res 324:101, 1984
149. Laptook AR: The effects of sodium bicarbonate on brain blood flow and O_2 delivery during hypoxemia and acidemia in the piglet. Pediatr Res 19:815, 1985
150. Bucciarelli RL, Eitzman DV: Cerebral blood flow during acute acidosis in perinatal goats. Pediatr Res 13:178, 1979
151. Lou HC, Lassen NA, Friis-Hansen B: Decreased cerebral blood flow after administration of sodium bicarbonate in the distressed newborn infant. Acta Neurol Scand 57:239, 1978
152. Purves MJ, James IM: Observations on the control of cerebral blood flow in the sheep fetus and newborn lamb. Circ Res 25:651, 1969
153. Hernandez MJ, Brennan RW, Bowman GS: Autoregulation of cerebral blood flow in the newborn dog. Brain Res 184:199, 1980
154. Toubas PL, Silverman NH, Heymann MA, et al: Cardiovascular effects of acute hemorrhage in fetal lambs. Am J Physiol 240 (Heart Circ Physiol 9):H45, 1981
155. Tweed WA, Cote J, Pash M, et al: Arterial oxygenation determines autoregulation of cerebral blood flow in the fetal lamb. Pediatr Res 17:246, 1983
156. Papile L-A, Rudolph AM, Heyman MA: Autoregulation of cerebral blood flow in the preterm fetal lamb. Pediatr Res 19:159, 1985
157. Laptook AR, Stonestreet BS, Oh W: Brain blood flow and O_2 delivery during hemorrhagic hypotension in the piglet. Pediatr Res 17:77, 1983
158. Ong BY, Greengrass R, Bose D, et al: Acidemia impairs autoregulation of cerebral blood flow in newborn lambs. Can Anaesth Soc J 33:5, 1986
159. Young RSK, Hernandez MJ, Yagel SK: Selective reduction of blood flow to white matter during hypotension in newborn dogs: A possible mechanism of periventricular leukomalacia. Ann Neurol 12:445, 1982
160. Hernandez MJ, Hawkins RA, Brennan RW, et al: Redistribution of regional cerebral blood flow during neonatal asphyxia. Acta Neurol Scand 60, Suppl. 72:288–289, 1979
161. Ment LR, Stewart WB, Duncan CC, et al: Beagle puppy model of perinatal cerebral infarction. Acute changes in cerebral blood flow and metabolism during hemorrhagic hypotension. J Neurosurg 63:441, 1985
162. Rice JE III, Vannucci RC, Brierley JB: The influence of immaturity on hypoxic-ischemic brain damage in the rat. Ann Neurol 9:131, 1981
163. Häggendal E, Johansson B: Effects of arterial carbon dioxide tension and oxygen saturation on cerebral blood flow autoregulation in dogs. Acta Physiol Scand 66, Suppl. 258:27–53, 1965
164. Freeman J, Ingvar DH: Elimination of hypoxia of cerebral blood flow autoregulation and EEG relationship. Exp Brain Res 5:61, 1968
165. Volpe JJ: Cerebral blood flow in the newborn infant: relation to hypoxic-ischemic brain injury and periventricular hemorrhage. J Pediatr 94:170, 1979
166. Goddard-Finegold J: Periventricular, intraventricular hemorrhages in the premature newborn. Arch Neurol 41:766, 1984
167. Hohimer AR, Richardson BS, Bissonnette JM, et al: The effect of indomethacin on breathing movements and cerebral blood flow and metabolism in the fetal sheep. J Dev Physiol 7:217, 1985
168. Leffler CW, Busija DW, Fletcher AM, et al: Effects of indomethacin upon cerebral hemodynamics in newborn pigs. Pediatr Res 19:1160, 1985
169. Cowan F: Indomethacin, patent ductus arteriosus, and cerebral blood flow. J Pediatr 109:341, 1986

7

^{31}P NMR Spectroscopy in the Newborn

Maria Delivoria-Papadopoulos
Britton Chance

INTRODUCTION TO SPECTROSCOPY

In recent years, nuclear magnetic resonance (NMR) spectroscopy has emerged as a noninvasive tool for observing both the biochemistry and structure of intact biologic tissues.[1–8] It is a form of spectroscopy based on the properties of nuclides that possess a net spin and associated magnetic moment, and so resonate at characteristic frequencies that can be detected with appropriately positioned magnetic fields and receiving coils. The resonance of the nuclides is detected by the electromotive force (emf) generated in a receiving coil at a particular frequency.

The nuclides that are detectable and of most interest in an NMR study are ^{1}H, ^{23}Na, ^{31}P, ^{43}Ca, ^{17}O, ^{13}C, ^{25}Mg, ^{35}Cl, ^{14}N, ^{15}N, ^{19}F, and ^{39}K. The naturally abundant isotopes among these are ^{1}H, ^{23}Na, ^{31}P, ^{14}N, ^{39}K, and ^{35}Cl, which do not usually require isotopic enrichment in intact cells.

Nuclear magnetic resonance (NMR) spectroscopy relies on the fact that atomic nuclei with an odd number of nucleons (protons and neutrons) have an intrinsic magnetism that makes each such nucleus a magnetic dipole: in essence, a bar magnet. Such nuclei include the hydrogen-1 proton (^{1}H), which is the nucleus in 99.98 percent of all hydrogen atoms occurring in nature; the carbon-13 nucleus (^{13}C), which is the nucleus in 1.1 percent of all carbon atoms; and the phosphorus-31 nucleus (^{31}P), which is the nucleus of all phosphorus atoms.

In NMR spectroscopy two fields are applied to cells, to tissue, or to parts of a living organism. The first field is a strong magnetic field. It causes the nuclear dipoles (that is, the ^{1}H, ^{13}C, and ^{31}P nuclei in the sample) to orient themselves so that the dipole of each nucleus is aligned either with the applied field or against it. Alignment with the field is a state in which the nucleus stores less energy than it does when it is aligned against the field. Following this, the second field is applied, which consists of electromagnetic radiation in the radiofrequency (RF) part of the spectrum.

For any particular strength of the magnetic field in which the sample is placed, there is a particular frequency of the electromagnetic radiation for which each photon, or quantum of the radiation, will carry precisely the right amount of energy to allow the alignment of a certain type of nucleus to "flip." Hence, if the magnetic field strength is held constant and the RF is varied (or conversely the RF is held constant and the magnetic field strength is varied), there comes a time when those

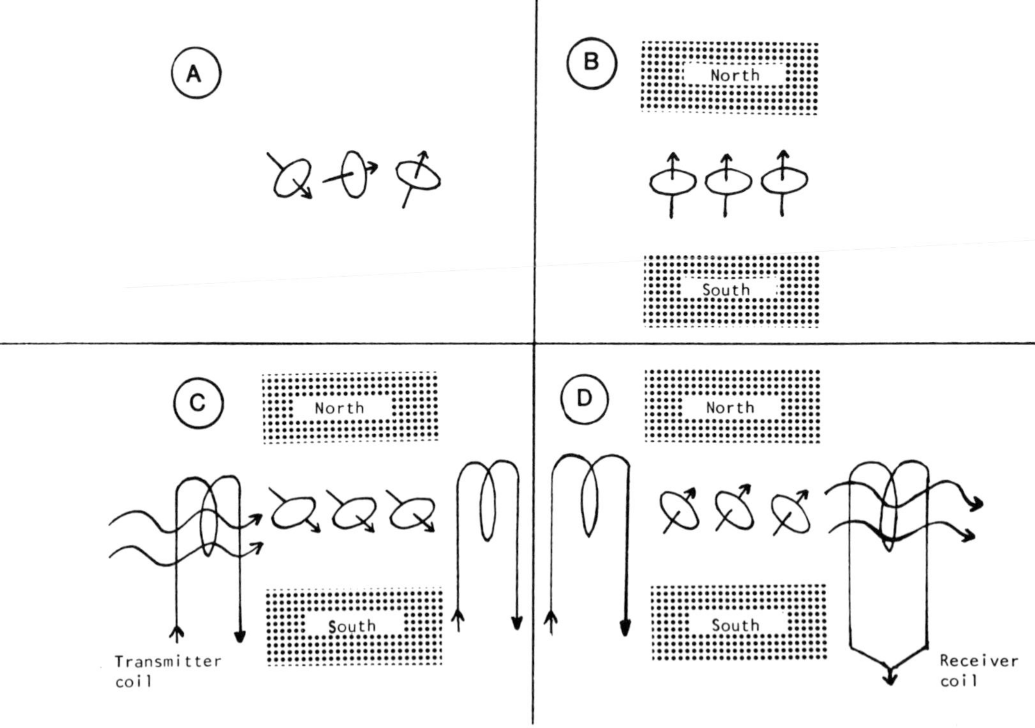

Fig. 7.1. Diagram of NMR principles. (**A**) Nucleons are distributed randomly in absence of magnetic field. (**B**) Placement in strong magnetic field produces alignment of nucleons with field. (**C**) Specific RF signal adds energy to system and displaces nucleons. (**D**) Nucleons realign on cessation of energy input. Emitted energy loss, RF signal, is then detected and processed.

nuclei of that particular type resonate: they absorb the radio photons. For example, in a magnetic field with a strength of 84,000 gauss, the ^{1}H nucleus resonates at a frequency of about 360 megahertz (360 million cycles per second), the ^{31}P nucleus at about 146 megahertz, and the ^{13}C nucleus at about 90 megahertz. The interested reader is referred to the excellent reviews that are available on this topic for more details.[9,10]

In summary, the basic process of NMR spectroscopy occurs because certain nuclei, including ^{1}H and ^{31}P, have an unequal number of nuclear protons or neutrons, and therefore behave in a manner analogous to that of a small bar magnet. Normally the nucleons are randomly aligned (Fig. 7-1A); however, when placed in a strong magnetic field, they align with it (Fig. 7-1B). When electromagnetic energy is added to this system—such as with a brief pulse of a specific frequency from an RF transmitter—the absorption of energy displaces the aligned nucleons (Fig. 7-1C). On cessation of the energy input, the nuclei return to their original alignment by losing the additional energy. This energy loss, an emitted RF signal, is detected by a receiver (Fig. 7-1D), and Fourier transformed from time to frequency by a computer to provide spectral or positional data about the nucleus.

The magnetic field of the earth is approximately 0.5 gauss; by comparison, the strength of the magnets used for nuclear magnetic resonance imaging ranges from 1500 to as high as 15,000 gauss (1.5 Tesla), and the fields generated by high-resolution spectroscopy units may be as strong as 110,000 gauss (11 Tesla).

The observation of this phenomenon—nuclear magnetic resonance—was first reported by Bloch and Purcell in 1946.[11,12] The spectrum of absorbed or emitted electromagnetic radiation depends on the nature of the nucleus of interest and its local chemical environment; these are expressed in terms of chemical shift, and provide information about the molecular structure of which the nucleus is a part.

The medical application of NMR spectroscopy was pioneered by Odeblad.[13,14] Several years later, Damadian and Weissman[15,16] proposed that there are abnormal NMR properties in animal tumors. In 1974, Hoult et al.[17] and Dawson et al.[17a] showed that ^{31}P NMR spectroscopy could be used to measure the concentration of adenosine triphosphate (ATP), phosphocreatine (PCr), and inorganic phosphate (Pi), as well as the intracellular pH in muscle.

Imaging with nuclear magnetic resonance began much later than spectroscopy; the first published image was produced by Lauterbur in 1973.[18]

^{31}P NMR SPECTROSCOPY

Phosphorus 31 has been the nuclide most extensively studied by NMR in intact tissues. Adenosine triphosphate (ATP), adenosine diphosphate (ADP), adenosine monophosphate (AMP), and Pi, as well as sugar phosphates, are intimately involved in the regulation of energy metabolism of cells. Thus, their relative and absolute intracellular concentrations are of great interest. The rapid turnover of these compounds and their compartmentation in the cell cytosol make classical extraction procedures difficult to interpret. By comparison, NMR can noninvasively measure the amount of these compounds in intact cells, and will generally detect only those compounds that are relatively free in the cytosol.

Theory for ATP Systems

The metabolic activity of cells and tissues is a tightly regulated phenomenon. At rest, the adenosine triphosphatase (ATPase) activity, particularly of skeletal muscle tissue, falls to low values,[19] as does the level of ADP.[20] In stimulated muscle the breakdown of ATP leads to the delivery of ADP and Pi to the mitochondria in approximately equal amounts,[21] and causes a stimulation of respiration. The concept that mitochondria are reversibly responsive to ADP and are the "regulated element" in cell respiration in experiments in vitro was introduced in 1952.[22] Chance and Williams, in experiments in vitro,[23] detailed five states of mitochondrial activity; two of these states (states 4 and 3) referred to the ADP activation of respiration following the function of skeletal muscle ATPase during the contraction/relaxation cycle. The same investigators[23] added discrete amounts of ADP and could therefore ascertain both the requirements for Pi and ADP for stimulation of respiration; in vivo, however, the activity of creatine kinase, together with the relatively large pool of PCr, maintains ATP at a nearly constant level, and ADP at levels difficult to determine by analytical biochemistry. They also estimated that low levels of ADP control muscle metabolism.[23a]

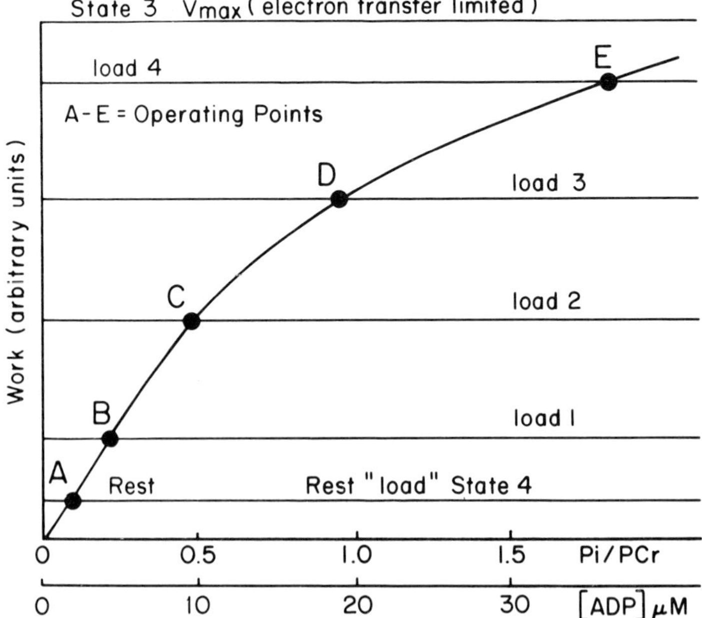

Fig. 7.2. Relationships between steady-state work (V) of the cell (ordinate) and the increase of ADP concentration necessary to activate metabolism to the appropriate value of V. The analysis shows that Pi/PCr is proportional to ADP and the proportionality constant is evaluated.

The control system of body processes follows the well-known Michaelis-Menten hyperbola, where the abscissa is the concentration of the control chemical, and the ordinate is the steady state velocity of the process[24] (Fig. 7-2). The abscissa is the ADP concentration (or Pi/PCr value), which controls ATP synthesis. It is useful to apply Figure 7-2 to the production of ATP by oxidative metabolism in the mitochondria.

If we further recognize that maintenance of the living state requires that the rate of ATP synthesis equal the rate of ATP breakdown (i.e. cellular work), we can see from the Michaelis-Menten hyperbola where stable and unstable states of metabolism exist. The required metabolic velocity (V) allows the tissue to operate in the lower portion of the hyperbola, where a small perturbation of metabolism is corrected by a small change in ADP concentration, and the V/V_{max} is small. If, however, the stress of metabolism requires V to approach V_{max}, much higher concentrations of the controlling ADP are required, and we operate near the asymptote of the hyperbola. Here, a small further change in metabolic stress will result in a loss of control; in fact, negative feedback control is no longer possible. The metabolic needs of the brain are no longer satisfied by its metabolic machinery.[25] In biochemical terms, the increase in ADP and Pi stimulates glycolysis, lactate acidosis rises, ATP is depleted, and ADP is lost through its conversion to AMP, inosine monophosphate (IMP), adenine, and finally, hypoxanthine and uric acid (see Fig. 7-3).

In this situation, insufficient ADP remains to allow the resynthesis of ATP. If therapeutic intervention produces a reflow of oxygen into previously ischemic re-

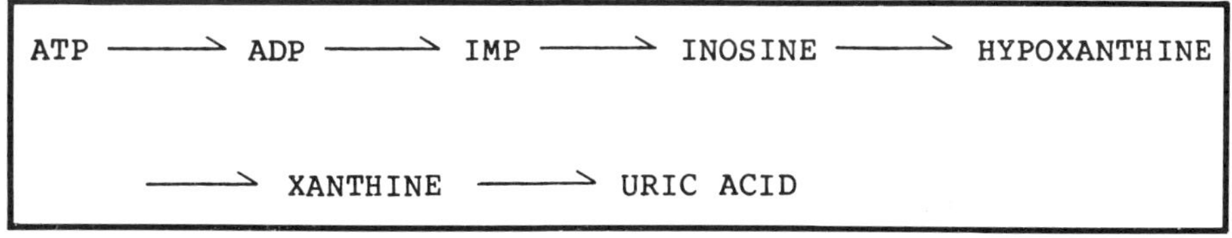

Fig. 7.3. Pathway for breakdown of ADP to uric acid, which may occur in ischemic hypoxic tissue.

gions, free-radical damage may further impair the capabilities for recovery. In short, when V and V_{max} become equal, control is lost and cellular life may be lost. This is a very simple concept that applies particularly to the brain of the preterm newborn infant, where oxygen delivery to tissues may be compromised by the many complications of the birth process and preterm neonatal life.[26] If indeed this hypothesis is correct, its applicability to the neonatal brain is of importance, since brain-damaged neonates may incur severe functional disabilities that handicap their later life (see Ch. 9).

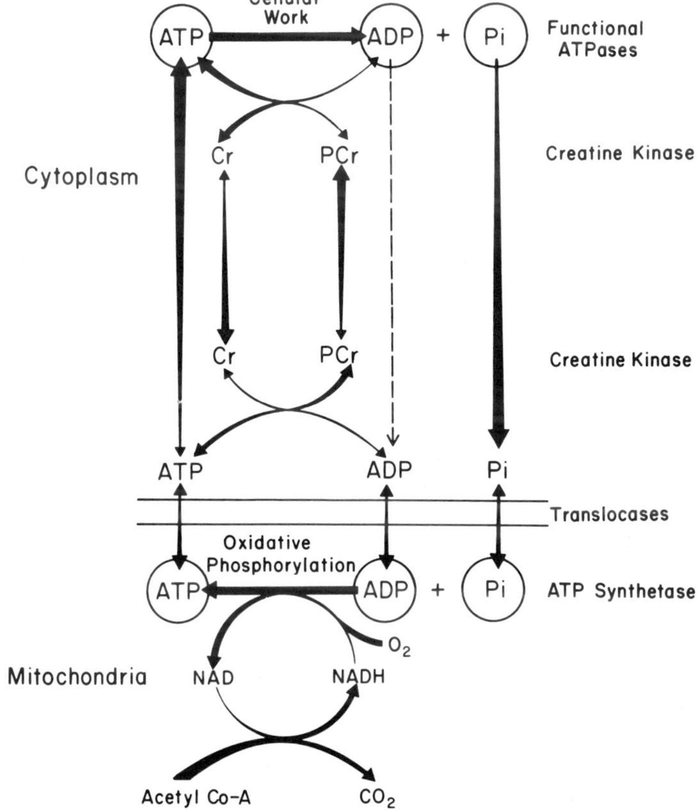

Fig. 7.4. Kinetic couplings of mitochondria and cellular ATPase(s) via shuttles and translocases. The bold arrows represent the main pathways of transfer of phosphate and adenine nucleotides via the creatine kinase shuttle.

In order to determine the V/V_{max} for the newborn brain in a noninvasive, safe, and quantitative procedure, we applied phosphorus 31 magnetic resonance spectroscopy (^{31}P MRS), a technique that measures ATP directly in living tissues together with its "backup" system, PCr and creatine kinase (Cr). In the cortical neuron there are mitochondria in the cytoplasm, and thus many places where ATP can be used at synaptic junctions, axons, and other loci, as well as in the cell body itself.[27] Loss of ATP immobilizes the ion pumps and allows the effusion of potassium and entry of sodium and water into the cell. At the same time, the release of large amounts of neurotransmitters, particularly glutamate, causes severe osmotic stress to the neuronal membrane,[28] resulting in osmotic forces that rupture it. Irreversible membrane structural damage follows this biochemical catastrophe.

The interplay of cell ATPases and mitochondrial ATP synthesis in a steady-state system (V less than V_{max}) is charted in Figure 7-4. The ATP utilized in the cytosol is immediately restored by the Cr equilibrium, resulting in the production of Cr and Pi, which diffuse to the mitochondria. This phosphate directly activates oxidative phosphorylation, and the ADP produced as a result of reconversion of Cr to PCr enters the mitochondria for rephosphorylation. This entire cycle is rapid, near equilibrium, and the key to maintaining the metabolic stability of the brain.[29,30]

^{31}P NMR SPECTROSCOPY IN NEWBORN STUDIES

The feasibility of NMR spectroscopy in newborn infants is based on multiple prerequisites, including safety features, continuous monitoring of all vital signs, and a knowledge of potential health hazards. Preparatory work protocols, including reviews and approval by the Human Subjects Committee of the University of Pennsylvania, as well as informed parental consent, preceded all of our newborn infant studies. The various technical aspects are discussed as follows:

Technical Aspects

Babies are transported by a physician to the NMR spectroscopy suite, which is located within the intensive care nursery. Once in the spectroscopy suite, each infant is removed from the transport isolette, swaddled in an infant blanket, and placed on a heated mattress in a specially designed spectroscopy isolette. The baby is stabilized in the prone position with the left temporal parietal region under a 4-cm-diameter RF surface coil; the coil is positioned just above the helix. When the baby is stable, quiet, and correctly positioned, an air bladder under the mattress is gradually inflated until the scalp is touching the Faraday shield surrounding the RF coil. The Faraday shield is used to dissipate electrostatic fields at the skin surface. The isolette is then closed and inserted into the bore of a 10-inch superconducting magnet (Oxford Instruments). The isolette is designed for easy removal and instant access to the baby should it be required.

Nuclear magnetic resonance studies are performed at 1.5 Tesla (^{1}H NMR frequency of 80.3 MHz; ^{31}P NMR frequency of 32.5 MHz). Double tuning of the rf coil tuning for ^{31}P or ^{1}H is achieved with a specially designed circuit. The surface coil samples a roughly hemispherical volume of tissue with a 2 cm radius.[31] Since the neonatal scalp and skull are thin and do not contain NMR-"visible" phosphorus compounds, most of the phosphorus spectrum comes from brain, and primarily cortical, tissue. Spectra are collected using a Phospho Energetics (PE 80-250 NMR) spectrometer. After the infant is placed into the magnet, the coil is tuned to 80.3 MHz and the magnetic field is shimmed for a proton spectral resolution of approximately 0.4 parts per million (ppm). The shimming process is the adjustment of the magnetic field to achieve maximum homogeneity of the sensitive tissue region in the superconducting magnet. The coil is also tuned to 32.5 MHz, and two ^{31}P NMR spectra, each with 200 free induction decays (FID) in 10 minutes, are obtained, with an optimum pulse length of 50 microseconds.

Test-retest comparisons are performed by analyzing each 5-minute, 75 FID spectrum separately. Because the signal-to-noise ratio in the spectrum is improved by longer periods of data collection, the final data analysis may be performed on the spectrum obtained by adding the 150 FID together (i.e., a 10-min accumulation). Since ^{31}P NMR spectra exhibit spectral overlap, the data are processed with a spectral analysis program. The validity of this program has been demonstrated by comparing the results from in vivo spectra with results of high-resolution NMR studies of extracts prepared after funnel-freezing the brain in situ.[32] The final graphic output of the examination consists of the original curve, a fitted curve, and the fitted individual elements of each curve (see Fig. 7-5). Final quantitative data include the peak location, the area under the curve, and the ratio of the various peaks to PME, Pi, and beta ATP.

Magnetic field

To test the safety of the magnetic field, numerous animal studies have been conducted, including our studies of a large number of mice that were conceived, reproduced, and grown to maturity in the 1.5 Tesla magnet that we are using. They were subjected to a battery of psychological tests to determine whether or not they were inferior with respect to control animals.[37] The experiments continued over several months; two groups of mice were even observed over several generations and no significant differences were observed (Gur R, Budinger T: personal communication). Thus, the static magnetic field is believed safe. Rapidly varying magnetic fields, however, can generate voltages across blood flowing in the major vessels, and may also effect some neurologic processes in the retina. At present, rapidly varying magnetic fields are not acceptable for neonatal studies, and the PE (Phospho Energetics) spectrometer is therefore not used for neonatal imaging.

Health hazards and safety of spectroscopy

Three potential health hazards have been associated with NMR studies: exposure to static magnetic fields, exposure to time-varying magnetic fields, and absorbance of energy from radiofrequency electromagnetic fields. The Bureau of Radiologic Health of the U.S. Food and Drug Administration has published guidelines for evaluating electromagnetic exposure in trials of clinical NMR systems.[33] The guidelines give levels below which there is no "significant risk" requiring an investigational-device-exemption application. Specifically, the FDA recommends static magnetic fields below 2.0 Tesla and exposure to RF fields resulting in a specific absorption rate below 0.4 W/kg. For infant studies, the magnet used produces a

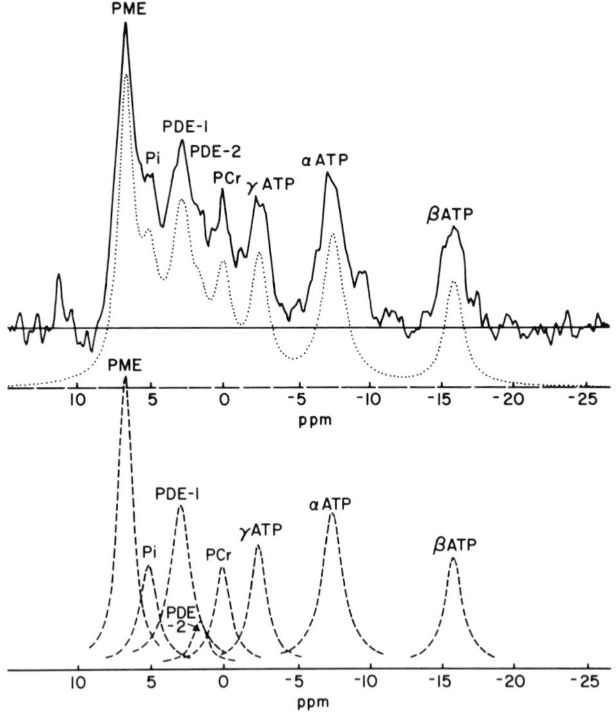

Fig. 7.5. Typical NMR spectrum of an infant brain. The solid line is the properly phased spectrum; the dotted line represents the fitted curve. Individual peaks for phosphorylated monoesters (PME), phosphodiesters (PD), inorganic phosphate (Pi), phosphocreatine (PCr), and gamma, alpha, and beta ATP are easily identified. Quantification of peak areas is difficult, however, because of spectral overlap, a broad unresolved tissue signal, and natural line widths. The utility of our spectral analysis software is demonstrated in the bottom half of the figure, showing resolution of the individual peaks.

field of 1.5 Tesla, and the average RF power deposition was estimated at less than 0.03 W/kg.

Numerous studies have failed to demonstrate any significant, harmful effects of NMR exposure on biologic systems.[34–36] Therefore, we believe that NMR spectroscopy is a safe procedure and does not expose the infant to any undue risk.

Safety of infants

Safety in the isolette during neonatal brain studies (Fig. 7-6) depends upon the use of monitoring equipment. All health-care monitoring apparatus must be available and employed in such a way that the use of one type of apparatus does not exclude or defeat the use of another. Thus, ECG, transcutaneous oxygen, and CO_2 monitors, together with the capability for blood sampling, may all be required. In addition, an endotracheal tube or an appropriately oxygenated atmosphere must be available.

It is most important to maintain the temperature at the correct value, and to ensure that no abrasion of the head occurs by contact with the electrostatic shield that prevents direct contact with the probe. For this reason, the baby is placed on an airbag and gently raised to contact the NMR coil shield. Infants of a gestational

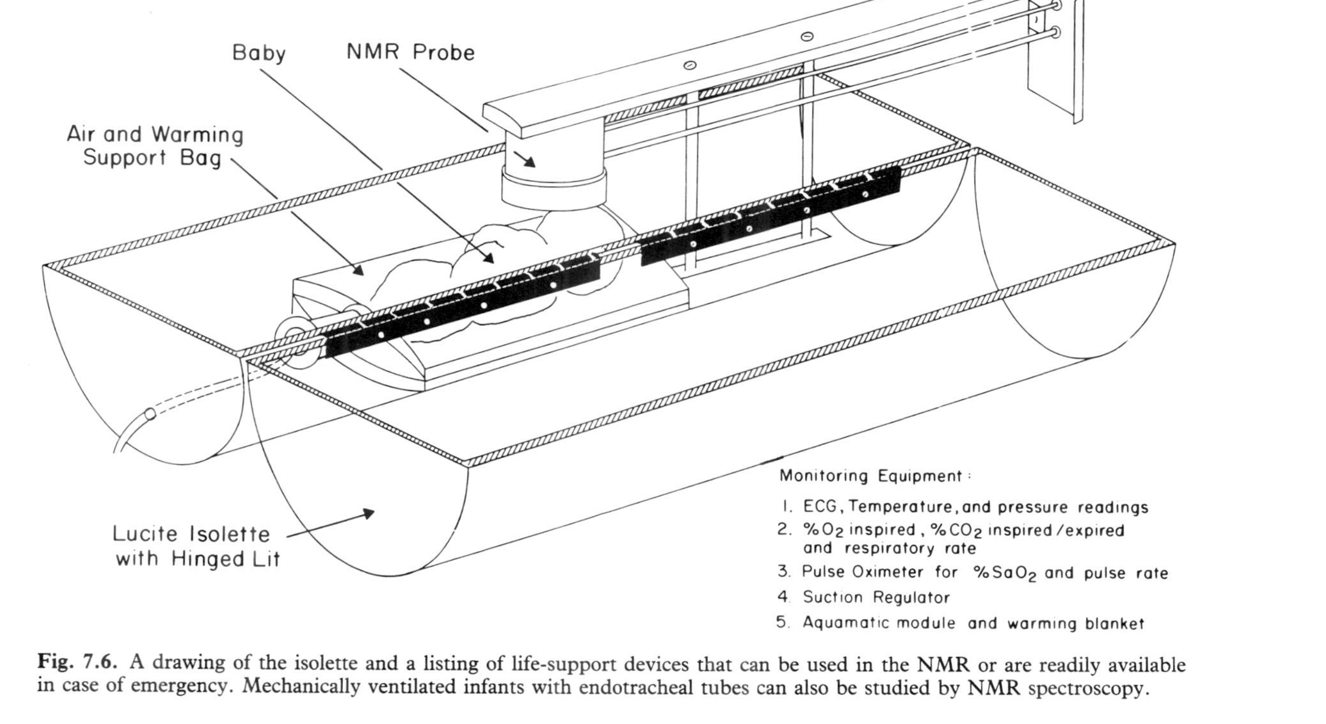

Fig. 7.6. A drawing of the isolette and a listing of life-support devices that can be used in the NMR or are readily available in case of emergency. Mechanically ventilated infants with endotracheal tubes can also be studied by NMR spectroscopy.

age of 25 to 30 weeks may weigh less than a kilogram, and are placed within the isolette shown in Figure 7-6 with all monitoring devices in operation, and with a Faraday shield.

Radiofrequency power deposition

Radio frequency (RF) power deposition may also pose a serious problem with proton imagers (some transmitters have 10 and 20 kilowatts available for rapid imaging). The acceptable power levels are based on the effects of electrostatic fields. A device that is used only for spectrometry generates power over electrostatic fields that are 10^{-4} of the permissible (10 mW/cm^2) limit. Our shielded surface coil[38] allows no electrostatic fields to penetrate body organs, but only magnetic fields do so, and the latter have no detectable effect on infants.

Duration of NMR examination in the newborn

It is a significant disturbance simply to move an infant from its nursery isolette into the isolette appropriate for NMR, and studies must therefore be carried out expeditiously and the results obtained promptly. Five to 7 minutes is usually adequate for the shim process, and the signal-to-noise ratio usually permits one to obtain NMR values of PCr/Pi to an accuracy of plus or minus 10 percent in 5 minutes. Usually both hemispheres of the brain are studied, however, the very nature of the undifferentiated neonatal brain makes NMR examination of the total volume adequate. Because of the shortness of time, imaging methods have seldom been applied to neonates, and they do not yet seem to have been studied for benefit/risk ratio. Furthermore, the complex structure of the adult brain is not expected in the undifferentiated preterm neonatal brain. Thus, the surface-coil evaluation of metabolism in one portion of the brain can be representative of metabolism elsewhere. However, as mentioned above, when time permits, several different regions of the brain are studied.[26,39] Depth selection in the neonatal brain has not been employed because the skull is thin, muscles are undeveloped, and a surface coil placed on the side of the head appears to give signals attributed wholely to brain tissues, as demonstrated by spectra of "dead brain" (see Fig. 7-17). The studies of other organs are also simplified.[40] The sternum is thin and in heart disease, the hypertrophic tissue gives large and clear signals attributed almost completely to cardiac tissue, a case distinctly different from that of the adult human, where significant difficulties have been reported.[41] In the case of neonatal liver carcinoma, signals identified with the tumor are obtained,[42] and obviously, studies of the arms and legs are possible.[43,44] To date, little has been done with the neonatal kidney, but indications are that the NMR signals from this organ may be clearer in the neonate than in the adult. In summary, ^{31}P NMR studies in the newborn are rapid and accurate. Both research and clinically useful information in the preterm and full-term population can be obtained.

Location of the spectrometer

Phosphorus NMR is a device for detecting the early phases of diseases that may lead to loss of the steady state of metabolism and the eventual death of tissue. For example, studies of newborn infants shortly after birth trauma make an early diagnosis of potential brain damage very important. Examinations of older infants in acute phases of disease are also highly significant. These examinations of endangered, unstable infants cannot involve extensive and complicated transportation procedures to distant NMR centers. Thus, we have found it essential to locate our spectrometer in the intensive care nursery, 10 to 20 feet away from the population of infants to be studied. In this setting, ^{31}P NMR is available at any time for neonatal study; transportation of the neonate is simplified; all emergency equipment is available as mentioned above, in case an emergency occurs during the neonatal examination; and the ^{31}P NMR equipment occupies a minimum of space.

For these reasons, we have designed a special neonatal spectrometer with a restricted fringe field, with an adequate magnet bore to take care of all preterm neonates. This magnet allows the isolette containing the neonate to be conveniently placed into the 7-inch bore of the magnet. It is unlikely, however, that a high field adult magnet (1 m bore) could be reasonably located within an intensive care nursery.

Newborn Infant ^{31}P NMR Spectra

A typical NMR spectrum from the brain of an infant is illustrated in Figure 7-5. There are distinctive peaks caused by each of the three phosphate groups of ATP (alpha, beta, and gamma); the alpha ATP peak has a slightly higher amplitude because of the contribution of NAD/NADH at that frequency. Adenosine diphosphate (ADP) can contribute to the alpha and gamma ATP peaks. The beta ATP peak does not include any other compounds known to be present in brain tissue in significant amounts, and is used as a reference for ATP concentration. The PCr peak occurs at 0 ppm; in this spectrum of brain the peak is low, lower than that of beta ATP. The peak caused by phosphodiesters (PDE), including glycerolphosphorylcholine, phosphatidylcholine, and phosphatidylethanolamine, occurs at 2.7 ppm. The Pi peak, which is small and not much greater than the background noise signal, occurs at 4.8 ppm; the Pi concentration is above the regulatory point of brain mitochondria.[30,43,46] The highest peak of the spectrum is at 6.6 ppm, and is attributed to phosphorylated monoesters (PME), particularly phosphorylethanolamine and phosphorylcholine, although sugar phosphates (glucose-6-phosphate and ribose-5-phosphate) may make a small contribution to the PME peak.

The location of the peaks defines the compounds they represent (Fig. 7-5), and is reproducible. With the PCr peak taken as 0 ppm, we obtained a PME peak at 6.5 ± 0.1, Pi 4.9 ± 0.1, PD 2.6 ± 0.3, gamma ATP -2.6 ± 0.1, alpha ATP -8.0 ± 0.2, and beta ATP -16.5 ± 0.2 (all values mean $\pm$ SD).[46]

Intracellular pH can be calculated from the chemical shift of the Pi peak relative to the PCr peak. The mean pH in newborn infants was 7.1 ± 0.1.

The concentration of NMR-detectable compounds is determined relative to ATP, which is most reliably determined by analytical biochemical methods because its level is maintained at a constant value by the decrease in PCr during the extraction procedure. In fetal and newborn animals, cortical ATP concentrations are approximately 2.5 mmol/kg.[47] Based on this value, we estimate the PME concentration to be approximately 3.9 mmol/kg; Pi to be approximately 2.2; PD to be approximately 3.8; and PCr to be approximately 1.8.[46]

TYPES OF TISSUES SURVEYED BY ^{31}P NMR SPECTROSCOPY IN NEWBORN INFANTS

Skeletal Tissue

As mentioned above, the favorable conditions for observation of the neonatal heart and brain make studies of these organs uniquely possible in the neonate.[40,41,48] Figure 7-7 compares the ^{31}P NMR spectra of skeletal tissue, of heart tissue, and of brain tissue, acquired within relatively short intervals. The quality of the spectra is good, the baseline noise being of little significance in interpreting the data. Secondly, arms and limbs show five characteristic peak spectra, with three due to ATP, one to PCr, and one to Pi. Since background corrections are unnecessary, the spectra are sufficiently accurate for quantification by peak height determination prior to computer fitting.

Heart

The cardiac region of the neonate shows, in addition to the three peaks of ATP, a smaller PCr peak and a higher Pi peak than does the skeletal muscle. The heart is working ($V/V_{max} \sim 0.5$), while the muscle is at rest ($V/V_{max} \sim 0.1$), and hence the ADP content is higher in the heart, and this is related to the Pi/PCr value. In addition to these peaks, two additional peaks appear. One, between Pi and PCr, is the PDE peak, usually phosphorylglycerolcholine. Beside the phosphate peak is a PME peak, which contains phosphoethanolamine and phosphocholine. The

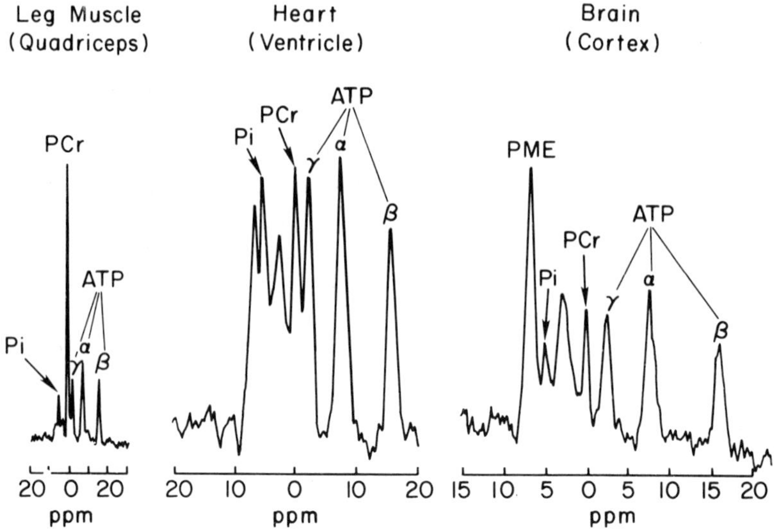

Fig. 7.7. A comparison of the spectra of skeletal tissue (leg muscle from a healthy young adult) with the heart of a 2-year-old child and brain of a normal term infant. Note the different Pi/PCr values of the resting muscle and the active heart and brain. Also, PME appears as a highly significant peak in the neonate brain.

thin sternum contributes little from its muscle content, and hence, the low Pi/PCr of resting tissue is not observed. Thus in the neonate, the thin overlying skeletal muscle interferes minimally with the observation of the much lower values of the cardiac tissue. Some contribution from 2,3-diphosphoglyceric acid in red blood cells within the ventricles may be observed as a peak at about 6 ppm.

Brain

Finally, and most important, is the ^{31}P NMR spectrum of the neonatal brain. As before, the three ATP peaks, PCr, and Pi are distinctly shown. The Pi/PCr value is high as in the heart because this is a working tissue ($V/V_{max} \sim 0.5$). The values for ADP and Pi/PCr must rise in order to sustain a metabolic rate equal that of ATPase. A unique, striking feature of the spectrum is the PME peak. Biochemical analysis of puppy brains shows this peak to be largely attributed to phosphorylethanolamine. The phosphoglycerolcholine peak lies between that of PCr and Pi.[49]

Species differences

The puppy and the human preterm neonate have very nearly identical ^{31}P NMR signatures, as indicated in Figure 7-8. The high PME/ATP value is presumably characteristic of the rapid growth phase of the neuronal tissues. The Pi/PCr value of the puppy brain is slightly lower than that of human preterm neonates, who are generally stressed in order to obtain adequate oxygen for their body tissues. We conclude that the newborn dog provides an acceptable model for the ^{31}P NMR study of the human neonate, and have found similar biochemical patterns in the brain of piglet and lamb.

In vivo ^{31}P NMR examination has been used to study cerebral metabolism in human infants[50,46] and several species of newborn animals.[49,51,52] In babies and newborn dogs, the mean PCr/Pi ratio is approximately 1.2 and the PME/PDE ratio is approximately 1.7. In lambs the PCr/Pi was higher and the PME/PDE was lower. Infant rabbit spectra have still higher PCr/Pi ratios (2.26). Serial studies in newborn rats and puppies[52,53] have demonstrated age-related changes in PCr, PDE, and PME. At birth, lambs are more mature than babies or puppies, and these spectral differences are presumably a metabolic reflection of different degrees of central nervous system (CNS) maturation.

Age Dependence of PME/ATP

The analysis of newborn spectra reveals a high concentration of PME and relatively low concentrations of PCr, Pi, and PDE.[54] Similar results have been reported by Cady and colleagues.[55]

Although Cady and colleagues identified the PME peak as a sugar phosphate, we believe that it represents phosphorylethanolamine and phosphorylcholine. This conclusion is based on several different items of information. The analysis of puppy brain shows the PME peak to be 90 percent of the total.[49] The PME peak is at 6.5 ppm, which is very close to that reported for phosphorylethanolamine (6.4 ppm) and phosphorylcholine (6.1 ppm), but relatively far from that for glucose-6-phosphate (7.2 ppm).[55] As the human brain matures, the size of the PME peak decreases and the PDE peak increases. Presumably phosphorylethanolamine and

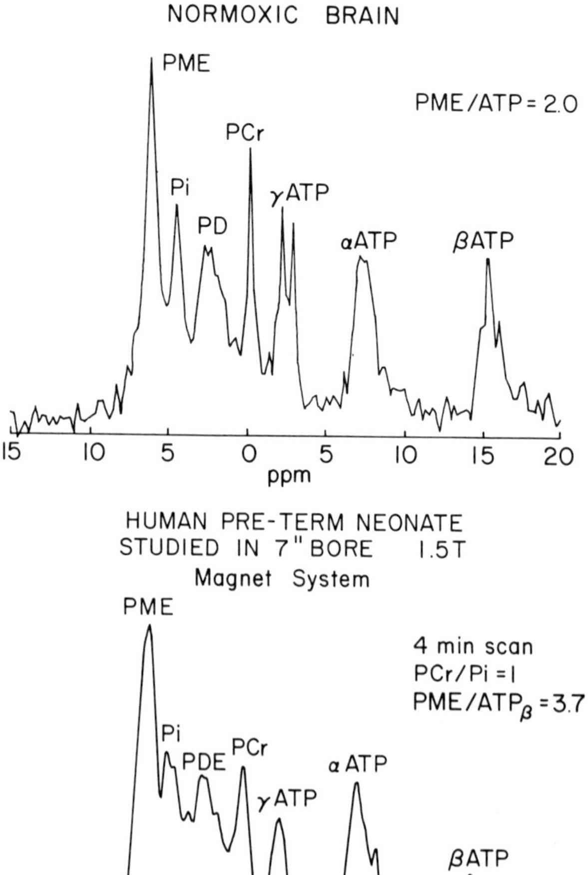

Fig. 7.8. Similarity of ^{31}P NMR signal of the neonatal dog and neonatal human. Note that the PME peak is distinctive, and in the full-term puppy the Pi/PCr is lower than in the human neonate. The neonatal spectrum is typical of an infant of 32 weeks gestation, 1840 g birthweight.

phosphorylcholine are present during infancy for the later synthesis of phospholipids; as this synthesis occurs, the PME concentration decreases and the PDE concentration increases.[57]

Figure 7-9 plots the logarithm of the PME/ATP value as a function of log time, and indicates that the PME peak moves toward its adult values upon maturation of the neuronal connections.[58] Thus, the PME peak is a marker of the rapidly maturing neuronal tissue. In rapidly growing neuroblastoma, the PME/ATP ratio is ~ 2.0.

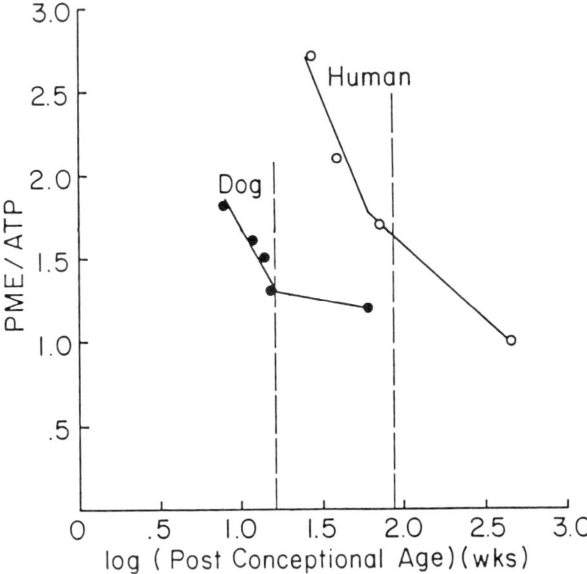

Fig. 7.9. "Maturation" of brain biochemistry in the neonatal dog and human as measured by ^{31}P NMR. The dashed vertical lines indicate time of structural maturation.

CLINICAL APPLICATIONS OF BRAIN ^{31}P NMR SPECTROSCOPY IN THE NEWBORN

Clinical Introduction

Over the past decade, there has been a significant reduction in morbidity and mortality among high-risk babies. Despite these improvements, neonatal neurologic problems are a major concern and frequent cause of long-term handicap (Ch. 9). Perinatal cerebral injury is probably related to changes in cerebral blood flow (CBF) and metabolism, but current methods for measuring these changes require radioactive materials and are not suitable for frequent studies in babies (see Ch. 6). Alterations in CBF and metabolism result in changes in cerebral metabolites[48] that can be assessed noninvasively in vivo with phosphorus 31 nuclear magnetic resonance spectroscopy (^{31}P NMR).[31]

Perinatal asphyxia occurs in from 1 to 5 percent of all births, and frequently results in a permanent neurologic handicap.[59] The extent of brain damage is probably related to the duration and degree of fetal hypoxia and ischemia, and to resultant changes in cerebral metabolism. Following hypoxic-ischemic insults, cortical metabolism changes from aerobic to anaerobic glycolysis due to a fall of PCr/Pi, a rise of ADP and V to the level of Vm as in Fig. 7.2, with secondary changes in phosphorus-containing metabolites, lactate accumulation, and acidosis.[60] These changes may represent the final common pathway of hypoxic cerebral damage that occurs after hypoxia or ischemia.[57]

Normal term and preterm infants

Phosphorus 31 spectra from healthy term and preterm infants are shown in Figures 7-10 and 7-11. The seven labeled peaks are evident in the spectra from both infants. The beta, gamma, and alpha components of ATP, magnesium complemented aden-

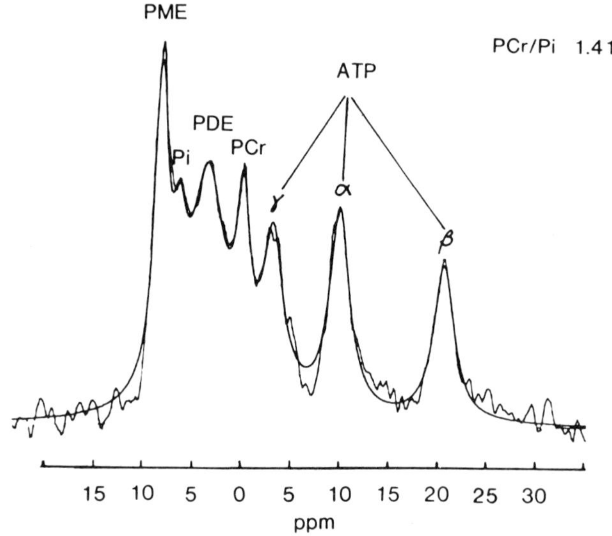

Fig. 7.10. Characteristic ^{31}P NMR spectrum from a full-term neonate using the 1.5 Tesla Phospho Energetics spectrometer. Spectral data were collected for 16 minutes using a 4-second pulse delay, which causes partial saturation of the phosphorylated monoester (PME) peak. Individual peaks are PME; inorganic phosphate (Pi); phosphorylated diesters (PDE); phosphocreatine (PCr); and alpha, beta, and gamma adenosine triphosphate (ATP).

osine triphosphate which probably include undetectable contributions from other nucleotides triphosphate. The peak labeled PDE is attributable to phosphodiesters and membrane phospholipids.[61] Both infants had normal neurologic examinations for their age. The components of the PME peak are mainly phosphorylethanolamine and phosphorylcholine.[49]

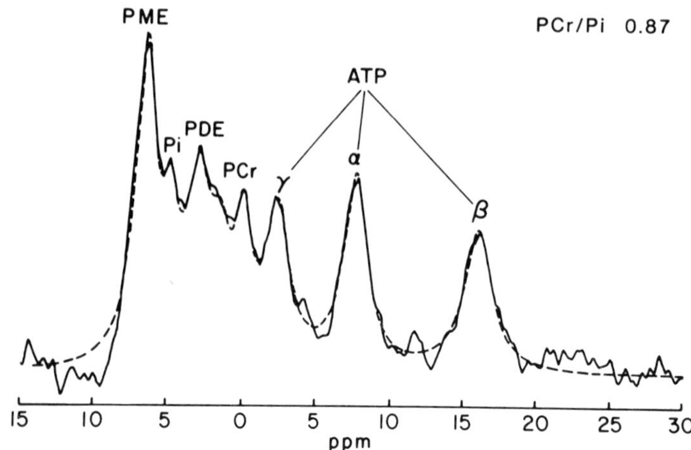

Fig. 7.11. Characteristic ^{31}P NMR spectrum from a normal growing preterm infant (34 week gestation) using the 1.5 Tesla Phospho Energetics spectrometer. Spectral data were collected for 16 minutes using a 4-second pulse delay, which causes partial saturation of the phosphorylated monoester (PME) peak. Individual peaks are PME; inorganic phosphate (Pi); phosphorylated diesters (PDE); phosphocreatine (PCr); and alpha, beta, and gamma adenosine triphosphate.

The mean values obtained by several investigators for PCr/P in term infants (Fig. 7-10) were 1.30 ± 0.27 and 1.35 ± 0.22.[50,62,63,64]

No significant difference was seen in the PCr/Pi values of healthy term infants with their heads in the supine and prone positions, respectively. The preterm infants had mean PCr/Pi ratios of 0.94 ± 0.18 (right) and 0.97 ± 0.24 (left). No significant changes in PCr/Pi ratios were noted with the head in the supine versus prone positions.

Focal seizures

Seizures are commonly associated with hypoxic encephalopathy, and frequently herald the onset of stroke in babies. In the case study depicted in Figure 7-12, the hemisphere with focal seizure activity showed major changes: ATP concentrations could not be maintained, and were less than half the values in the unaffected hemisphere. The PCr was decreased and is just barely detectable; the Pi was increased and the PCr/Pi ratio less than 0.5. The pH in the affected hemisphere of the patient was slightly below that in the normal hemisphere; in addition, phosphomonoesters and phosphodiesters were reduced.

In focal seizures, the combination of a very low PCr/Pi ratio and significant reduction in ATP concentration strongly suggests that the metabolic needs of the seizing hemisphere were greater than the substrate supply.[65] However, intracellular pH does not change significantly, suggesting that blood flow is sufficient to remove the lactate being generated by anaerobic glycolysis.

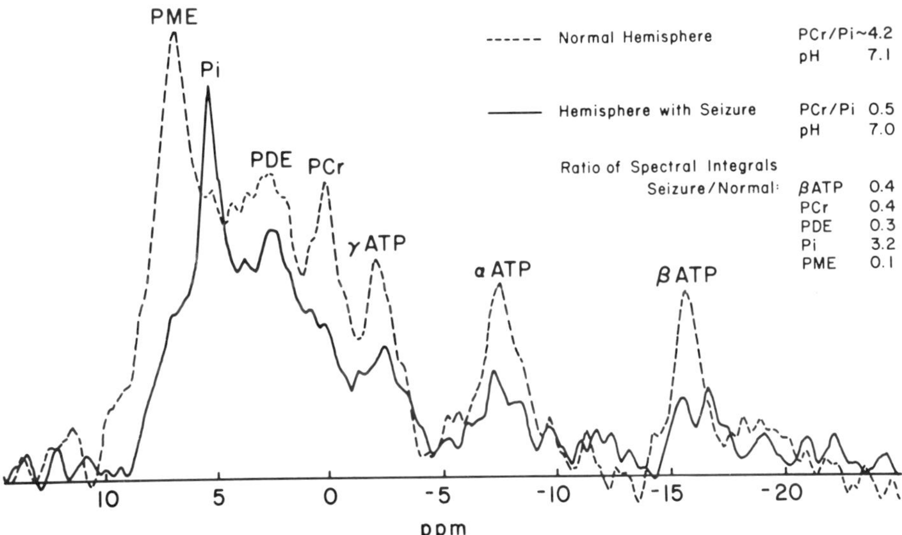

Fig. 7.12. Phosphorus NMR spectrum in focal seizures, obtained at 24 hours, showing major spectral differences. Subtle seizure activity occurred during the study. The spectrum from the nonictal hemisphere (dotted line) is normal; the ictal hemisphere (solid line) shows major changes in PCr, Pi, and PME levels. The ATP concentration in the ictal hemisphere is approximately 40 percent of that of the nonictal hemisphere. The intracellular pH is not significantly different between hemispheres (7.1 ictal; 7.2 nonictal).

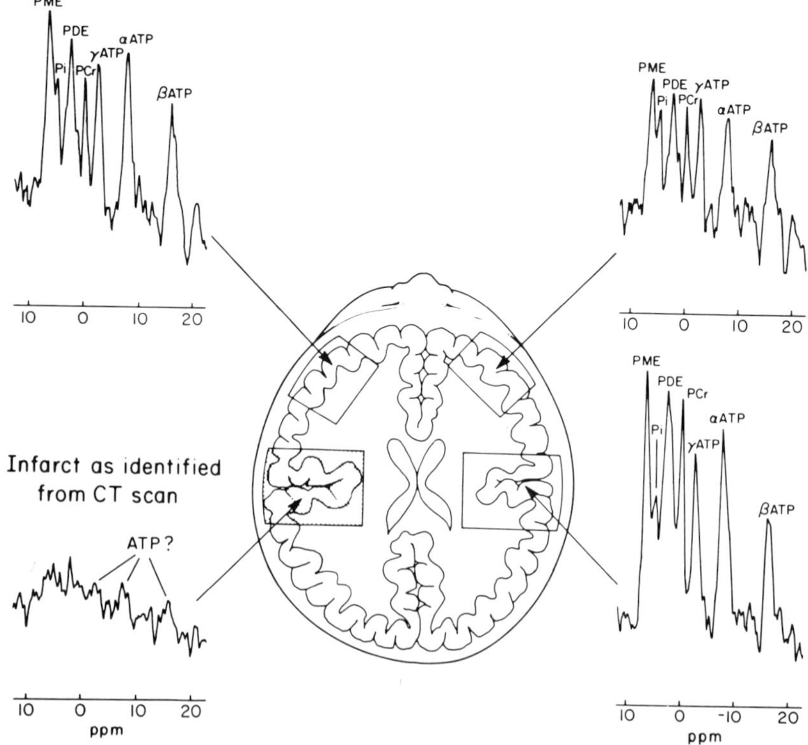

Fig. 7.13. Use of surface coil to compare ^{31}P NMR signal in different quadrants of the brain, one of which includes an infarct identified by computerized tomography (CT), which showed no recognizable biochemicals. This full-term infant had a cyanotic right arm at birth; arteriography showed occlusion of the right brachial artery as well as occlusion of a carotid artery, causing chronic ischemia of the left frontal lobe. A CT scan showed a left hemisphere infarct.

Brain Infarct

Localized damage

The infant whose spectra are shown in Figure 7-13 had a localized infarct in the left hemisphere which has a distinctive NMR signature different from that of three other brain regions which gave approximately equal and normal values of ATP and of PCr/Pi. The infarct is characterized by the lack of any phosphate compound and, presumably, has been filled with cerebrospinal fluid. The region of the infarct identified by ^{31}P NMR corresponds to the region identified in the CT scan.

Prognosis of infarct

Since ^{31}P NMR permits safe and repetitive monitoring of the neonatal brain, many of the infants studied with this technique have been followed longitudinally in time. An example similar to the previous one (Fig. 7-14) shows that the region deficient in ATP and PCr will show no recovery, while the contralateral hemisphere will show an increasing PCr/Pi, characteristic of the normally developing brain. If there is a difference present initially, it disappears with growth and development of the neonate.

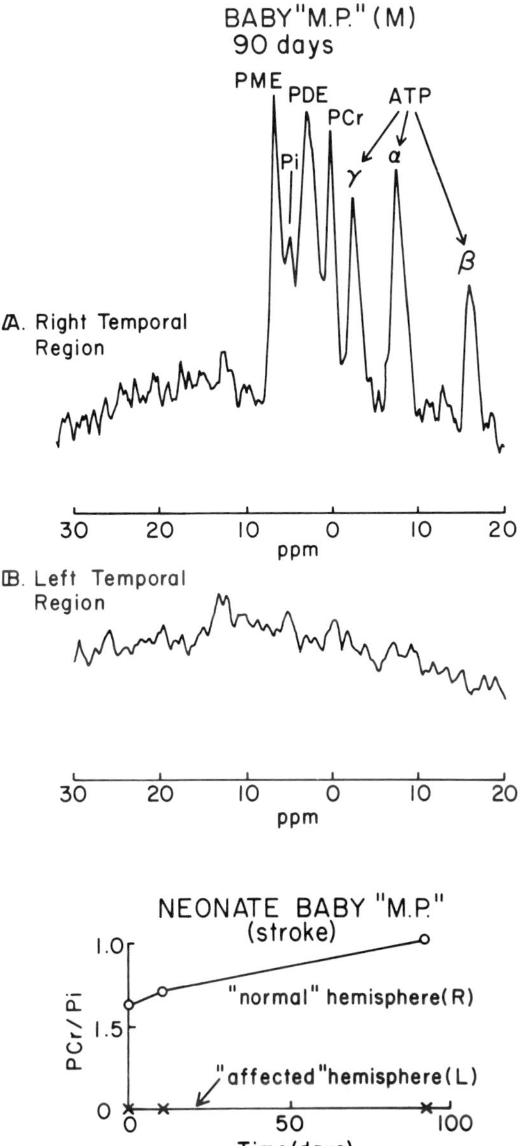

Fig. 7.14. Time course of ^{31}P NMR signals in a brain-damaged hemisphere (lower trace) and the contralateral hemisphere. The longitudinal study shows no improvement of the damaged hemisphere.

Relation to adult infarcts

As indicated by Figure 7-13, infarcted regions may show no detectable biochemicals, and presumably are filled with cerebrospinal fluid (CSF). This contrasts significantly with adult stroke patients, in whom studies of affected brain regions[41] indicate the presence of survivor cells, presumably glia.

Relation to functional deficits

It is expected that many of the infarcted regions observed early in preterm neonates will develop into functional brain deficits in later life. The direct correlation may be complicated by the plasticity of the neonatal brain and by the variety of regions that can be affected. Matured infarcts detectable by magnetic resonance imaging (MRI), computerized tomography (CT), and ultrasound may exist in the brains of neonates that mature to functional deficits.

Phosphorus NMR spectroscopy is a valuable new investigative tool for neurologic problems in human newborns raising a number of important, unanswered questions concerning brain metabolism. The results of our neonatal studies to date suggest that newborn cortical metabolism is significantly different from that in mature animals and previous neonatal animal models.

Hypoxic-Ischemic Encephalopathy

Hypoxic-ischemic encephalopathy: CBF and metabolism

Hypoxic-ischemic encephalopathy is the most common neurologic problem in the perinatal period, and a thorough understanding of the physiologic control of CBF and metabolism during hypoxia-ischemia is essential for the rational clinical management of asphyxiated infants.[66] Due to its importance, this problem has been extensively investigated in newborn animals. In two studies, CBF correlated inversely with PaO_2, increased two- to threefold over baseline values at a PaO_2 below 30 mmHg, and was able to increase further at a lower PaO_2.[66,67] When the PaO_2 was lowered to 35 mmHg, increased CBF maintained a constant cerebral O_2 uptake and cerebral O_2 delivery.[67] In lambs, cerebral glucose uptake was constant at a PaO_2 of 30 mmHg,[68] but in newborn dogs the cerebral metabolic rate of glucose increased in cortical gray and subcortical white matter during severe hypoxia (PaO_2 less than 12 mmHg), presumably due to anaerobic glycolysis.[69] These studies indicate that the newborn undergoes physiologic changes in CBF and metabolism during hypoxia, but leave unanswered the question of when these responses are inadequate to protect the nervous system from hypoxia (see Ch. 6).

Biochemical changes have also been studied. In asphyxiated newborn animals, cerebral PCr, ATP, glycogen, and glucose were found to decrease and lactate to increase.[47,70–72] Compared with mature animals, newborns had a longer survival and slower ATP depletion.[73,74] In mature animals, PCr and ATP concentrations were constant with a PaO_2 below 30 mmHg.[75,76] Our data fit a logarithmic regression line, suggesting progressive changes in PCr/Pi or pHi with hypoxemia. However, an analysis done separately on ^{31}P NMR results obtained at PaO_2 values below 45 mmHg or below 30 mmHg resulted in linear correlations which intersected at a PaO_2 of 33 mmHg for PCr/Pi. Below these critical levels of PaO_2, protective mechanisms reach their limit and cerebral bioenergetics change; above these values, the linear regression line has a slope of 0, suggesting that PCr/Pi is independent of PaO_2. Our results are consistent with similar studies in infant rabbits, which did not demonstrate changes in PCr or ATP when PaO_2 was lowered to 27 mmHg.[51]

We measured cerebral PCr, Pi, ATP, and pHi with in vivo phosphorus NMR during 10- to 15-minute periods of reversible hypoxic hypoxia in 20 newborn lambs (1 to 11 days old). There was a significant correlation between PaO_2 and the PCr/

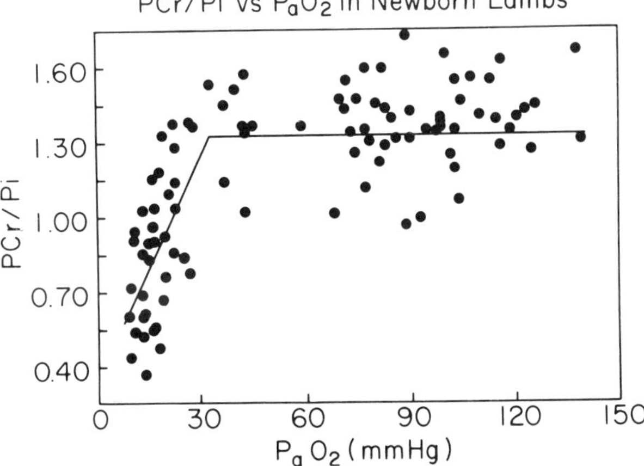

Fig. 7.15. The PCr/Pi ratio is a function of PaO_2 in newborn lambs. The analysis was done separately for PaO_2 values below 30 mmHg and PaO_2 values above 45 mmHg. For PaO_2 below 30 mmHg, $Y = 0.34 + 0.03 * X$, $r = 0.56$, $P < 0.01$. For PaO_2 above 45 mmHg, $Y = 1.33 + 0.0006 * X$, $r = 0.06$, P = NS. The lines intersect at 33 mmHg.

Pi ratio or pHi; however, at a PaO_2 between 130 and 33 mmHg, metabolite changes were not significant. The PCr/Pi and pHi decreased significantly when the PaO_2 was lowered below 33 and 28 mmHg respectively (see Fig. 7-15). Following recovery, metabolite ratios and pHi returned to baseline values within 5 minutes. During the early phases of hypoxia and recovery, there were large fluctuations in metabolites and pHi, indicating that mitochondrial reactions were not in a steady state. After several minutes of hypoxia or recovery, PCr/Pi and pHi stabilized, suggesting steady-state kinetics for mitochondrial respiration. Nuclear magnetic resonance spectroscopy is extremely sensitive to changes in tissue oxygenation, and stable PCr/Pi and pHi values indicate that the cerebral oxygen tension of the newborn lamb is adequate at a PaO_2 between 30 and 140 mmHg.

Partial loss of neuronal population

The most frequently encountered state of a population of neurons with hypoxia is a heterogeneous one in which neurons capable of steady-state activity ($V/V_{max} \sim 0.5$) exhibit normal values of PCr and ATP, while others (V greater than V_{max}) demonstrate rapidly deteriorating concentrations of PCr and ATP.[77] Steep oxygen gradients may occur in rapidly respiring tissues such as the neonatal brain. As a result, neurons that are in a steady state may be only a few hundred microns from others in an unsteady state, leading to diffuse brain damage of a scale impossible to image by available MRI and CT techniques. However, with ^{31}P NMR spectroscopy, such regions are identified as having a global loss of ATP, which we propose is proportional to the fraction of the endangered steady-state neurons. An example of this is afforded by Figure 7-16, which shows on its right hand side a near normal hemisphere, and on the contralateral side an afflicted hemisphere in which half of the ATP has been hydrolyzed. This results in a very high phosphate peak due to the contribution to phosphate from the breakdown of ATP and PCr. Analysis of these results indicates that the PCr/Pi value of the surviving cells (50

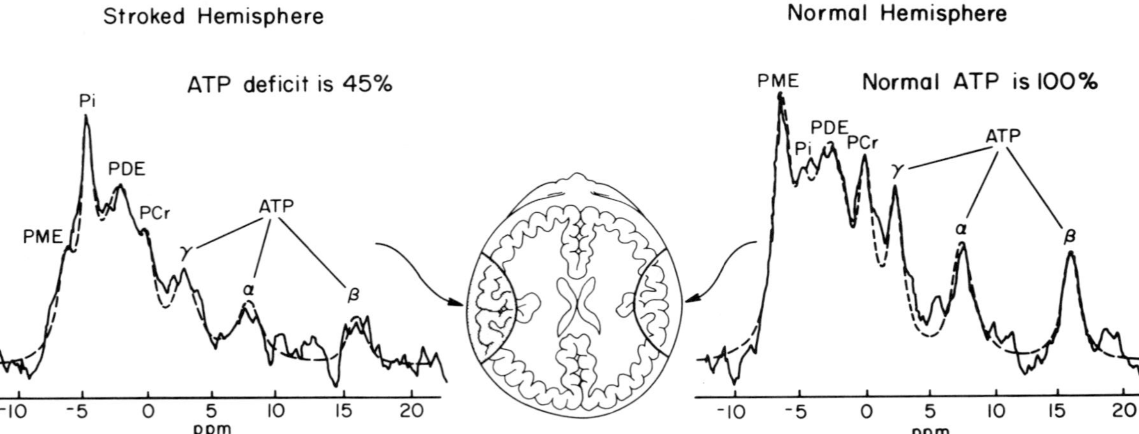

Fig. 7.16. An illustration of NMR signals from two hemispheres of the neonatal brain, in which hypoxia and ischemia selectively affected the left hemisphere; the right hemisphere appears to be normal compared with other age-matched neonates. The significant feature of the spectrum is that hydrolysis of ATP has occurred in one hemisphere. Two types of traces are presented, the original data and the computer fitting of the same data. This full-term infant had fetal distress and on day 1, seizure activity was present; the EEG showed focal status left hemisphere; the CT scan showed an infarct in the left hemisphere.

percent of the total in that hemisphere) is less than 1.0. Animal experiments simulating this phenomenon suggest that in a brain endangered by hypoxia and ischemia, as much as 10 percent per hour of the neuronal population may make a transition from a viable steady-state to a nonviable, nonsteady state. Thus, time is critical in detecting such a state and correcting it with aggressive therapeutic measures.

Brain Death

Two examples of ^{31}P NMR spectra of the neonatal brain manifest global and local cell death.[77] The biochemical changes that occur immediately upon death of the neonate show that ATP and PCr are no longer detectable. The Pi accumulation appears as a single peak in Figure 7-17, with PME remaining as a metabolically inactive component. The absence of PCr and of ATP in a tissue signifies that the steady state is no longer maintained, that V is greater than V_{max}, and that cell death ensues.

SUMMARY AND FUTURE DIRECTION OF NMR SPECTROSCOPY

Nuclear magnetic resonance is a technique that permits the noninvasive evaluation of cellular function from the distribution of protons and other selected elements. We have presented a basic description of NMR and addressed ^{31}P NMR spectroscopy in infants. The applications of this technique are diverse, and this chapter has attempted to give an overview of this new technology and its potential role in patient management.

Although NMR does not involve the use of high energy radiation such as gamma or x-rays, magnetic resonance uses electromagnetic fields that are 10^{13} times less in energy. Studies of NMR in several biologic systems and follow-up studies in humans have found no evidence of radiation effects. In addition, instruments currently available operate below the levels established by the Bureau of Radiologic Health of the U.S. Food and Drug Administration, to ensure patient safety.[33] These recommendations establish guidelines for both static magnetic field strength and energy deposition during NMR studies. This new technique will enhance diagnostic capabilities while increasing the understanding of physiologic processes in infants, and will thereby optimize infant care.

A multitude of studies and experience is defining those clinical applications of ^{31}P NMR spectroscopy in which metabolic studies may prove beneficial. To date, a number of pathologic conditions, including stroke, brain tumors, reduced brain perfusion, glycogen storage diseases, fructose intolerance, hepatitis, and meningitis, as well as infant cardiomyopathies, liver tumors, neuroblastomas, birth asphyxia, and neonatal neurologic disorders have been observed. In the case of neonate brain, the loss of PCr and ATP signals in hypoxic/ischemic brain may be very useful in clinical management and solve some problems outlined recently by Coulter.[78] Present trends seem to indicate that NMR centers are likely to feel financial and clinical pressures to perform studies on large numbers of patients to establish empirical correlations between metabolic patterns, clinical diagnoses, and patient management. There is no doubt that past performance lends credence to this valid and practical approach, as NMR imaging and spectroscopy is fast be-

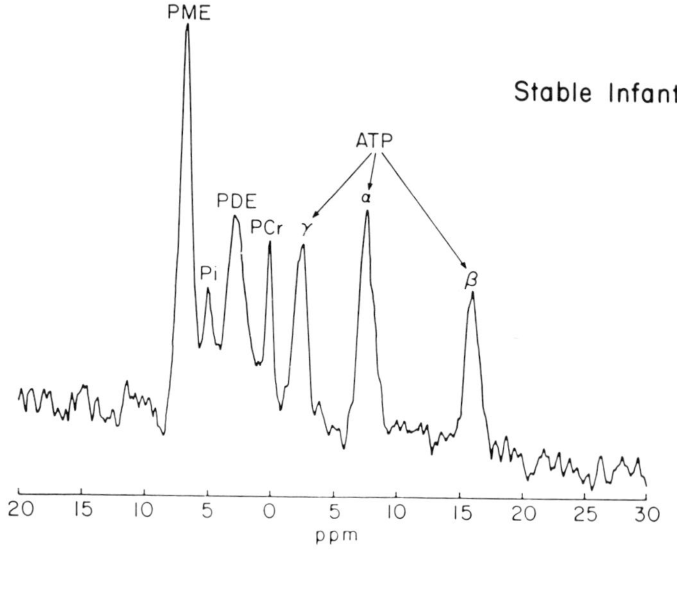

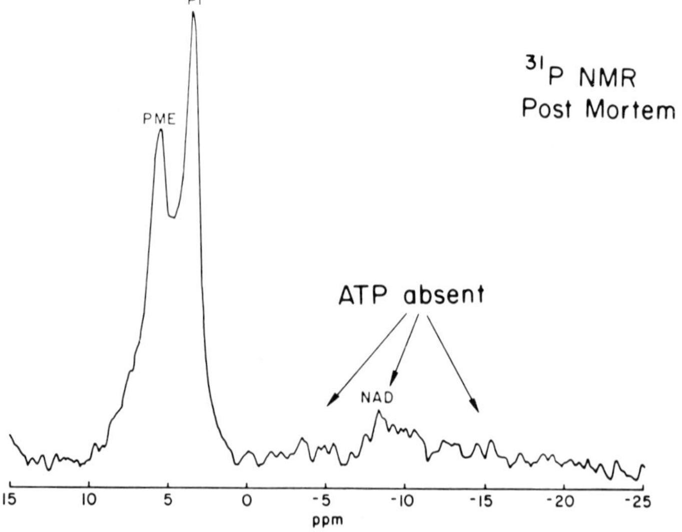

Fig. 7.17. Comparison of ^{31}P NMR spectra in stable and unstable states of brain metabolism. Adenosine triphosphate and PCr are not seen, and Pi is very high in the dead brain; the PME peak remains.

coming a technique that fosters a better understanding of biochemical relevance in clinical practice.

REFERENCES

1. Balaban RS: Nuclear magnetic resonance studies of epithelial metabolism and function. Fed Proc 41:42, 1982
2. Burt CT, Cohen SM, Barany M: Analysis of intact tissue with ^{31}P NMR. Annu Rev Biophys Bioeng 8:1, 1979

3. Delayre LJ, Ingwall JS, Malloy C, Fossel ET: Gated ^{31}Na NMR images of an isolated perfused working heart. Science 212:935, 1980
4. Gadian DG: Nuclear Magnetic Resonance and Its Application to Living Systems. Clarendon, Oxford, UK 1982
5. Gadian DG, Radda GK: NMR studies of tissue metabolism. Annu Rev Biochem 50:215, 1980
6. Meyer RA, Kushmerick MJ, Brown TR: Application of ^{31}NMR spectroscopy to the study of striated muscle metabolism. Am J Physiol 242 (Cell Physiol 11):C1, 1982
7. Scott AI, Baxter RL: Applications of ^{14}C NMR to metabolic studies. Annu Rev Biophys Bioeng 10:151, 1981
8. Shulman RG, Brown TG, Ugurbil K, et al: Cellular applications of ^{31}P and ^{13}C NMR. Science 205:160, 1979
9. Selzer PM: Understanding NMR imaging with the aid of a simple mechanical model. Resident and Staff Physician 31(6):30, 1985
10. Pykett IL: NMR imaging in medicine. Sci Amer 246(5):78, 1982
11. Bloch F: Nuclear induction. Phys Rev 70:460, 1946
12. Purcell EM, Torrey HC, Pound RV: Resonance absorption by nuclear magnetic moments in solids. Phys Rev 69:37, 1946
13. Odeblad E, Bahr BN, Lindstrom G: Proton magnetic resonance of human red blood cells in heavy water exchange in experiments. Arch Biochem Biophys, 63:221, 1956
14. Odeblad E: Micro NMR in high permanent magnetic fields. Acta Obstet Gynecol Scand, suppl. 2:1, 1966
15. Damadian R: Tumor detection by nuclear magnetic resonance. Science 171:1151, 1971
16. Weissman ID, Bennett LH, Maxwell LR, et al: Recognition of cancer in vivo by nuclear magnetic resonance. Science 179:1288, 1972
17. Hoult D, Busby S, Gadian D, et al: Observation of tissue metabolites using ^{31}P nuclear magnetic resonance. Nature 252:285, 1974
17a. Dawson MJ, Gadian DG, Wilkie DR: Muscular fatigue investigated by phosphorus nuclear magnetic resonance. Nature 274:861, 1978
18. Lauterbur PC: Image formation by induced local interactions: examples of employing nuclear magnetic resonance. Nature 242:190, 1973
19. Kushmerick MJ, Larson RE, Davies RE: Proc R Soc Lond [B], 174:293, 1969
20. Veech RL, Lawson JWR, Cornell NW, Krebs HA: Cytosolic phosphorylation potential. J Biol Chem 254:6538, 1979
21. Davies RE: A molecular theory of muscle contraction: Calcium-dependent contractions with hydrogen bond formation plus ATP-dependent extensions of part of the myosin-actin cross-bridges. Nature 199:1068, 1963
22. Lardy HA, Wellman H: Oxidative phosphorylation: Role of inorganic phosphorylation and acceptor systems in control of metabolic rates. J Biol Chem 195:215, 1952
23. Chance B, Williams H: Respiratory enzymes in oxidative phosphorylation. III The Steady State. J Biol Chem 217:409, 1955
23a. Chance B, Mauriello G, Aubert X: ADP arrival at muscle mitochondria following a twitch. p. 128. In: Rodahl K, Horvath SM (eds): Muscle as a Tissue. McGraw–Hill, New York, 1962
24. Michaelis L, Menten M: Die Kinetic der Intervertasewirkung. Biochem Z 49:333, 1913
25. Chance B, Leigh JS Jr, Nioka S: P MRS as a sensor of oxygen in the heart or brain tissue. Soc Mag Res in Med, Fifth Ann Mtg, Montreal, 4:1368, 1986
26. Younkin DP, Delivoria-Papadopoulos M, Maris J, et al: Cerebral metabolic effects of neonatal seizures measured with in-vivo 31-P NMR spectroscopy. Ann Neurol 20:513, 1986
27. Lentz TL: Cell Fine Structure: An Atlas of Drawings of Whole Cell Structure. W.B. Saunders, Philadelphia, 1971
28. Rothman S: Synaptic release of excitatory amino acid neurotransmitter mediates anoxic neuronal depth. J Neurosci 4:1884, 1984
29. Chance B, Leigh JS Jr, Clark BJ, et al: Control of oxidative metabolism and oxygen delivery in human skeletal muscle: A steady-state analysis of the work/energy cost transfer function. Proc Natl Acad Sci USA 82:8384, 1985
30. Chance B, Leigh JS, Kent K, et al: Multiple controls of oxidative metabolism of living tissues as studied by 31-P MRS. Proc Natl Acad Sci USA, 83:9458, 1986
31. Ackerman JJH, Grove Th, Wong GG, et al: Mapping of metabolites in whole animals by ^{31}P NMR using surface coils. Nature 283:167, 1980
32. Younkin DP, Wagerle LC, Chance B, et al: ^{31}P NMR studies of cerebral metabolic changes during graded hypoxia in newborn lambs. J Appl Physiol In press, 1986
33. Bureau of Radiologic Health, U.S. Food and Drug Administration: Guidelines for evaluating electromagnetic exposure for trials of clinical NMR systems. Federal Register 47, No. 54, March 1982

34. Cooke P, Morris PG: The effects of NMR exposure in living organisms. II. A genetic study of human lymphocytes. Br J Radiol 54:622, 1981
35. Saunders RD, Orr JS: Physiologic effects of NMR. p. 383. In Partami CL, James AE, Rollo FO, Price RR (eds): Nuclear Magnetic Resonance Imaging, W.B. Saunders, Philadelphia, 1983
36. Thomas A, Morris PG: The effects of NMR exposure on living organisms. I. A microbial assay. Br J Radiol 54:615, 1981
37. Maris J, Argov Z, DaMico L, et al: 31-P NMR in hamster dystrophy: Skeletal muscle bioenergetics in an animal model of inherited myopathy. Soc Mag Res Med, Fifth Ann Mtg, Montreal, 2:442, 1986
38. Chance B, Eleff S, Leigh JS Jr: Noninvasive, nondestructive approaches to cell bioenergetics. Proc Natl Acad Sci USA 77:7430, 1980
39. Delivoria-Papadopoulos M, Guillet R, Lawson B: Sequential cerebral metabolic studies in preterm appropriate for gestational age (AGA) low birth weight infants. Proc Soc Mag Res, 1986
40. Chance B, Clark BJ, Nioka S, et al: Phosphorus NMR spectroscopy in vivo. Circulation 72, suppl 4:103, 1985
41. Bottomley PA, Smith LS, Brazzamano S, et al: The fate of Pi and pH in regional myocardial infarction: A noninvasive 31-P NMR study. Fifth Ann Mtg, Montreal, Soc Mag Res in Med, 3:608, 1986
42. Maris JM, Evans AE, McLaughlin AC, et al: 31-P Nuclear magnetic resonance spectroscopic investigation of human neuroblastoma in situ. N Engl J Med 312:1500, 1985
43. Chance B, Eleff S, Leigh JS Jr, et al: Mitochondrial regulation of phosphocreatine/inorganic phosphate ratios in exercising human muscle: A gated 31-P NMR study. Proc Natl Acad Sci USA 78:6714, 1981
44. Arnold DL, Matthews PM, Radda GK: Metabolic recovery after exercise and the assessment of mitochondrial function in-vivo in human skeletal muscle by means of 31-P NMR. Mag Res in Med 1:307, 1984
45. Chance B, Eleff S, Bank W, et al: 31-P NMR studies of control of mitochondrial function in phosphofructokinase-deficient human skeletal muscle. Proc Natl Acad Sci USA 79:7714, 1982
46. Younkin DP, Delivoria-Papadopoulos M, Leonard JC, et al: Unique aspects of human newborn cortical metabolism evaluated with phosphorus nuclear magnetic resonance spectroscopy. Ann Neurol 16:581, 1984
47. Vannucci RC, Duffy TE: Cerebral metabolism in newborn dogs during reversible asphyxia. Ann Neurol 1:528, 1977
48. Whitman GJ, Chance B, Bode H, et al: Diagnosis and therapeutic evaluation of a pediatric cardiomyopathy using 31-P NMR. J Am Coll Cardiol 5:745, 1985
49. Gyulai L, Bolinger L, Leigh JS Jr, et al: Phosphorylethanolamine—The major constituent of the phosphomonoester peak observed by ^{31}P NMR on developing dog brain. FEBS Lett 178:137, 1984
50. Hope PL, Cady EB, Tofts PS, et al: Cerebral energy metabolism studied with phosphorus NMR spectroscopy in normal and birth-asphyxiated infants. Lancet 2:366, 1984
51. Gonzalez-Mendex R, McNeill A, Gregory GA, et al: Effects of hypoxic hypoxia on cerebral phosphate metabolites and pH in the anesthetized infant rabbit. J Cereb Blood Flow Metab 5:512, 1985
52. Tofts P, Wray S: Changes in brain phosphorus metabolites during postnatal development of the rat. J Physiol 359:417, 1985
53. Donlon E, Sinnwell T, Younkin DP, Chance B: Maturational changes in cerebral phosphorus metabolites in the puppy. (abstr) Mag Res in Med Mtg, Fifth Ann Mtg, Montreal, In press. 1986
54. Younkin DP, Delivoria-Papadopoulos M, Leonard JC, et al: Unique aspects of human newborn cortical metabolism evaluated with phosphorus nuclear magnetic resonance spectroscopy. Ann Neurol 16:581, 1984
55. Cady EB, Dawson MJ, Hope PL, et al: Noninvasive investigations of magnetic resonance spectroscopy. Lancet 1:1059, 1983
56. Pettegrew JW, Copp SJ, Dacok J, et al: ^{31}P nuclear magnetic resonance spectroscopy of phosphoglycerol in developing and generating brain. J Neuropathol Exp Neurol 46:419, 1986
57. Thulborn KR, du Boulay GH, Duchen LW, Radda G: A 31-P nuclear magnetic resonance in vivo study of cerebral ischemia in the gerbil. J Cereb Blood Flow Metab 2:299, 1982
58. Nioka S, Mayevsky A, Chance B, et al: Age dependent metabolic control parameters in the neonate puppy brain from birth to 21 days. Soc Mag Res in Med, Fifth Ann Mtg, Montreal, 3:674, 1986
59. Nelson KB, Ellenberg JH: Neonatal signs as predictors of cerebral palsy. Pediatric, 64:225, 1979
60. Holowach-Thurson J, Hauhart RE, Jones EM, et al: Decrease in brain glucose in anoxia in spite of elevated plasma glucose levels. Pediatr Res 7:691, 1973
61. Glonek T, Kop ST, Kot E, et al: P-31 nuclear magnetic resonance analysis of brain: The perchloric acid excretion spectrum. J Neurochem 39:1210, 1982

62. Younkin DP, Delivoria-Papadopoulos M, Subramanian H, et al: Studies of cortical metabolites in potasphyxiated newborn infants. Pediatr Res 18(4):357A, 1984
63. Younkin DP, Delivoria-Papadopoulos M, Wagerle LC, Chance B: In vivo ^{31}P NMR spectroscopy in neonatal neurologic disorders. p. 149. In Plum F, Pulsinelli W (eds): Cerebrovascular Diseases. Raven Press, New York, 1985
64. Hamilton PA, Cady EB, Wyatt JS, et al: Impaired energy metabolism in brains of newborn infants with increased cerebral echodensities. Lancet 2:1242, 1986
65. Wagerle LC, Delivoria-Papadopoulos M, Younkin DP, et al: Cerebral bioenergetic reserve and blood flow compensation in hypoxic newborn lambs. Pediatr Res 19(4):370A, 1985
66. Volpe JJ: In Neurology of the Newborn. p. 141. W.B. Saunders, Philadelphia, 1981
67. Jones MD, Traystman RJ, Simmons MA, Molteni RA: Effects of changes in arterial O_2 content on cerebral blood flow in the lamb. Am J Physiol 240 (Heart Circ Physiol 9):H209, 1981
68. Gardiner RM: Cerebral blood flow and oxidative metabolism during hypoxia and asphyxia in the newborn calf and lamb. J Physiol (Lond) 305:357, 1980
69. Duffy TE, Cavazzuti M, Cruz NF, Sokoloff LL: Local cerebral glucose metabolism in newborn dogs: Effects of hypoxia and halothane anesthesia. Ann Neurol 11:233, 1982
70. Holowach-Thurston J, McDougal DB: Effect of ischemia on metabolism of the brain of the newborn mouse. Am J Physiol 216:348, 1969
71. Halowach-Thurston J, Hauhart RE, Jones EM: Anoxia in mice: Reduced glucose in brain with normal or elevated glucose in plasma and increased survival after glucose treatment. Pediatr Res 8:238, 1974
72. Vannucci RC, Duffy TE: Carbohydrate metabolism in fetal and neonatal rat brain during anoxia and recovery. Am J Physiol 230:1269, 1976
73. Duffy TE, Kohle SJ, Vannucci RC: Carbohydrate and energy metabolism in perinatal rat brain: Relation to survival in anoxia. J Neurochem 24:271, 1975
74. Duffy TE, Vannucci RC: Metabolic aspects of cerebral anoxia in the fetus and newborn. p 316. In Barenberg SR (ed): Brain–Fetal and Infant. Nyhoff Medical Division, The Hague, 1977
75. Hilberman M, Subramanian VH, Haselgrove J, et al: In vivo time-resolved brain phosphorus nuclear magnetic resonance. J Cereb Blood Flow Metab 4:334, 1984
76. Lien RI, Sinwell T, Chance B, Delivoria-Papadopoulos M: Analysis of cerebral metabolism in a neonatal population. Soc Mag Res, Fifth Ann Mtg, 2:293, 1986
77. Delivoria-Papadopoulos M, Lawson B, Lien R, et al: In vivo brain oxidative metabolism in preterm and term infants. Pediatr Res In press, 1987
78. Coulter DL: Neurologic uncertainty in newborn intensive care. New Engl J Med 316:840, 1987

8

Cerebral Neurophysiologic Assessment of the High-Risk Neonate

Mark S. Scher
Michael J. Painter
Robert D. Guthrie

Advances in neonatal intensive care have dramatically improved the survival of high-risk infants. Concomitant with improvements in the neonatal survival rate has been an increasing awareness of a "new morbidity." Although neurologic disorders occasionally occur in asymptomatic children without obvious prenatal or neonatal medical difficulties, pediatricians and pediatric specialists have focused special attention on the acutely ill newborn who requires intensive medical care. Long term follow-up studies of high-risk infants over the last 10 years have indicated that between 10 and 50 percent of these babies suffer variable degrees of long term neurodevelopmental sequelae.[1–9] The spectrum of clinical problems ranges from hearing loss in 3 percent, and visual loss in 5 percent to delay in psychomotor development or neurologic damage in as many as 50 percent of the survivors.[9] Longer term studies of very low birthweight infants suggest that one-fifth to one-third need special educational assistance upon reaching school age, despite normal intelligence and no clearly defined neurologic handicap.

Although long term central nervous system (CNS) damage can be identified in many infants from prenatal epidemiologic factors or perinatal clinical factors, others may lack these "identifiers" of high-risk status, and appear neurologically intact on clinical neonatal examination. The need for more sensitive and specific methods of CNS evaluation has therefore gained emphasis. New methods must be developed to identify infants at risk for cognitive impairment if we are to accomplish a major goal in neonatal intensive care in the next decade: to decrease or ameliorate the long term morbidity suffered by many of these high-risk infants.

NEW METHODS OF ASSESSING NEWBORN BRAIN STRUCTURE AND FUNCTION

Important brain imaging techniques have been developed over the last 15 years that have revolutionized the diagnosis of major structural diseases of the brain. Cranial ultrasonography and cranial computerized tomography (CT)[10–13] have both added important dimensions to the diagnosis of congenital malformation, intraventricular hemorrhage, hydrocephalus, and cerebral infarction. More recently, the development of magnetic resonance imaging (MRI)[14–16] and positron emission tomography (PET)[17,18] has further extended our ability to detect specific areas of the brain with either acquired or congenital anatomic abnormalities. The potential diagnostic value of MRI and PET for the newborn is just beginning to be appreciated.

In addition to these advances in anatomic diagnosis, newborn brain abnormalities may also be reflected in *functional disturbances*, with or without demonstrable structural abnormalities. Recent advances in the neurophysiologic assessment of newborn brain function offer a unique opportunity for more sophisticated evaluation of the normal and abnormal central nervous system (CNS). These new techniques include paper-recorded EEG, synchronized-video EEG recordings, evoked-potential analyses, computerized EEG analyses, topographic EEG mapping, and monitoring of chronobiologic rhythms in the neonate and infant.

Any significant improvement in assessment of the long term prognosis for and neurologic care of the high-risk infant will depend on the development and implementation of innovative methods for measuring brain structure and function, which complement and extend our clinical observations. The reliable and rapid identification of infants at risk for neurodevelopmental sequelae will provide an opportunity for early intervention programs that may improve the outcome in some infants. Timely diagnosis will give the clinician the opportunity for cerebral resuscitation at a time when cerebral injury is potentially reversible.

ELECTROENCEPHALOGRAPHY

General Considerations

Neonatal electroencephalographic studies have been reported for nearly four decades.[19] Pioneering investigations by several independent researchers have offered a wealth of information about the developmental neurophysiology of the immature brain.[20–30] Some of these studies predated the creation of the modern neonatal intensive care unit (NICU) and, as a consequence, the neonatal electroencephalographer had an understandably limited role in the diagnostic assessment and ongoing clinical care of the sick neonate. Nonetheless, improvements in the recording apparatus and standardization of recording techniques paralleled the establishment of the present-day tertiary-level NICU. Electroencephalographic machines and recording techniques have evolved as a result of sophisticated technologies; 8-channel recordings have been replaced by 21-channel recordings; improved filtering systems and electrode construction minimize physiologic and environmental sources of artifact; synchronized video and EEG recordings permit more accurate comparisons of electroencephalographic and clinical changes; and an internationally-accepted system of electrode placement adapted for the newborn and infant permits standardization of recordings between laboratories.[31]

Several basic premises for neonatal EEG can serve as a preamble to understanding its principal clinical uses. There are expected changes in the scalp-generated EEG patterns for neonates of different gestational ages. The experienced electroencephalographer can approximate the electrical maturity of the neonatal brain within 2 weeks of the gestational age.[20,26,32,33] Changing electrical patterns reflect the postconceptual age of an infant independent of his or her birthweight. The development of the newborn's sleep-wake cycle follows the maturation of the CNS, and the EEG patterns and sleep cycling behaviors of preterm neonates, when corrected to full-term, post-conceptional age, should be similar to those of full-term, appropriate-for-gestational-age newborns.

Assessment of Central Nervous System Maturation

Since Dreyfus-Brisac and her associates[20] demonstrated that the features of the normal EEG are related to the gestational age of the neonate, other neonatal electroencephalographers have independently confirmed and refined this concept for both the preterm and full-term neonate. It is now generally accepted that a combination of regional and bihemispheric electrical patterns can be correlated with CNS maturation within 2 weeks of the clinically derived gestational age.

Regional changes in electrical activity clearly occur in the EEG of the premature neonate when recordings are obtained after 24 to 25 weeks' estimated gestational age (EGA) and at weekly intervals.[30,32,33] Central and midline fast and slow rhythms predominate, with inactivity in the frontal and temporal regions and a discontinuous background. Specifically, delta slow waves and delta brushes are seen only in the midline-central regions. As the neonate matures from 28 through 32 weeks, greater amounts of occipital activity appear, followed by temporal EEG activity, including theta bursts and delta brushes. Periods of quiescence decrease in duration and number[34] and a greater degree of interhemispheric synchrony emerges[35] as the infant approaches 38 to 40 weeks. At a full-term gestational or postconceptual age, specific EEG patterns define states of rapid eye movement and non-rapid eye movement sleep. Delta brushes and temporal theta patterns are only occasionally noted, and the organization of an ultradian sleep cycle of 40 to 60 minutes is clearly established. Examples of these different maturational electrical patterns are illustrated in Figures 8-1 through 8-4.

Current standard methods for the assessment of CNS maturation include gestational age calculated from the mother's last menstrual period, fetal ultrasonographic changes in head and body size, and a variety of clinical obstetrical signs that can usually be correlated with overall fetal maturation. Clinical examination of the neonate at birth can add to the estimation of CNS maturity.[36,37] A variety of clinical scoring techniques emphasizes neurologic parameters of CNS maturation.[24,26,28,32] However, these current standard methods may be inaccurate and misleading in specific clinical situations. The neonatal EEG estimation of CNS maturation can be especially helpful if such situations arise, or to verify presumably accurate clinical gestational age assessments. Detailed electroanatomic correlations, in which changes in sulcation and gyral development are assessed against evolving electrical patterns, are now being compared with clinical information about gestational maturity. Neuropathologic studies of convolutional measurements have been a reliable guide to maturation.[38,39] Preliminary findings in our laboratories have correlated different EEG patterns with anatomic brain studies.[40] Estimations of gestational age based on the first EEG tracing obtained during the first 8 days of life in 25 neonates who later expired have been compared with subsequent neuropathologic examinations. In 92 percent of the infants there was agreement (within 2 weeks) between maturational stage and electrical patterns and convo-

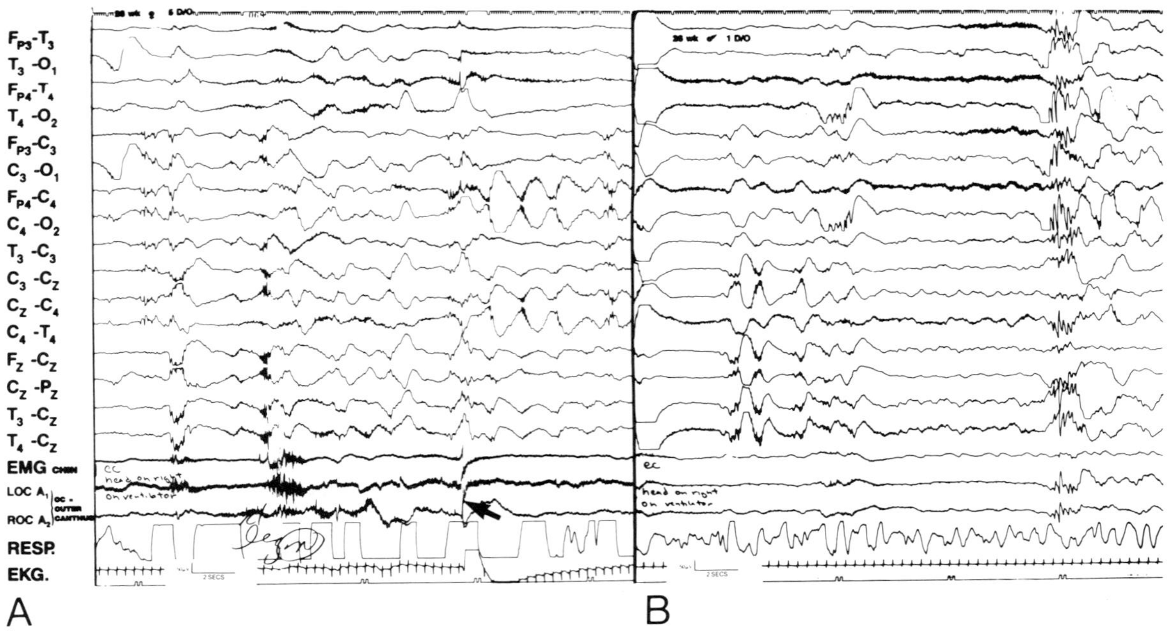

Fig. 8.1. (**A**) A 26-week, 5-day-old female. Relatively continuous background of slow and fast frequencies. Rhythmic central delta is noted with superimposed delta brushes in the same region. Asymmetric/asynchronous occipital delta activity is also noted. Prominent temporal attenuation is also seen. Myoclonic movement is indicated (arrow). (**B**) A 26-week, 1-day-old male. Discontinuous background activity consisting of central and vertex delta slow activity with super-imposed delta brushes. Diffuse theta bursts with occasional occipital theta bursts are also noted.

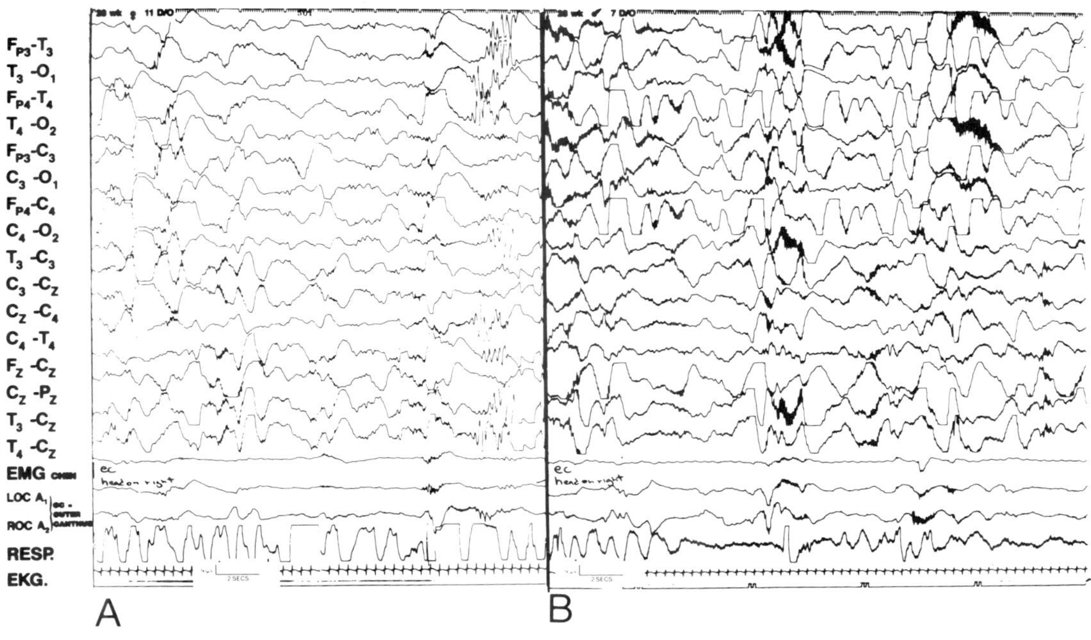

Fig. 8.2. (**A**) A 28-week, 11-day-old female (ca. 29.5 weeks). Largely continuous background activity with predominant delta slowing. More active temporal activity including prominent temporal theta bursts. Delta brushes are seen in the occipital and vertex regions as well. (**B**) A 28-week, 7-day-old male (ca. 29 weeks). Rhythmic occipital delta in different head regions, with prominent temporal delta brushes. Periodic breathing is noted in the respiratory channel.

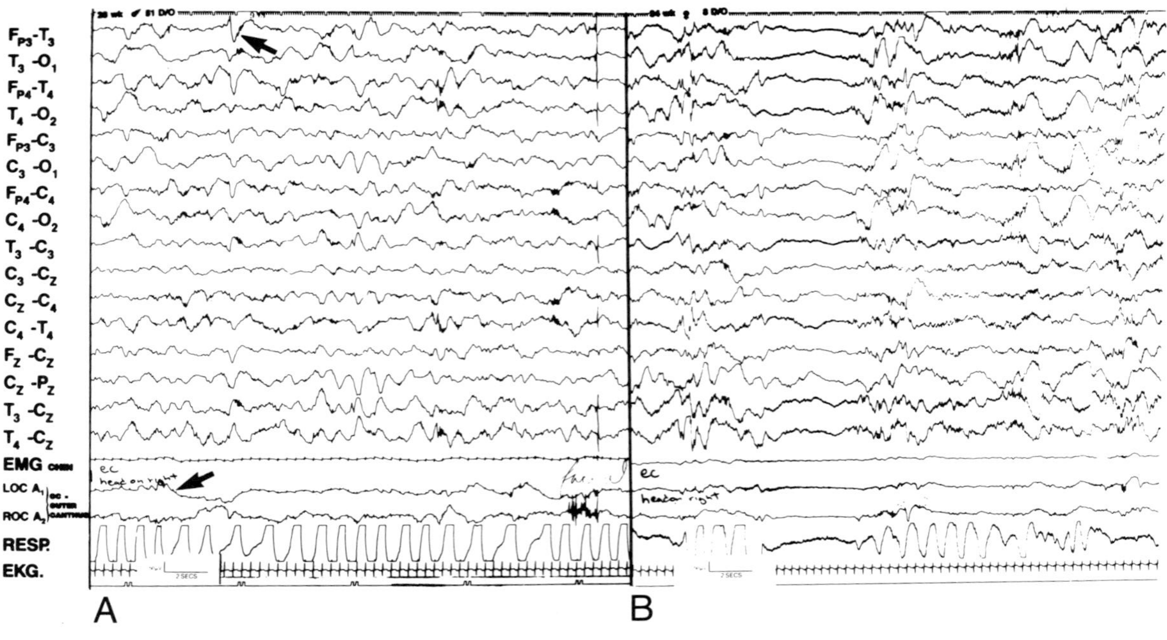

Fig. 8.3. (**A**) A 28-week, 51-day-old male (ca. 35 weeks). Continuous background activity which is appropriately lower amplitude for the corrected age. This activity consists of fast frequencies with delta brushes in multiple head regions. An isolated frontal sharp wave is present, as well as rapid eye movements. (**B**) A 34-week, 8-day-old female (ca. 35 weeks). Discontinuous background with age-appropriate, short interburst intervals. Very rhythmic occipital delta with good interhemispheric synchrony. Periodic breathing noted in the respiratory channel.

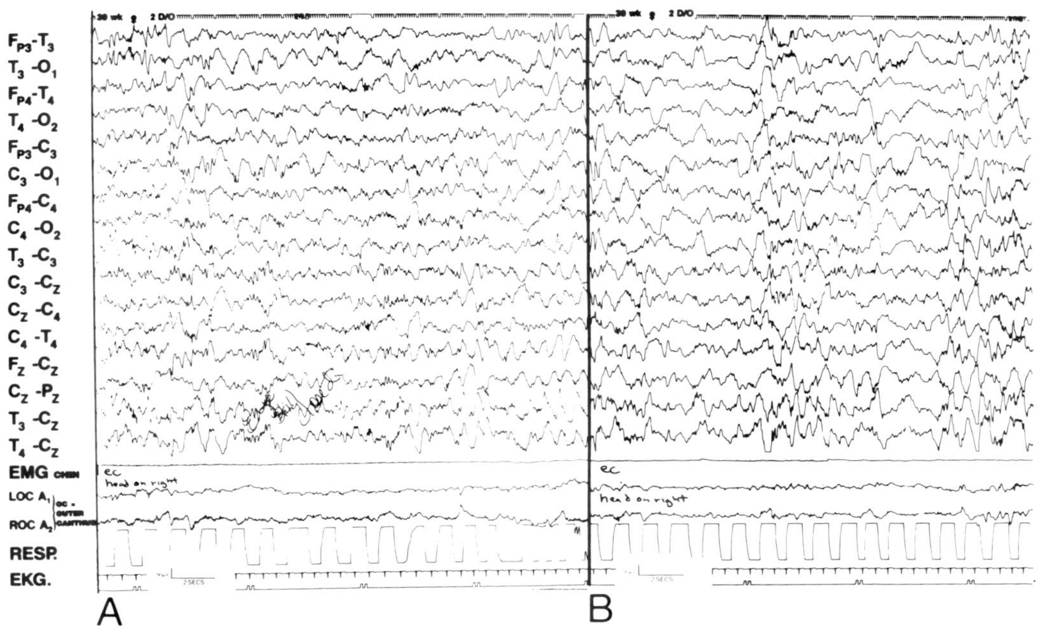

Fig. 8.4. (**A**) A 39-week, 2-day-old female. High-voltage slow (HVS) pattern of quiet sleep with scattered sharp waves, particularly in the temporal regions. Regular respirations with no movements are noted in the polygraphic channels. (**B**) A 39-week, 2-day-old female. Trace' alternant (TA) pattern of quiet sleep with synchronous high-amplitude bursts, age-appropriate brief interburst intervals, and a well-developed background. Agreement with the polygraphic criteria of sleep for respirations and movements.

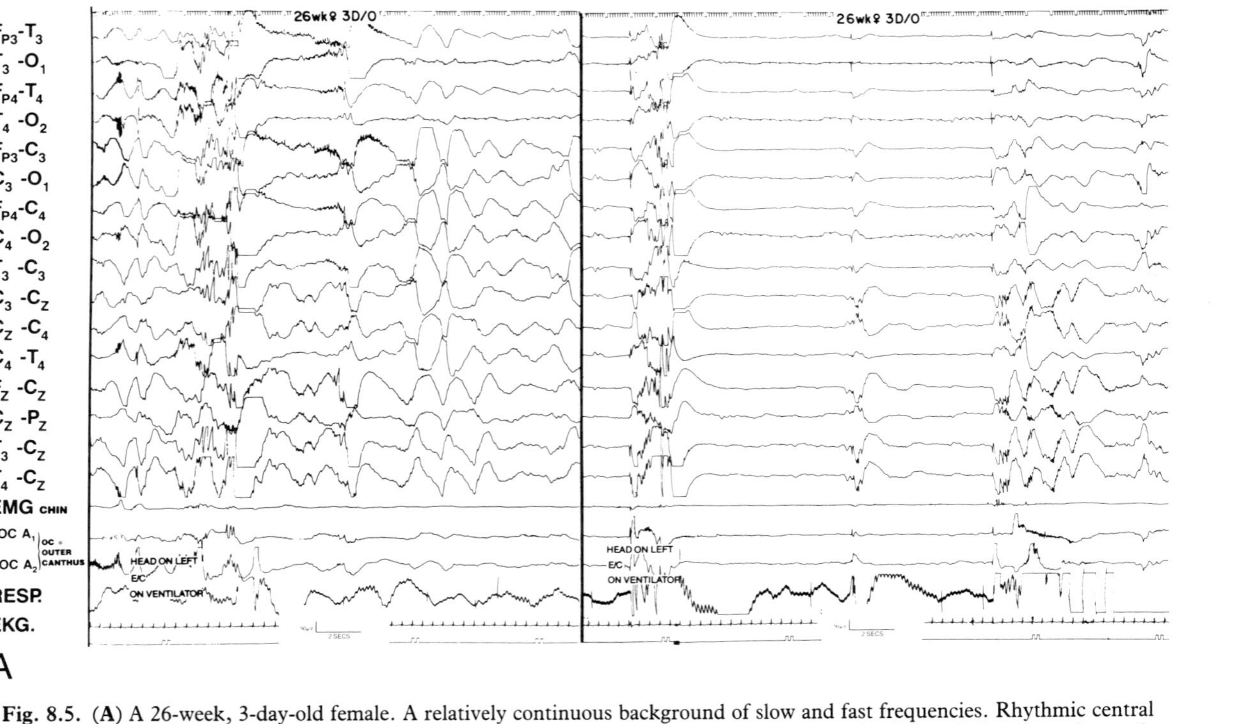

Fig. 8.5. (**A**) A 26-week, 3-day-old female. A relatively continuous background of slow and fast frequencies. Rhythmic central delta is prominent, with superimposed, widespread theta bursts. Prominent temporal attenuation is noted. Interburst intervals do not exceed 40 seconds, and there is good interhemispheric synchrony. Delta brush patterns are seen at the vertex and central regions. (*Figure continues.*)

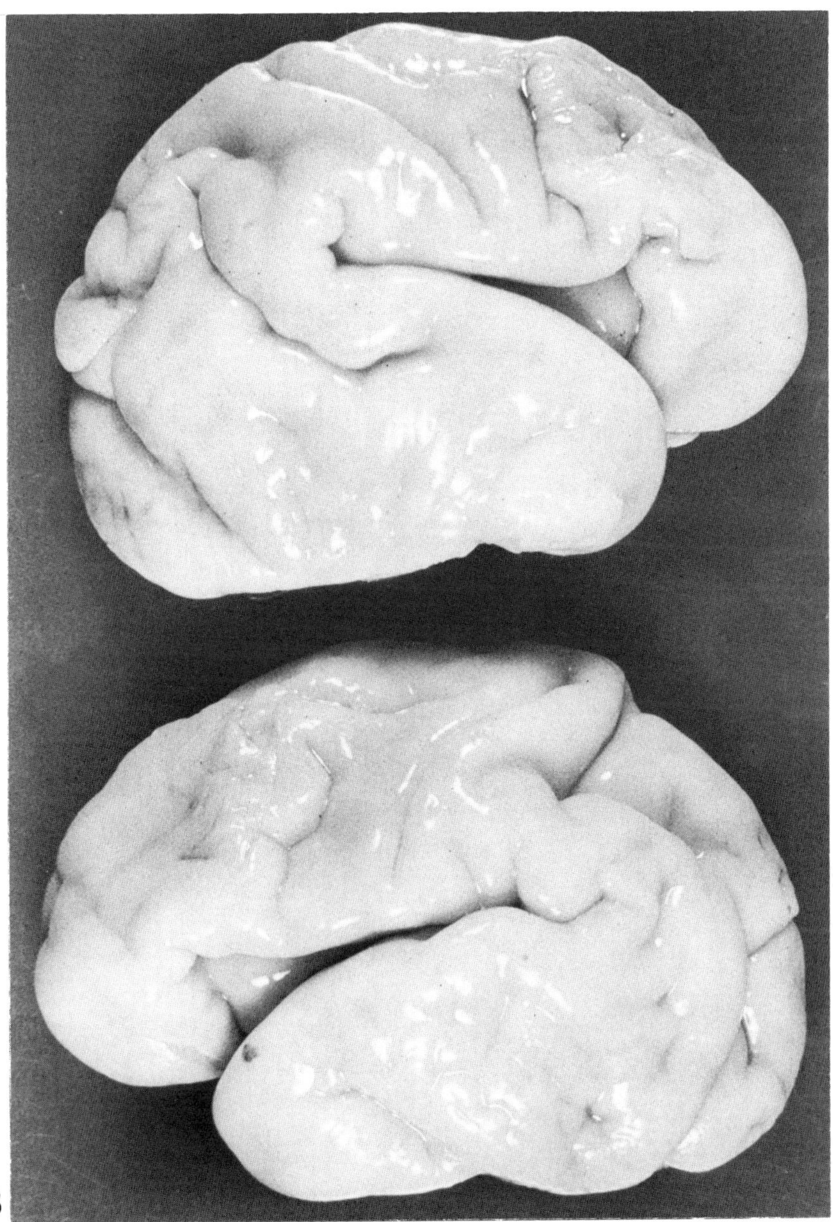

Fig. 8.5 (*Continued*). (**B**) Lateral view of brain of the patient in **A**. Prominent appearance of the insula with underdevelopment of the temporal pole and inferior frontal lobe. Age-appropriate underdevelopment of the major gyral landmarks, including rolandic, superior temporal, and calcarine gyri.

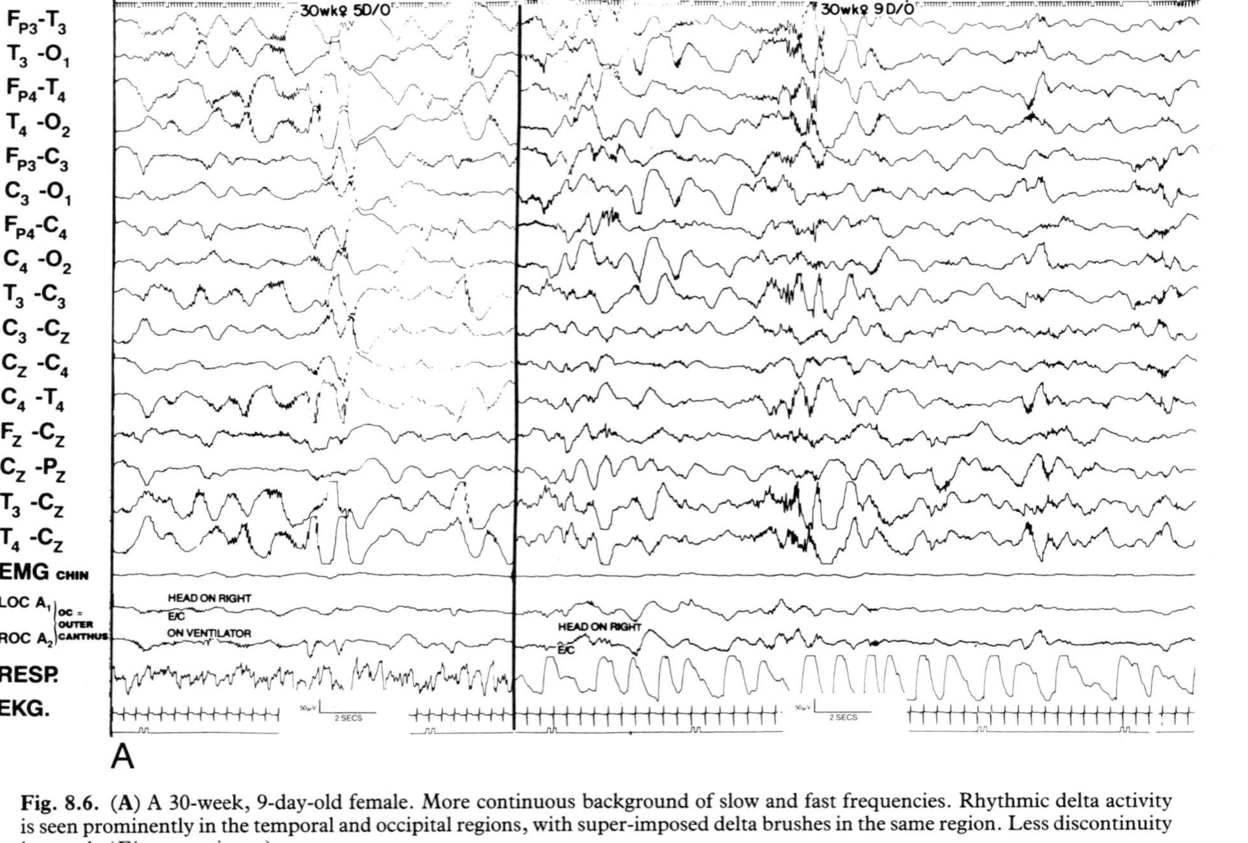

Fig. 8.6. (**A**) A 30-week, 9-day-old female. More continuous background of slow and fast frequencies. Rhythmic delta activity is seen prominently in the temporal and occipital regions, with super-imposed delta brushes in the same region. Less discontinuity is noted. (*Figure continues.*)

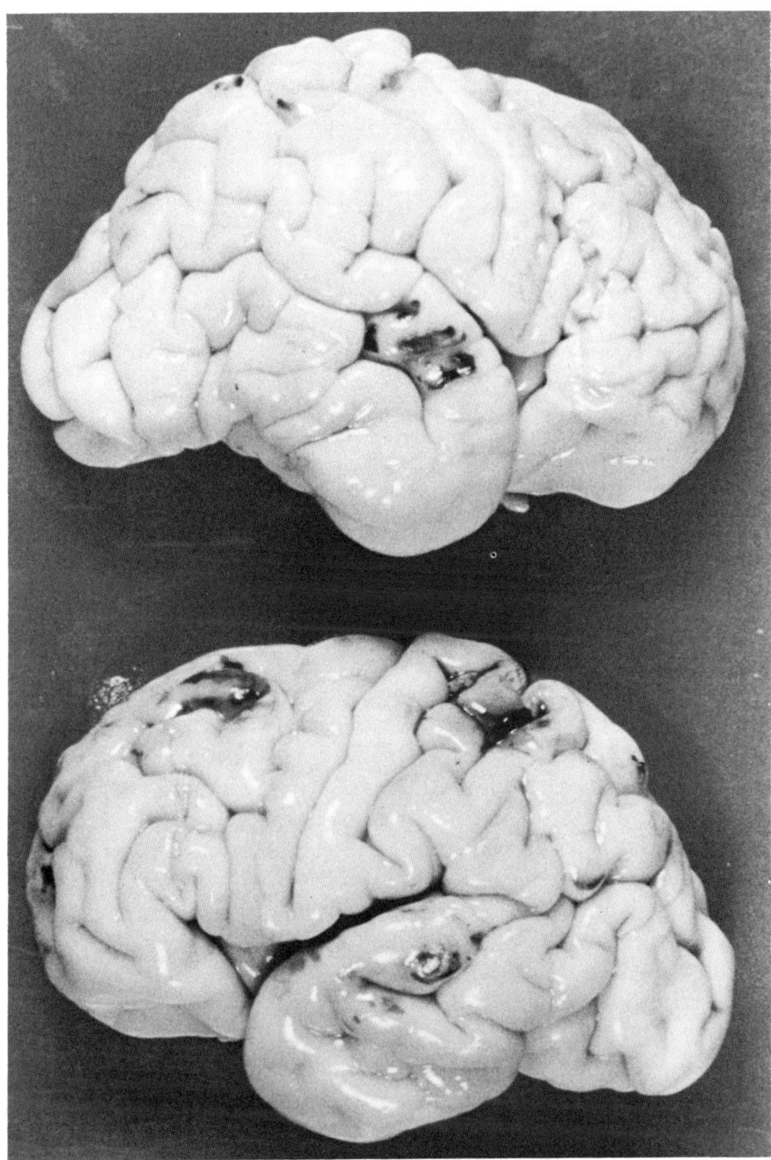

Fig. 8.6. (*Continued*). (**B**) Lateral view of brain of the patient in **A**. Increased gyral markings with less prominent view of the insula and significant elaboration of gyral pattern.

lutional measurements of the inferior frontal, superior temporal, and calcarine gyri, as well as the cytoarchitecture of various brain regions. This is compared to a 70 percent agreement between three clinical parameters for estimating gestational age (i.e., last maternal menstrual period, fetal ultrasonography, and neonatal examination criteria suggested by Ballard) and convolutional measurements. Examples of changing EEG patterns and anatomic changes are illustrated in Figures 8-5 and 8-6.

Table 8-1. Major EEG Abnormalities

	Near Term and Full Term[a] (36–41+ weeks)	Preterm[b] (30–36 weeks)
Inactive[c]	X	X
Burst suppression	X	X
Slow[d]	X	X
Low-voltage[e]	X	
Monorhythmic	X	
No spatial/temporal organization	X	
Asymmetry	X	X (>50%)
Interhemispheric asynchrony	X	X
Abnormal superimposed patterns	X	
Focal spikes	X	X
Seizures	X	X

[a] Monod N, Pajot N. Guidasci S: The neonatal EEG: Statistical studies and prognostic value in fullterm and preterm babies. Electroencephalogr Clin Neurophysiol 32:529, 1972

[b] Tharp BR, Cukier F, Monod N: The prognostic value of the electroencephalogram in premature infants. Electroencephalogr Clin Neurophysiol 51:219, 1981

[c] Below 5 uv or isoelectric.

[d] 0.5 to 1 Hertz.

[e] Maximal 25 uv.

Assessment of Encephalopathy

Determination of the sick neonate's level of consciousness is an enormously difficult task. The limited clinical repertoire for the assessment of arousal in an immature infant, as well as the practical limitations to accurate examination of a sick patient who is confined by intubation, indwelling catheters, neuromuscular blockade, and(or) an isolette environment impede a true assessment of the state of arousal and responsiveness. Moreover, sleep states predominate for the neurologically intact neonate, with only transient periods of wakefulness. Yet it is essential to assess the level of neurologic state stability and regulation in the sick neonate. An improving or worsening trend in these mental status parameters may have important diagnostic as well as prognostic ramifications.

Numerous medical conditions can contribute to an encephalopathic state in the sick newborn, which may involve bicortical, diffuse, or multifocal brain dysfunction. Metabolic abnormalities principally related to asphyxia, seizures, intracranial hemorrhage, CNS infections, or malformations all contribute to encephalopathies in the neonate. Electroencephalographic findings can add substantially to both single and serial clinical assessments of these causes of encephalopathy. Comparison of the infant's electrical background patterns with those expected for a particular gestational or conceptional age can permit a rapid estimate of the severity of the encephalopathy. Severe electrographic disturbances have been described for preterm and full-term infants, and help establish a reference point for the neonatologist (Table 8-1). Serial EEG studies can help monitor the resolution or persistence of a particular abnormality in state, particularly in the paralyzed infant.

Persisting or worsening EEG abnormalities must be correlated with the available medical history of an infant. Both acute and chronic medical conditions can be expressed by similar EEG abnormalities. For example, a hydropic infant with significant intrauterine asphyxia secondary to placental infarction has an abnormal

EEG recording resembling that of a newborn with acute exsanguination from rupture of a velamentous insertion. Although the EEG recording is particularly sensitive to CNS effects of disease states, such electrographic findings are not pathognomonic for any specific medical condition. Accurate clinical correlations must always accompany the electrical interpretation of an EEG.

Diagnosis of Seizures

Neonatal seizures reflect significant neurologic dysfunction in the immature brain, which can be caused by a variety of factors.[41,42] Neonatal seizures remain one of the most common manifestations of neurologic disease of the newborn. Their occurrence represents a medical emergency[43] and is associated with significant morbidity and mortality.[42–45]

Despite the need for a rapid diagnosis, there are several unique aspects of this neurologic problem that impede its prompt recognition.[46] Difficulty with the diagnosis of neonatal seizures may reflect the variable and less organized clinical expression of seizures in this patient population.[44,46–49] Accepted clinical criteria[41,49] may not adequately distinguish seizure movements from pathologic but non-seizure-related movements. New classifications are being developed[46] that will hopefully improve the clinical accuracy of observation in such cases.

It has also been recognized that neonates may have seizures that go undetected unless the EEG is utilized. Some of these patients have been pharmacologically paralyzed in order to optimize their respiratory care,[50–53] while others fail to demonstrate clinical seizures despite having electrical seizures even in the absence of a paralytic agent.[46,54]

Few EEG laboratories have compared the diagnostic accuracy of the electroencephalographic and clinical identification of neonatal seizures. Seven hundred and sixty-three neonatal records were obtained on 330 neonates in our level III NICU over an 18-month period. One-hundred-and-eight records were specifically requested because of abnormal movements. During 79 percent (85/108) of the records, infants exhibited their aberrant clinical episode during an EEG recording, but only 16 percent of the records (14/85) exhibited coincident electrographic seizures. Sustained clonic movements were the most predictive clinical parameter of coincident electrographic seizures, while tremors, tonic, or myoclonic movements were the least helpful.

This problem in recognition suggests the possibility of both underestimating and overestimating the incidence of this neurologic condition. Previous studies found the incidence of clinical seizures to be from 0.2 to 1.4 percent in live-born infants.[55,56] There have been no reports of the incidence rates of EEG-confirmed seizures among neonatal patients admitted to an NICU. For this reason, the EEG diagnosis of seizures at Magee-Womens Hospital (MWH) was monitored for a 3-year period to assess the contribution made by EEG to the overall diagnosis of neonatal seizures.[54] During this period, 30,823 live-born infants were delivered at MWH, with 3,463 admissions to our level III NICU. Seventy-one neonates, or 2.1 percent of all admissions to the NICU (0.2 percent of all live births), were diagnosed as having at least one electrographic seizure during their hospitalization.

There were 101 EEG records with neonatal seizures for these 71 neonates (48 preterm; 23 full-term). Thirty-seven records showed both EEG and clinical seizures. Twenty-two records showing electrical seizure were seen in neonates re-

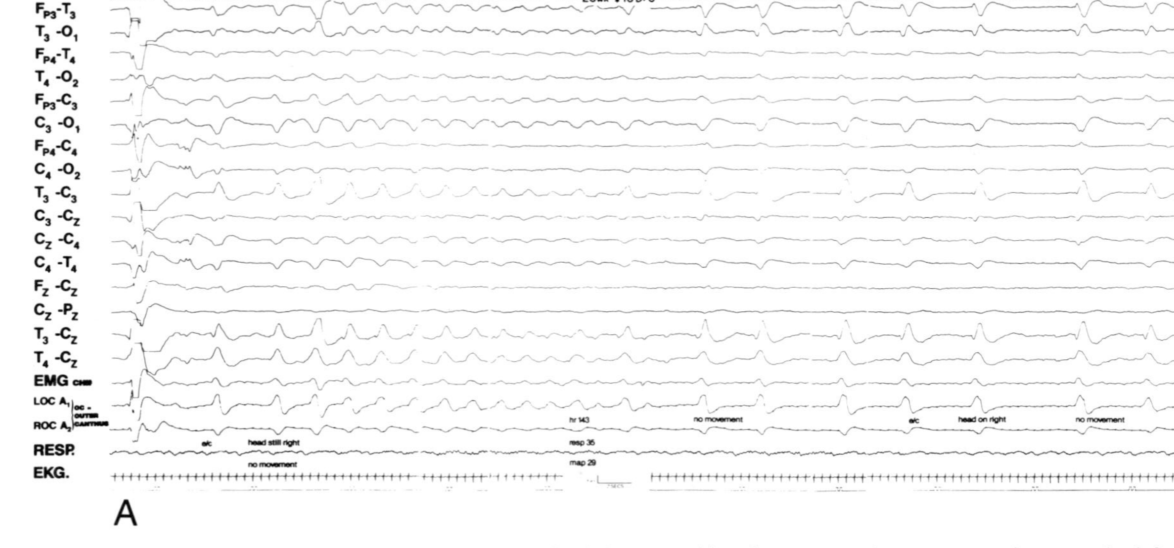

Fig. 8.7. (**A**) A 27-week, 10-day old female. A generalized electrographic seizure, somewhat more prominent on the left as compared with the right hemisphere, and of approximately 1 minute duration, consisting of rhythmic, sharply contoured delta and sharp-wave activity. (*Figure continues.*)

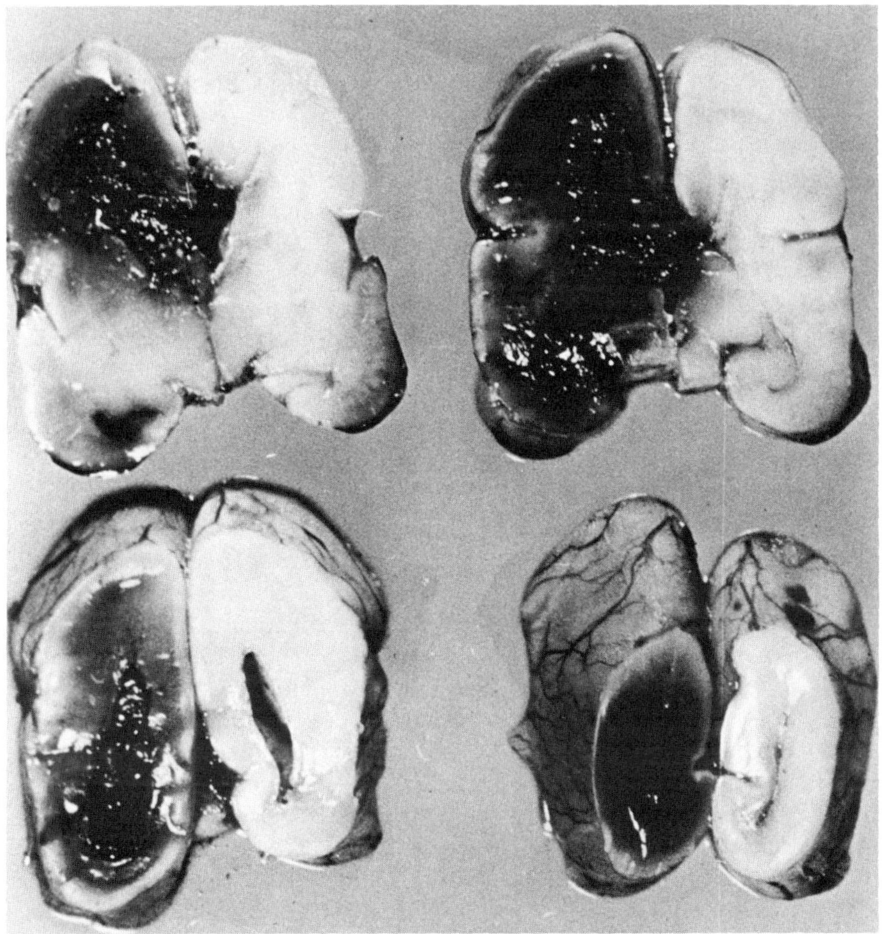

Fig. 8.7 (*Continued.*) (**B**) Coronal sections of brain of patient in **A**, showing an extensive hemorrhagic infarction involving the left hemisphere, with extravasation of blood into the ventricular space.

ceiving neuromuscular blockade. Forty-four records demonstrated electrographic seizures without clinical signs, with a majority of this last group of neonates having received at least one anticonvulsant medication. Frequent use of neonatal EEG is clearly essential for the diagnosis of seizures since, in our experience, clinical criteria are helpful in only one-third of cases for which the EEG records show electrical seizures.

It is also apparent that an EEG diagnosis of seizures correlates significantly with high morbidity and mortality based at least in part on the underlying brain injury. Over the past 3 years, 72 percent of neonates with seizures (51 neonates) at MWH had brain lesions documented by cranial CT or neuropathologic analysis.[54] More than 50 percent of these patients had unifocal or multifocal cerebral infarctions (see Fig. 8-7). Other cerebral lesions include intracerebral hemorrhage, brain abscess, and malformation. Seizures may be confined to one region of the brain, such as the midline, requiring the careful placement of electrodes. One-quarter of our records showing seizures demonstrated midline EEG findings, often as electrical seizures without clinical accompaniment.[57] Regardless of the location, neonates with seizures are more likely to expire. Thirty-five of our 71 neonates with seizures (49 percent) died during the neonatal period.[54]

Prompt recognition of seizures and other cerebral abnormalities in high-risk neonatal patients is essential because of the high probability of death and later neurodevelopmental difficulties in this group. Without the application of EEG analysis, many potentially treatable conditions of this type will not be rapidly and accurately diagnosed. Prospective, randomized clinical trials are necessary to ascertain: (1) whether anticonvulsant therapy for infants with electrical seizures alters the outcome, and (2) the anticonvulsant regimen that gives the optimal neurodevelopmental outcome.

Selected Diagnostic Considerations: Acquired versus Congenital Cerebral Lesions

Certain neonatal neurologic conditions may be associated with specific EEG patterns. These associations may assist in the neurodiagnostic evaluation of the high-risk neonate. Several excellent reviews of neonatal electroencephalography have previously discussed the importance of specific EEG abnormalities in various clinical situations.[32,33] This report will emphasize recent clinical correlations.

With the development of cranial ultrasonography (US) and computed tomography (CT), acquired as well as congenital lesions of the brain can be more readily detected. Ultrasound is of value in detecting these abnormalities in the antepartum period. Ultrasonographic studies have also been instrumental in the rapid bedside diagnosis of intracranial hemorrhage, ventriculomegaly, and other acquired or congenital lesions that occupy the intraventricular space or periventricular regions. Computed tomographic scans can further delineate parenchymal structures above and below the tentorium as well as in the ventricular regions. Magnetic resonance imaging further refines and extends the anatomic description of a variety of structural abnormalities.

However, these various imaging procedures may fail to detect or inadequately delineate diffuse, multifocal, or focal brain dysfunctions (with or without structural damage) because of the limits of imaging resolution, inadequate timing of the examination, or inability to transport an acutely-ill neonate to the radiology suite. Portable bedside neurophysiologic analysis equipment can therefore complement the diagnostic anatomic evaluation of the immature brain, particularly when the infant is too sick to transport outside the NICU.

Neonatal EEG has only recently been shown to be helpful in the evaluation of focal, regional, or hemispheric abnormalities of the brain.[32,58] Unfortunately, studies of this type have been primarily reported anecdotally or in single case reports. Most reports describe full-term infants; the preterm infant is discussed less frequently. Neurophysiologic and structural correlations have been offered for a variety of pathologic situations, including infarction,[32,33,59–63] intraparenchymal hemorrhage,[58,64,65] subdural hemorrhage,[33,66] cystic brain lesions,[67] meningitis,[68,69] and CNS malformations.[32,33]

Asymmetries of the EEG background are the most commonly encountered abnormalities in both congenital and acquired brain lesions. These hemispheric or regional asymmetries have been reported as either slowing[68,70–72] or attenuation[60,61,66] of the background rhythms. Some asymmetries have been contralateral to the focal radiographic abnormality, and have raised the question of whether high-amplitude slowing or attenuation is the more accurate electrographic marker. Other reports describe no EEG asymmetries[68,73] in patients with structural lesions, but the EEG recordings in these cases were either obtained at a time remote from the time of the insult, or involved recording techniques that were limited by an inappropriate paper speed and filter settings. Some observers emphasize only the occurrence or electrical location of seizures.[59,61–65] One report describes transient asymmetries in reportedly healthy neonates,[74] but no imaging studies were obtained for the verification of normal brain structure.

Despite these disagreements, careful serial EEG recordings can assist the clinician in an electroanatomic correlation with clinical findings. One report[75] describes 271 EEG studies on 58 neonates (28 preterm, 30 full-term), with 52 patients

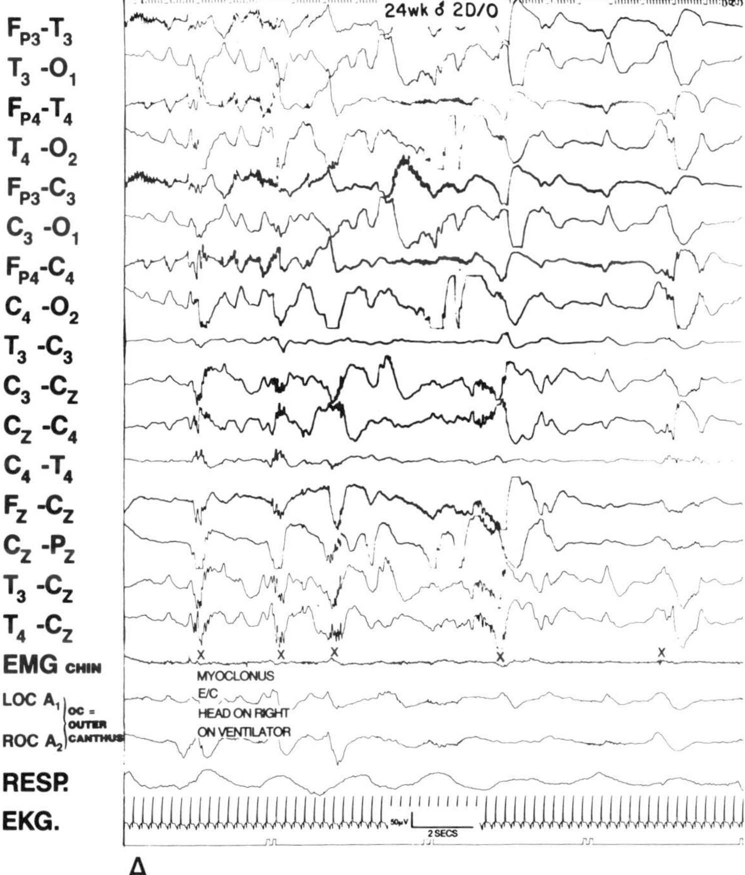

Fig. 8.8. (**A**) A 24-week, 2-day-old male. Attenuation of background in the left hemisphere (channel T_3C_3). An excessive myoclonic movement disorder was noted, as indicated by the X marks. (*Figure continues.*)

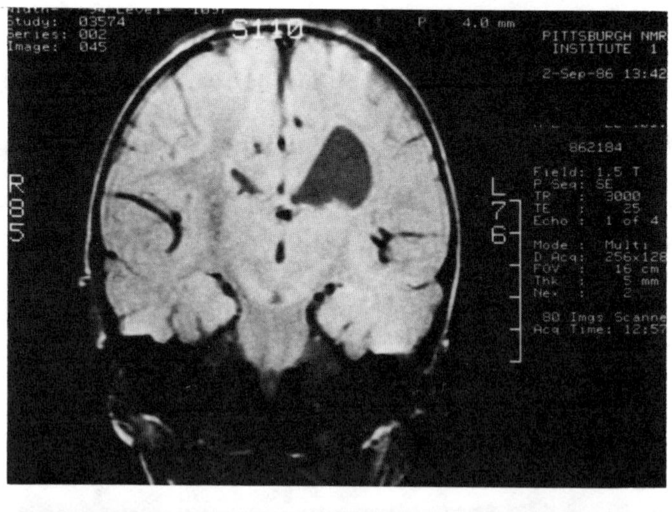

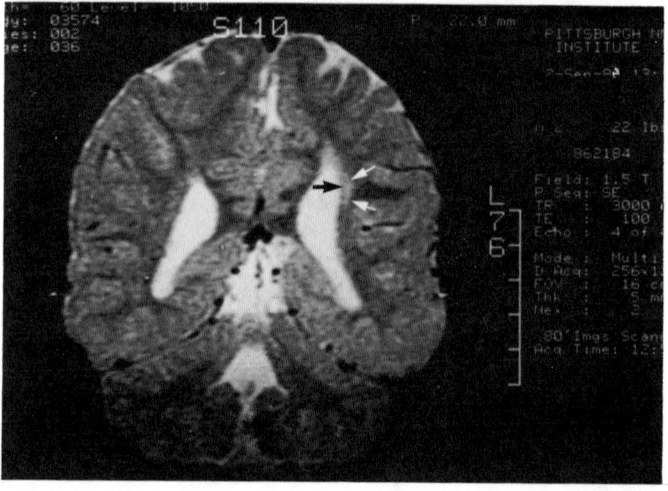

Fig. 8.8 (*Continued*). **(B)** Magnetic resonance imaging scan for the patient in **A**. Two coronal sections are shown. The upper image (a T_1 image) indicates a porencephalic cyst continuous with the left lateral ventricle. The lower image (T_2 weighted image) shows slight enlargement of the ventricular space in addition to a periventricular halo suggesting altered myelin development in the deep white matter, characteristic of periventricular leukomalacia (see arrows). (MRI images provided by Dr. James Brunberg.)

having three or four recordings over their NICU experiences. Nearly 90 percent of infants with hemorrhage or infarction had the maximum EEG abnormality on the side of the focal injury. The predominant EEG abnormality was an attenuation of background frequencies, amplitude, or both (see Fig. 8-8). The attenuation disappeared in one-fifth of these EEGs within 3 weeks, without subsequent asymmetry in some records, while increased slowing of the background developed in the same region or hemisphere in other records.

Midline EEG attenuation also indicates a cerebral lesion localized to the corresponding parasagittal or periventricular region. In a population of 60 neonates (47 preterm, 13 full-term) with midline EEG abnormalities and cerebral lesions identified on imaging tests or by neuropathologic examination, intraventricular hemorrhage was the most common hemorrhagic lesion, while periventricular leukomalacia and cerebral infarction were the most common ischemic lesions associated with a midline electrographic attenuation[57] (see Fig. 8-9).

Several patterns of electrographic abnormality in this study were correlated with midline destructive or congenital lesions. Other studies have also demonstrated the association of positive-vertex sharp waves with either intraventricular hemorrhage[57,58,76,77] (see Fig. 8-10) or periventricular leukomalacia[57,58,78] (see Fig. 8-11), and midline electrographic seizures with infarction.[57,79]

Because of the high association of cerebral lesions with these lateralized or midline electrographic abnormalities, the clinician faced with these findings is strongly advised to consider cranial imaging studies for the accurate anatomic localization of a possible lesion.

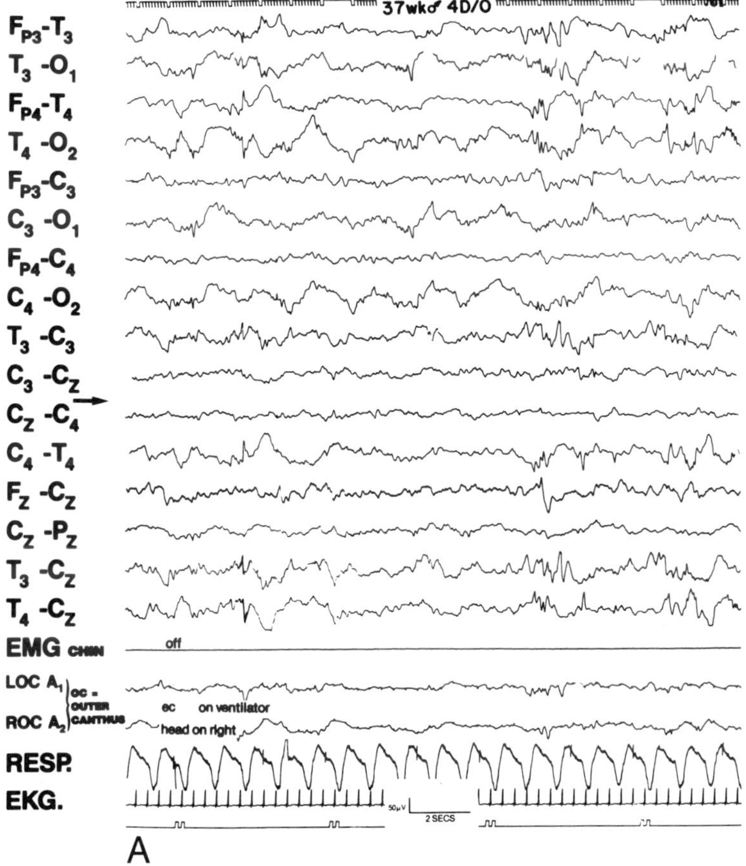

Fig. 8.9. (**A**) Electroencephalographic record of a 37-week, 4-day-old male, with attenuation of the background prominently noted at the midline (see arrow at C_Z). (*Figure continues.*)

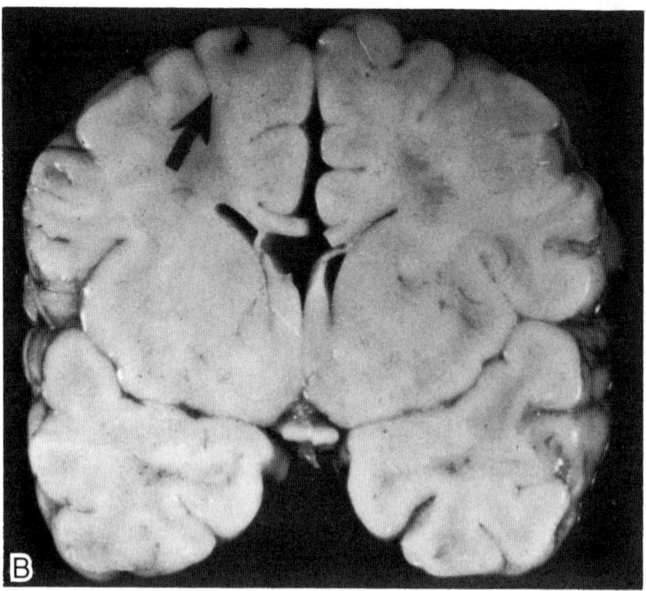

Fig. 8.9 (*Continued*). (**B**) Coronal section of brain from the patient in **A**, indicating infarction in the parasagittal region. (Scher M, Beggarty M: The value of midline electrodes in neonatal electroencephalography. Am J EEG Technol 25:24, 1985.)

Video-EEG Correlation of Seizures and Other Neonatal Behavior

Synchronized video-EEG monitoring has been applied to pediatric populations at risk for different neurologic disorders.[80] The rapid diagnosis of seizures and their subsequent therapeutic management remain the principal purpose for this technique. However, other applications include documentation of both normal and abnormal non-seizure behaviors of the child. Video-EEG analysis can better elucidate maturational issues of sleep and arousal, and assist in the description of movement disorders and the behavioral correlates of encephalopathies. It is of particular value in the long term monitoring of infants for electrographic seizures.[54]

The difficulties in rapid diagnosis of neonatal seizures are compounded by the need to verify the efficacy of their treatment. Several reports have already indicated that the recommended loading doses of phenobarbital may not stop all clinical seizure activity.[81,82] This observation is complicated by the persistence of electrical activity during neuromuscular blockade or without accompanying clinical seizure activity. One study emphasizes the large discrepancy between the clinical and EEG diagnosis of seizures in asphyxiated full-term infants who were not paralyzed.[83]

Because of the issues involved in subclinical seizure diagnosis and difficulties in the interpretation of observed clinical signs, Mizrahi and Kellaway[46] have proposed a new classification for both seizure and non-seizure behaviors with video-EEG correlations. Recent investigations utilizing bed-side electroencephalographic/polygraphic/video monitoring techniques have provided the basis for a reinterpretation of various abnormal clinical signs. Not all clinical phenomena currently considered to be seizures require electrocortical seizure activity for their initiation or elaboration. Similarities between animal models that demonstrate reflex physiology and infants with motor automatisms and opisthotonos imply that such clinical activity may not be seizure activity, but due to lack of brainstem inhibition. Although these abnormal signs may not be amenable to treatment, they reflect neurologic dysfunctions that may be relevant for diagnostic and prognostic considerations.

In addition to improved seizure detection, video-EEG monitoring offers the clinician a more accurate assessment of sleep behavior in the infant. Sleep is a complex, coordinated biologic system of different electrographic and behavioral patterns. Rapid eye movement (REM or active) and non-rapid eye movement (NREM or quiet) sleep can be clearly illustrated with synchronized video-EEG recordings. The neonatal sleep cycle, defined by two active and two quiet sleep electrographic states, involves complex behavioral alterations of eye motility and muscle tone. Important transient phenomena, including arousal, allow a transition between these states over the 40 to 60 minute sleep cycle.[24,26,32] Video-EEG monitoring can visually document the proportions of each state in a cycle, and help distinguish alterations in sleep cycling that may be related to environmental in-

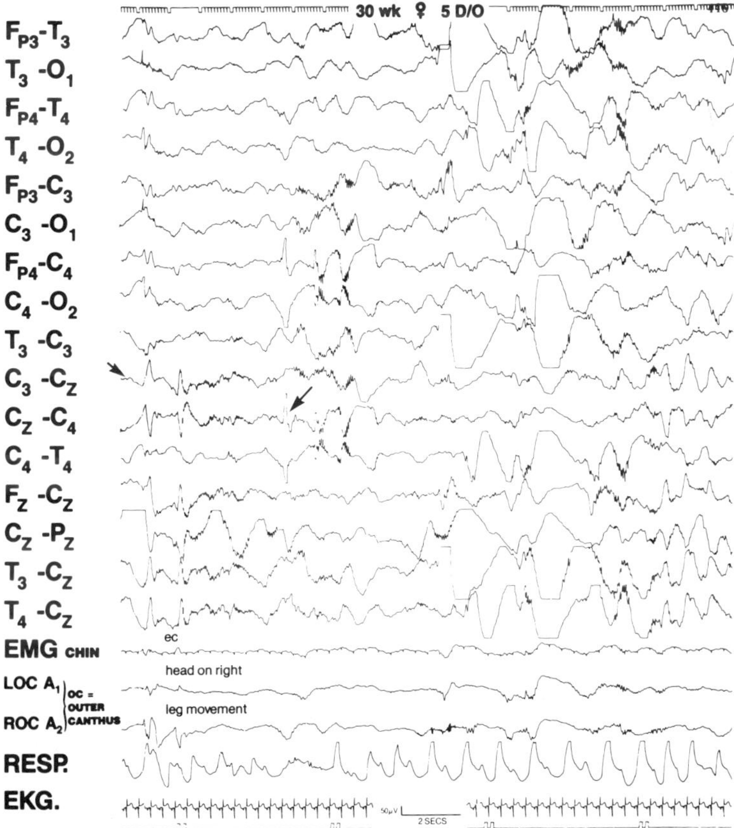

Fig. 8.10. (**A**) Electroencephalographic record of a 30-week, 5-day-old female with both vertex and rolandic positive sharp waves. (*Figure continues.*)

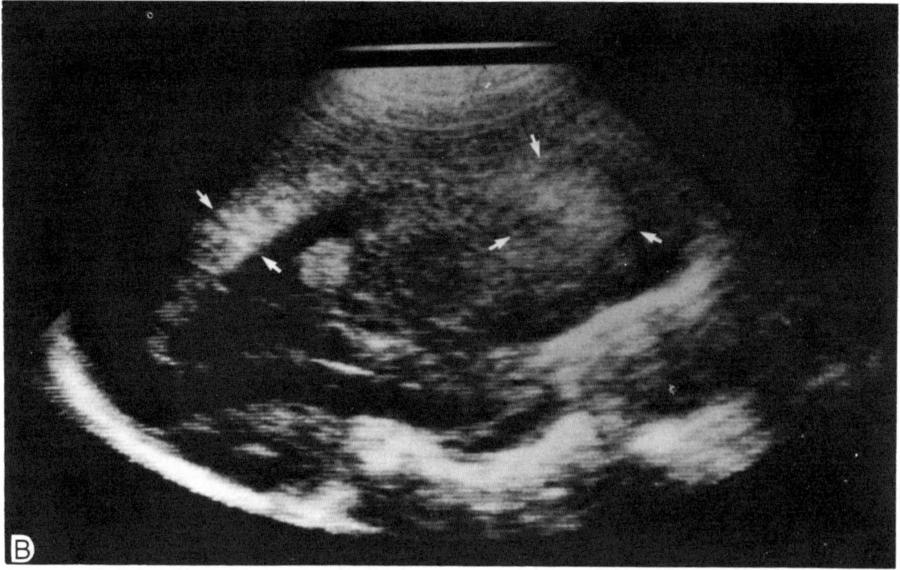

Fig. 8.10 (*Continued*). (**B**) Cranial ultrasound coronal view of the patient in **A** at 9 days of age, indicating a right intraparenchymal hemorrhage (arrows) with bilateral ventriculomegaly.

fluences, maturation, or disease states. In general, quantitative measures have now become relevant for assessing the degree and persistence of sleep-state patterns. Consequently, video-EEG monitoring will yield accurate and reproducible records for clinical review and quantitative analysis.

Assessment of Prognosis

Single or serial EEGs

Electroencephalographic studies at weekly or bimonthly intervals during the neonatal period offer greater information than can be obtained from an isolated recording session. Some reports note the prognostic significance of single recordings showing severely abnormal features in newborns with prenatal illnesses or perinatal cerebral insults,[84–86] and other reports suggest that serial studies can provide the clinician with a sensitive prognostic indication of subsequent neurodevelopmental outcome. Monod et al.[87] analyzed 691 neonatal EEGs done on 270 children whose clinical condition was documented when they were from 3 to 14 years of age. Certain EEG features were related to subsequent development. Tharp and coworkers[29] later revised these findings with respect to preterm infants. In a retrospective analysis of 184 neonatal EEGs from 81 infants born at or before 36 weeks' gestation, and subsequent clinical assessments done on 64 survivors, a single, severely abnormal record with specific pattern abnormalities was shown to be of prognostic value, while moderately abnormal records were not thought to be helpful in assessing outcome. Table 8-1 summarizes the major EEG abnormalities described in these two studies.

The value of the serial investigation of electrographic maturation has already been emphasized. Several authors have reported that persistent severe dysmaturity in relation to postconceptual age during the first months of life was associated with subsequent mental retardation or motor dysfunction.[29,88,89] Such abnormalities may be present without documented clinical abnormalities, but these same EEG findings may resolve and EEG patterns normalize, thus depriving the clinician of needed diagnostic information. Lombroso[90] has recently emphasized this issue of EEG normalization. Dunn et al.[91] prospectively studied 501 children with birthweights of 2,041 g or less and 203 control children of similar social-class distribution and birthweight. "Late neonatal" EEG records near term were compared with EEG records at 1 year and at 6¾ years of age. Since the neonatal recordings were obtained during the convalescent period after normalization of the EEG, only 27 percent remained borderline or abnormal. Only a few grossly abnormal neonatal EEG findings were considered to have grave prognostic significance. On the other hand, the abnormal EEG at 1 year of age was more useful prognostically with regard to future neurologic status and intelligence. Had the clinician been given

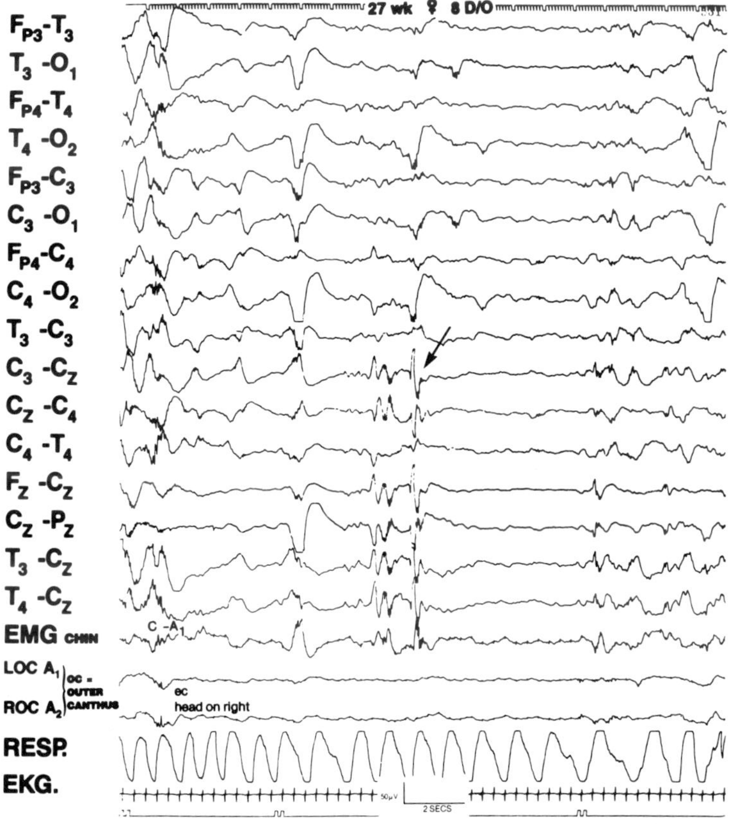

Fig. 8.11. **(A)** Electroencephalographic record of a 27-week, 8-day-old female with a vertex positive sharp wave seen at the vertex and an additional electrode (C′) 1 cm anterior to C_z (see arrow). (*Figure continues.*)

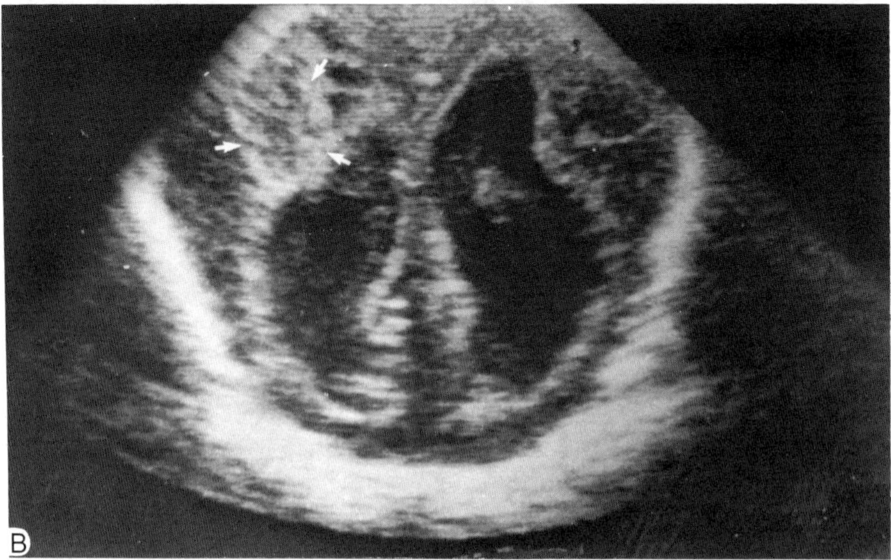

Fig. 8.11 (*Continued*). (**B**) Cranial ultrasound sagittal view of the patient in **A** indicating periventricular echogenicity diagnosed as leukomalacia (arrows).

a choice between useful interpretation of a single "late neonatal" recording or one obtained at 1 year, the latter would have been more helpful for predicting outcome. Minor EEG abnormalities documented in infants in the convalescent period who have overcome early, acute medical problems seem to have less prognostic value. The converse is also possible, in that an apparently normal newborn EEG record may not predict neurologic abnormalities at an older age.[92] In this particular study, 26 percent of 46 children who had normal neonatal EEGs were found to have neurologic sequelae on follow-up examination.

It has already been emphasized that neonatal recordings obtained early in the NICU experience should be supplemented by appropriately obtained serial studies. An additional consideration is the need for suitable normative data for the very premature neonate (less than 32 weeks and under 1,500 g), to allow appropriate comparisons with specific high-risk neonates. Earlier studies of the EEG in the very premature neonate had serious limitations: (1) they either predated the establishment of the current level III neonatal intensive care unit[93–97]; (2) lacked specific clinical data regarding accurate gestational age assessment[92–94]; (3) studied very limited numbers of preterm neonates[35,96,98,99]; or (4) lacked appropriate follow-up data with detailed cognitive and behavioral testing compared to an appropriate control group.[100]

Sleep cycling

The few comparison studies between sleep organization in preterm and term infants highlight similarities such as the shift from active to quiet sleep onset over the first 6 months of life, the disappearance of certain regional patterns in the neonatal period (e.g., frontal sharp waves), and the overall attainment of an infant sleep cycle.[99]

Yet important differences have also been noted between the structure and organization of sleep in preterm neonates followed to a full-term postconceptual age, as compared to the sleep of term infants: longer bursts during tracé alternant, the earlier appearance of sleep spindles, and more immature patterns and better phase stability in specific frequency bands than in full-term neonates.[98] The behavioral criteria of sleep are also different between the two groups.[101] These aspects suggest that sleep organization in the preterm neonate maturing to term and beyond is not entirely equivalent to that in the full-term newborn.

The traditional method of assessing sleep in the full-term newborn primarily utilizes behavioral criteria,[102] although electrical patterns have also been extensively studied.[26,27,30,32,33] This presents multiple dilemmas for the neonatal electroencephalographer interested in longitudinal, EEG-based sleep studies of healthy as compared to sick premature neonates. First, the assumption that the sleep patterns of full-term infants are the "gold-standard" of normality does not address the degree to which EEG sleep organization exists before 36 weeks of estimated gestational age. Second, failure to examine the electrical patterns of neonates prevents the interpretation of abnormal EEG patterns that may be diagnostically or prognostically relevant despite seemingly normal behavioral criteria for sleep. Finally, sufficient follow-up data do not yet exist for both seemingly healthy versus high-risk, very premature neonates (less than 32 weeks gestational age) to permit assessing the validity of EEG sleep analysis as a prognostic tool.

In summary, the current state of neonatal electroencephalography is characterized by a need for suitable normative data for the very premature neonate, so that appropriate comparisons can be made with specific high-risk groups of neonates. Longitudinal EEG studies as the neonate matures to a full-term postconceptual age will lead to more representative EEG sleep data for the premature neonate who matures to term outside the confines of the uterine environment. Well-organized, longitudinal cognitive and behavioral testing of survivors is needed to assess both intellectual deficits and behavior problems in this group of patients. With these studies, the full prognostic value of the neonatal EEG can be assessed.

EVOKED POTENTIAL ANALYSIS

An evoked potential (EP) is the electrographic response of the brain to an environmental stimulus. Each EP is represented by a sequence of waves, the amplitudes and latencies of which represent both conduction and the neuronal processing of sensory information through the CNS. Stimulus-evoked potentials have been used to assess auditory, visual, and somatosensory function. The technique involves computer averaging of the electrical potentials evoked by sound, a visual, or a somatosensory stimulus. Scalp-recorded EPs are much less apparent on paper records than on spontaneous EEGs, and the averaging technique allows the summation of numerous EPs to be time-locked to the sensory stimuli that evoke them. All random EEG activity that is not stimulus-related will cancel itself over time.

Individual component waves are identified both by polarity convention, which usually depicts negativity as an upward deflection, and by either their peak latency in milliseconds after a stimulus or their numerical order in the EP complex.

The present discussion pertains only to neonates and describes only early components of EPs, that occur within the first 50 msec after a stimulus. Intermediate components (up to 200 msec) and very slow component waves (greater than 200 msec) will not be discussed at this time because of their uncertain clinical relevance in the newborn. A more general review of these elements is available.[104]

Auditory Evoked Potentials

Since the demonstration that brainstem activity can be reproducibly recorded from the scalp,[105] various studies have solidified the concept that the series of EPs that constitute the auditory brainstem response are localized primarily in anatomically separate areas along the auditory pathway in the brainstem.

These auditory EPs can be elicited by a brief click stimulus delivered to each ear at a rate of 5 to 30/second, and the responses recorded with a single pair of scalp electrodes, often on the vertex. Seven positive wave-forms are typically generated by these stimuli; the first wave corresponds to the auditory nerve itself, while the fifth positive wave is the most easily measurable response, generated at or near the inferior colliculus.

Attempts have been made to define maturational changes in brainstem responsivity in terms of auditory EPs.[106] Analyses of various studies[107–110] allow the following generalizations: (1) the waveform and amplitude of auditory EP components depend on chronologic age, with increasing amplitudes over time; (2) while the peripheral transmission reflected by wave I matures before the subsequent waves, which represent central transmission, latencies do not reach adult values until 12 to 18 months; (3) the threshold for auditory responsivity is lower than that for auditory cortical events or that observed in behavioral testing, and similar to that for adults; and (4) different waveform components become more distinct at slower rates of stimulation, until 1 month of age.

Given these maturational correlates, auditory EPs can be judiciously applied clinically to the evaluation of suspected gross hearing impairment resulting from high-risk situations in newborns. The Joint Committee on Infant Hearing of the American Academy of Pediatrics has identified infants at risk for hearing loss. The principal clinical situations responsible for this loss include asphyxia, hyperbilirubinemia, intracranial hemorrhage, and developmental disorders. Such infants require close auditory and neuro-developmental follow-up. Auditory EPs can be a powerful tool for testing the integrity of the brainstem in this patient population, especially in the comatose neonate or the infant receiving neuromuscular blockade. One illustrative example demonstrates prolonged intra-axial latencies for auditory EPs in a comatose infant with nonketotic hyperglycinemia (see Fig. 8-12). Spongy leukodystrophy was noted on gross and microscopic examination of the infant's brain, and involved all myelinated traits, including structures subserving the auditory pathway.[111]

Visual Evoked Responses

Assessment of visual function constitutes another important aspect of neurologic evaluation of the neonate. Besides the specific information it yields about the integrity of the visual pathway, such assessment can help predict later intellectual

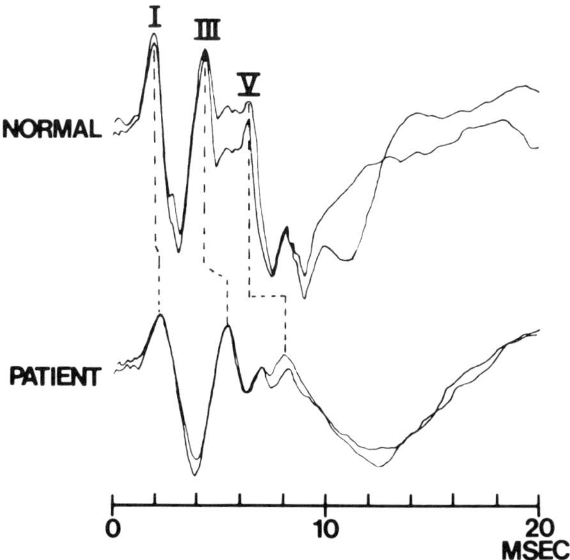

Fig. 8.12. Auditory brainstem responses to 70 dBnHL click stimuli for a normal, 38-week postconception newborn (top trace) and a patient with glycine encephalopathy (bottom trace) who was also tested at 38 weeks postconception. Dashed lines denote the difference in component wave latencies for the two infants.

performance.[112] Three techniques can assess visual processing: (1) behavioral testing,[113] (2) pattern preference testing,[114] and (3) the study of visual evoked responses (VER).[115] Only VERs will be discussed.

Visual evoked responses can be elicited by a light stimulus delivered either as a flash from a stroboscope or by a patterned checkerboard. The responses are recorded from the occipital regions of the scalp over the primary visual cortex. The checkerboard stimulus requires maintenance of fixation during testing, and flash responses have therefore been used in infants under 3 months of age. The earliest response to flash VERs is at 24 weeks' gestational age,[116] and the subsequent maturational changes in the VER waveforms have been described.[117,118] This earliest waveform is initially surface negative, and becomes surface positive only after 35 weeks' gestational age.

The most stable and readily identifiable component of the neonatal VER is a major positive waveform with a latency of approximately 190 msec. A number of investigators have verified the latency of this P2 peak, which has a rapidly decreasing latency by 2 months post-term, followed by slower changes throughout childhood.[119] Waking and sleep state may alter the latency of VERs, and it is generally recommended that VER testing be done during non-REM (quiet) sleep in newborns. Latencies can be expected to be 50 msec shorter during the waking state.[119]

Abnormal VERs can be encountered in rarely occurring, generalized neurodegenerative disorders that may involve the visual system[120] as well as in the more commonly encountered generalized brain insults such as asphyxia. Specific ischemic cerebrovascular disorders, such as cavitary periventricular leukomalacia, may result in abnormal VERs.[121] Under such clinical circumstances, crude correlations have been suggested between the severity of VER disruption and long-term neurodevelopmental outcome.[121,122] Normal flash VER results can be seen in patients with abnormal visual function. It is therefore generally recommended that patients at risk be re-evaluated with pattern VER at an older age, when their visual acuity and attention have matured. Pattern VER can be performed at 3 months of age.

Somatosensory Evoked Potentials

Somatosensory evoked potentials (SEPs) are elicited by the percutaneous electrical stimulation of peripheral nerves. The median nerve is principally used, with cerebral recording over the contralateral parietal somatosensory cortex. A complex sequence of waveforms results, with significant differences in their early components between groups of infants of different gestational age, reflecting the postnatal myelination of the sensory fibers of the central somatosensory pathway. Peripheral conduction velocities are largely within the adult range by 3 years of age, while spinal cord velocities do not attain adult values until 5 years.[124] The SEP studies that have been done in neonates and infants indicate that the first negative waveform, with a peak latency of 20 msec, is remarkably consistent in its changes over 8 years into the adult pattern. Although recording techniques and results can vary between authors, short latency SEPs in infants appear to be easily recorded and well tolerated.[125]

The SEP may assist in the localization of brain dysfunction by reflecting the integrity of the dorsal column-medial lemniscal system. Abnormal SEPs may suggest impairment and a less favorable prognosis for specific high-risk groups, such as children at risk for hemiplegia[126] or preterm neonates surviving periventricular hemorrhage.[125] In addition, SEP abnormalities associated with lesions of the spinal cord, brain lesions due to malformation,[127,128] or neurodegenerative disease[129] may prove helpful in formulating a prognostic statement.

COMPUTER ANALYSES

Computer techniques have recently been applied to clinical neurophysiologic testing. The principal purpose for this has been to extend the information derived from the visual interpretation of scalp-generated EEG activity. Spectral analysis is the technique most often used. Computerized spectral analysis distinguishes wavelength components in the EEG background by the use of Fourier analysis and the fast Fourier transform algorithm. This frequency-specific automated data can then be analyzed in a variety of ways.

Topographic EEG Mapping

One computer technique makes use of the different, topographically represented EEG frequency ranges for distinct regions of the scalp. Power or voltage distributions can be displayed for these frequency ranges, as represented by the overlying scalp-generated EEG activity. Either spontaneous or evoked EEG activity can be topographically represented on a computer-generated printout as a color-coded contour map of EEG power. Preliminary studies of topographic EEG analyses in diverse clinical populations have recently been discussed.[130] The pediatric target groups for such analyses include both normal premature and high-risk neonates.

In one report,[131] apparently healthy infants were subjected to detailed behavioral assessments outside the hospital setting. Differences in behavioral characteristics were found between healthy premature infants and control infants. The premature group also had altered topographical EEG activity when aroused from a drowsy to an alert state. An excessive abundance of delta-range slow activity persisted in the frontal and central regions among the premature infants. This group also demonstrated less ability to maintain attention in the alert state. These observations led the authors to speculate that preterm birth in some infants alters regional EEG mapping in frontal brain regions, leading to a higher risk for attentional deficits at an older age.

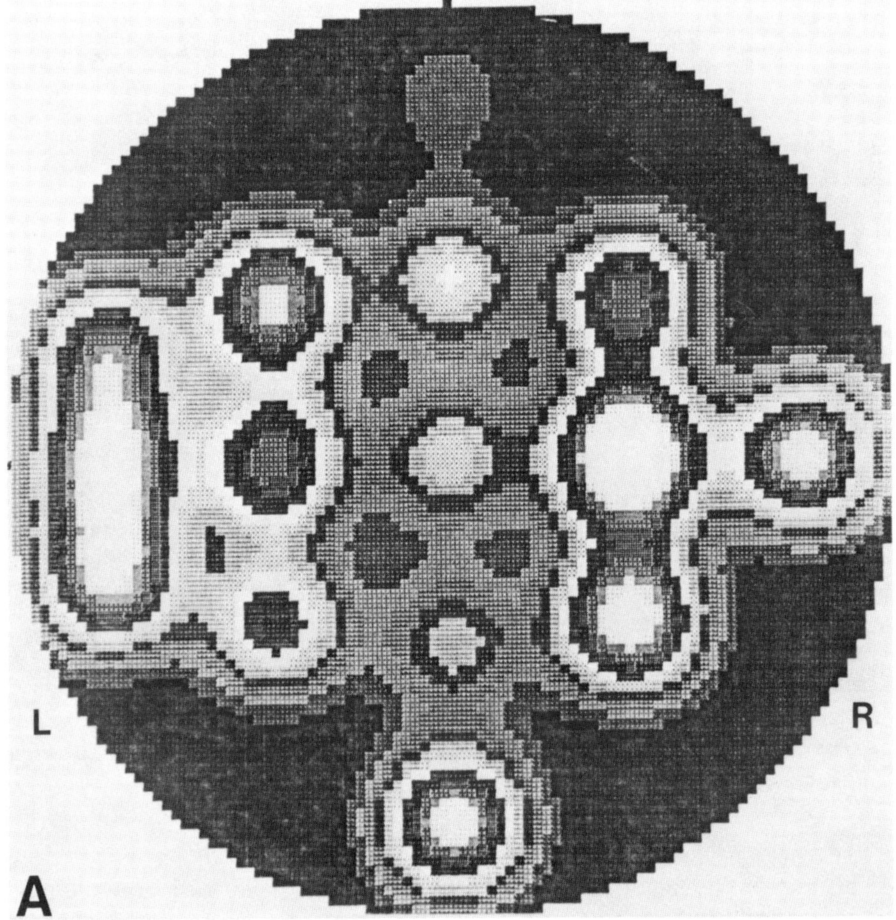

Fig. 8.13. A A 25-week, 97-day-old female. A black-and-white representation of a color-coded EEG computed tomography scan. Significant asymmetry of delta frequency power with a signal in the left temporal region greater than in the frontal region. There is a decreased delta signal in the central parietal region (*Figure continues.*)

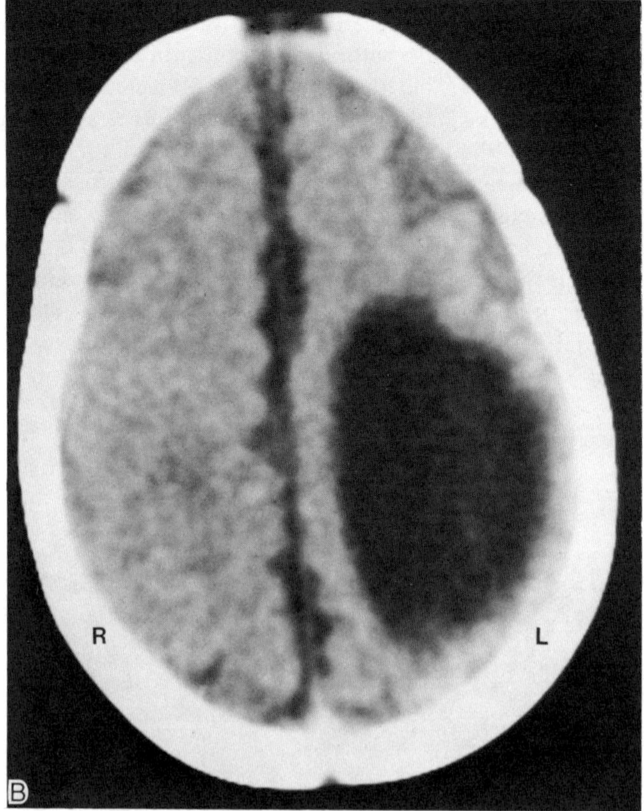

Fig. 8.13 (*Continued*). (**B**) Computed tomographic scan of the patient in **A** at 120 days of life, indicating extensive encephalomalacia of the left hemisphere.

Another report[132] describes topographic EEG mapping applied to electroencephalographic maturational studies at postconceptual ages ranging from 31 to 44 weeks in healthy infants, and compares the findings to those in abnormal infants. An anterior-posterior difference in EEG development was observed in newborns, with dominant patterns in the occipital region at 31 weeks, whereas frequencies were dominant in central regions at 44 weeks. The authors suggest that EEG analyses of this type in infants will correspond with documented brain lesions on imaging studies. Figure 8-13 illustrates such a comparison. An asymmetric topographic EEG map for a newborn, with increased slow activity in the left hemisphere, correlates with an extensive area of encephalomalacia.

Coherence and Periodicity Analyses

Other uses for the computer analysis of neonatal EEG activity include investigations of biorhythm data in which EEG activity is compared with other physiologic signals. Coherence and periodicity analyses are techniques utilizing power spectral analysis in studying developmental aspects of EEG and sleep organization. Although this technique has to date been largely confined to full-term neonates and young infants,[133–138] it appears to be a potentially useful approach in premature infants.

The periodicity of sleep cycles within a sleep session and the concept of coalescence between physiologic signals have emphasized the importance of maturational relationships of EEG sleep in healthy infants.[135] Coalescence means that each member of a pair of signals reflects the periodic activity of the other either directly or reciprocally. Using coherence analysis, this relationship can be quantified. These relationships are not readily apparent by visual analysis, but may be definable using mathematical algorithms such as time-series, cluster, or coherence analyses. It would seem appropriate to use these measures to study EEG sleep patterns in the preterm neonate maturing to a full-term postconceptual age.

Existing EEG data and behavioral criteria for sleep state definition suggest that in the premature neonate younger than 36 weeks estimated gestational age, agreement is lacking between the EEG and behavioral characteristics of active and quiet sleep.[102] More specifically, the polygraphic signals of muscle tone, REMs, respiration pattern, and body movements more accurately define active and quiet sleep than does the EEG signal.[102] This lack of agreement or "coalescing" between EEG and behavioral criteria may prove more apparent than true if computer measures are applied to the evolving EEG-sleep rhythms of the preterm neonate as the infant matures. An ultradian cycle of 40 to 60 minutes may exist in the premature neonate, beginning at 36 weeks estimated gestational age, much as in the full-term neonate.[26,96,137] Computer analysis may help confirm spatiotemporal patterns within and between hemispheres over one or more of these cycles in the preterm neonate, as has already been demonstrated in the full-term neonate.[98,136] In a recent study, Scholten[139] applied periodicity and coherence principles to the analysis of EEG, motility, and other physiologic signal for the newborn.

DEVELOPMENTAL CHRONOBIOLOGY

The ontogenic study of different biorhythms in the neonate and young infant has recently been reviewed[134,140]; interesting interrelationships exist between EEG measures of sleep state, rapid eye movements, arousal, and motility over a single sleep cycle and longitudinally, when compared with age. Although the circadian timing is not established for these and other rhythmic functions for several months beyond birth,[141,142] important phase and amplitude relationships may exist as ultradian rhythms in the preterm neonate.

Rapid eye movements

Rapid eye movements (REMs) represent one of the main identifying features of active sleep. Active sleep constitutes most of the 1-hour sleep cycle for both preterm and full-term neonates, although REMs apparently do not become "timelocked" to the continuous EEG activity of active sleep until 36 weeks estimated gestational age. In the full-term neonate, REMs do not represent a random rhythm,[143] but have predictable intervals of occurrence.[144] Although both active sleep and the duration of REM periods shorten with age, the number of REMs does not decrease but rather increases.[145] This also occurs in fetal life, independently of extrauterine influences, even at a premature age.[146] There may be different classes of REMs in the preterm infant, as has been already noted for the full-term infant.[147] In the full-term neonate, the burst duration of REMs, or the appearance of REM activity during a specific portion of active sleep, helps classify different types of REMs. No studies of neonatal sleep in preterm infants have attempted to study rapid eye movements with respect to their temporal distribution during the maturation of sleep patterns.

Arousal and motility

Attention to movement patterns as well as to arousal patterns in the newborn is an intricate part of the sleep state assessment for these infants.[24] Different motility patterns appear at successive neonatal ages up to a full-term age, with myoclonic and whole-body movements predominating in the preterm infant.[148–150] Smaller, slower body movements predominate in the full-term infant. Attention to the specific portion of the sleep cycle in which movements occur is important, since movements will differ in different portions of the cycle for the same infant.[150] Predictive motility patterns have also been noted in ultrasonographic fetal studies showing a similar developmental pattern prior to birth.[151] Spontaneous behaviors, including motility and arousal, appear to have gender differences, at least in the full-term infant,[152] and such behaviors may reflect the developing autonomic nervous system.[153] While motility is a biorhythm closely linked to the REM portion of the sleep cycle,[154] it also has an intrinsic periodicity of its own.[155] The clinical application of motility and arousal measurements is still both recent and quite limited in terms of the number of newborns studied. Quantitative as well as qualitative differences in the number of arousals have been seen in patients with severe neurologic damage as compared to a control group.[156,157] Furthermore, the development of spontaneous arousal and the responsiveness of arousal to stress appear to be important protective mechanisms during sleep, and may be deficient in certain disorders, such as near-miss sudden infant death syndrome.[158] Clearly, more systematic investigation is needed of the development of motility and arousal as they relate to the evolution of the EEG sleep cycle in preterm infants maturing to full-term postconceptual age.

Sleep organization may exist in unique ways in the preterm neonate maturing towards term as compared to the full-term infant. This organization may be better understood through the study of ultradian (high-frequency) rhythms. Since rapid eye movements, arousal, and motility all appear to fluctuate significantly relative to the high-frequency neonatal sleep-wake cycle of 40 to 60 minutes, there may be unique interrelationships of phase, amplitude, and period between various physiological components within the sleep cycle prior to the later establishment of circadian rhythms of sleep. These biorhythms appear to be more easily identified and expressed through computer analysis.[135]

Applications of biorhythm analysis to specific groups of high-risk infants have only recently been investigated. Seven-hour waking and sleep periods were assessed in infants awaiting adoption,[159] in order to evaluate the degree of stability of EEG-state organization as a possible predictive measure of neurologic outcome. Infants with less well organized state stability profiles later demonstrated poor neurodevelopmental outcome, while well-organized state profiles were noted for infants who were normal on follow-up. Lombroso[159] strongly suggests that waking as well as sleep states must be evaluated to more fully assess the infant's behavioral states.

Other reports have analyzed specific segments of the neonatal ultradian sleep cycle in order to assess sleep architecture and continuity as well as sleep-state stability in this population. Beckwith and Parmelee,[160] in an elegant prospective longitudinal study, followed 53 preterm infants with transient respiratory difficulties to a corrected term age. Analysis of their sleep data indicated that the amount of quiet sleep segment, tracé alternant (TA), may help predict neurodevelopmental outcome at 8 years of age. The authors, however, emphasized that decreased amounts of TA activity correlated with lower IQ scores only in those children who had a less enriched social environment. A reduced TA activity may indicate either a transient or more persistent deviation in neurodevelopment, depending on the individual's interactions with its environment, consisting largely of its parent-fam-

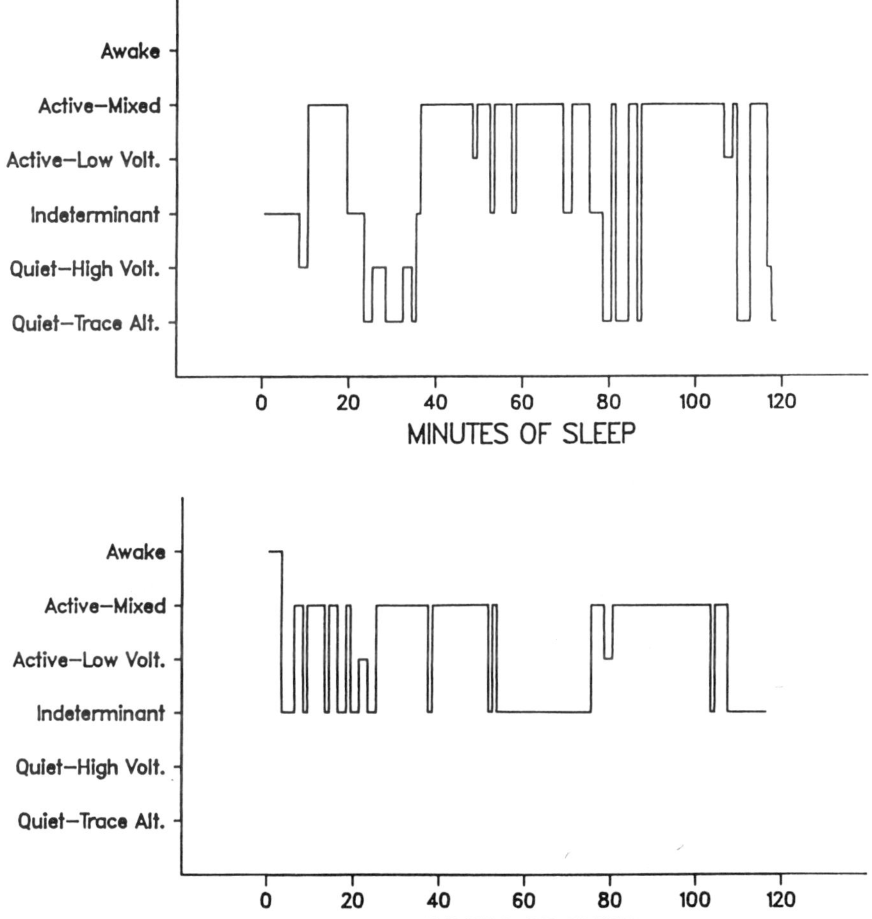

Fig. 8.14. (**A**) A normal sleep cycle for a term infant, illustrating smooth cycling between active and quiet sleep segments. (**B**) An abnormal example of a sleep cycle for a term infant, illustrating no quiet sleep and excessive transitional or indeterminate sleep.

ily support system. A reduced TA activity may be a biologic marker for potential neurodevelopmental delay if environmental conditions are suboptimal. This concept is indeed provocative, and continues to suggest the important influence of early environmental stimulation for the infant, within the limits of CNS plasticity and specific brain insults (see Ch. 9).

Similar findings have been reported in other groups of infants who have suffered either antepartum or postpartum stress to the brain.[161,162] Detailed scorings of 120 minutes of EEG sleep have been analyzed using standardized coding forms that document EEG sleep state, arousal, motility, and REM density in two groups of full-term infants born to mothers who used alcohol or marijuana during pregnancy. Another group of preterm neonates, with broncho-pulmonary dysplasia (BPD), was also studied with the same EEG-based sleep analysis system at a corrected term age. Significant correlations were noted between maternal substance abuse or BPD and an increased percentage of time spent in indeterminate (or transitional) sleep and a decreased percentage of time in tracé alternant, as compared to controls. In addition, an increased total number and duration of arousals were also observed for these two diverse groups of high-risk infants as compared to control infants. Examples of both normal and abnormal sleep cycles for two full-term neonates (see Fig. 8-14) contrast the smooth cycling between active and quiet sleep for the normal infant with the lack of quiet sleep and excessive indeterminate sleep for the abnormal infant. Long term neurodevelopmental follow-up of these infants is now in progress, to determine whether these sleep-state abnormalities persist and are predictive of poor neurodevelopmental outcome. Although disruptions of sleep architecture are not pathognomonic for specific disease states, their study can be adapted to many types of clinical situations because of its sensitivity. Clearly, the analysis of sleep-state organization, both in terms of stability and continuity, could assist the clinician in planning appropriate, early stimulation programs for children considered at risk for neurodevelopmental problems.

SUMMARY AND CONCLUSIONS

Tremendous strides in the care of high-risk neonates have resulted in their improved survival. Appropriate concern for neurodevelopmental sequelae in these survivors is increasing. The establishment of developmental neurophysiology laboratories within neonatal intensive care units offers an opportunity to better identify infants at risk for neurodevelopmental sequelae, and a chance to design new methods of treatment and prevention. The study of evoked potentials and the analysis of biorhythms complement sophisticated brain imaging by MRI and PET, by refining our descriptions of brain structure and function. A high quality of continuous diagnostic and therapeutic care for high-risk infants remains the highest priority in both their acute and convalescent care.

ACKNOWLEDGMENTS

Supported in part by The Twenty-Five Club of Magee-Womens Hospital, the Richard King Mellon Foundation, grants NIAAA 06666-01, NIDA 03874, and NINCDS 01110-01A1 to Mark S. Scher. Ms. Diane Minsterman typed the manuscript.

REFERENCES

1. Drillien CM, Thompson AJM, Burgoyne K: Low-birthweight children at early school-age: A longitudinal study. Dev Med Child Neurol 22:26, 1980
2. Nickel RE, Bennett FC, Lamson FN: School performance of children with birth weights of 1,000 g or less. Am J Dis Child 136:105, 1982
3. Hack M, Caron B, Rivers A, Fanaroff AA: The very low birth weight infant: The broader spectrum of morbidity during infancy and early childhood. Dev Behav Pediatr 4:243, 1983
4. Michelsson K, Lindahl E, Parre M, Helenius M: Nine-year follow-up of infants weighing 1500 g or less at birth. Acta Paediatr Scand 73:835, 1984
5. Ford GW, Rickards AL, Kitchen WH, et al: Handicaps and health problems in 2 year old children of birth weight 500 to 1500 g. Aust Paediatr J 21:15, 1985
6. Vohr BR, Garcia Coll CT: Neurodevelopmental and school performance of very low-birth-weight infants: A seven-year longitudinal study. Pediatrics 76:345, 1985
7. Rantakallio P, von Wendt L: Prognosis for low-birthweight infants up to the age of 14: A population study. Dev Med Child Neurol 27:655, 1985
8. Eilers BL, Desai NS, Wilson MA, Cunningham MD: Classroom performance and social factors of children with birth weights of 1,250 grams or less: Follow-up at 5 to 8 years of age. Pediatrics 77:203, 1986
9. Coolman RB, Bennett FC, Sells CJ, et al: Neuromotor development of graduates of the neonatal intensive care unit: Patterns encountered in the first two years of life. Dev Behav Pediatr 6:327, 1985
10. Edwards MK, Brown DL, Muller J, et al: Cribside neurosonography: Real-time sonography for intracranial investigation of the neonate. AJNR 1:501, 1980
11. Hill LM, Breckle R, Gehrking WC: The prenatal detection of congenital malformations by ultrasonography. Mayo Clin Proc 58:805, 1983
12. Pape KE, Bennett-Britton S, Szymonowicz W, et al: Diagnostic accuracy of neonatal brain imaging: A postmortem correlation of computed tomography and ultrasound scans. J Pediatr 102:275, 1983
13. Rumack CM, Manco-Johnson ML, Manco-Johnson MJ, et al: Time and course of neonatal intracranial hemorrhage using real-time ultrasound. Radiology 154:101, 1985
14. Johnson MA, Pennock JM, Bydder GM, et al: Clinical NMR imaging of the brain in children: Normal and neurologic disease. AJR 141:1005, 1983
15. Gooding CA, Brasch RC, Lallemand DP, et al: Nuclear magnetic resonance imaging of the brain in children. J Pediatr 104:509, 1984
16. Hope PL, Cady EB, Tofts PS, et al: Cerebral energy metabolism studied with phosphorus NMR spectroscopy in normal and birth-asphyxiated infants. Lancet 1:366, 1984
17. Volpe JJ, Herscovitch P, Perlman JM, Raichle ME: Positron emission tomography in the newborn: Extensive impairment of regional cerebral blood flow with intraventricular hemorrhage and hemorrhagic intracerebral involvement. Pediatrics 72:589, 1983
18. Doyle LW, Nahmias C, Firnau G, et al: Regional cerebral glucose metabolism of newborn infants measured by positron emission tomography. Dev Med Child Neurol 25:143, 1983
19. Okamato Y, Kirikae T: Electroencephalographic studies on brain of foetus, of children of premature birth and new-born, together with a note on reactions of foetus brain upon drugs. Folia Psychiatr Neurol Jap 5, 1951
20. Dreyfus-Brisac C, Samson-Dreyfus D, Fischgold H: Activité électrique cérebrale du prematuré et du nouveau-né. Ann Pediatr 31:1, 1955
21. Kellaway P, Petersen I: Neurological and Electroencephalographic Correlative Studies in Infancy. Grune & Stratton, New York, 1964
22. Parmelee AH, Jr: Changes in sleep patterns in premature infants as a function of brain maturation. p. 459. In Minkowski A (ed): Regional Development of the Brain in Early Life. F.A. Davis, Oxford, 1967
23. Prechtl HFR, Weinmann H, Akiyama Y: Organization of physiological parameters in normal and neurologically abnormal infants. Neuropaediatrie 1:101, 1969
24. Anders T, Emde R, Parmelee A: A Manual of Standardized Terminology, Techniques and Criteria for Scoring of States of Sleep and Wakefulness in Newborn Infants. NINDS Neurological Information Network, Los Angeles, 1971
25. Watanabe K, Iwase K: Spindle-like fast rhythms in the EEGs of low birth-weight infants. Dev Med Child Neurol 14:373, 1972
26. Werner SS, Stockard JE, Bickford RG: Atlas of Neonatal Electroencephalography. Raven Press, New York, 1977
27. Ellingson RJ, Peters JF: Development of EEG and daytime sleep patterns in low risk premature

infants during the first year of life: Longitudinal observations. Electroencephalogr Clin Neurophysiol 50:165, 1980

28. Lombroso CT: Normal and abnormal EEGs in full-term neonates. p. 83. In Henry CE (ed): Current Clinical Neurophysiology. Update on EEG and Evoked Potentials. Elsevier/North Holland, Amsterdam, 1980
29. Tharp BR, Cukier F, Monod N: The prognostic value of the electroencephalogram in premature infants. Electroencephalogr Clin Neurophysiol 51:219, 1981
30. Torres F, Anderson C: The normal EEG of the human newborn. J Clin Neurophysiol 2:89, 1985
31. American Electroencephalographic Society. Guidelines in EEG, 1–7 (Revised 1985). J Clin Neurophysiol 3:131, 1986
32. Tharp BR: Neonatal electroencephalography. p. 31. In Korobkin R, Guilleminault C (eds): Progress in Perinatal Neurology, Vol. 1. Williams & Wilkins, Baltimore, 1981
33. Dreyfus-Brisac C: Neonatal electroencephalography. p. 397. In Scarpelli EM, Cosmi EV (eds): Reviews in Perinatal Medicine, Vol. 3. Raven Press, New York, 1979
34. Hughes JR, Fino J, Gaghon L: Periods of activity and quiescence in the premature EEG. Neuropediatrics 14:66, 1983
35. Lombroso CT: Quantified electrographic scales on 10 pre-term healthy newborns followed up to 40–43 weeks of conceptional age by serial polygraphic recordings. Electroencephalogr Clin Neurophysiol 46:460, 1979
36. Ballard JL, Kazmaier O, Novak K, Driver M: A simplified score for assessment of fetal maturation of newly born infants. J Pediatr 95:769, 1979
37. Dubowitz MS, Dubowitz V, Goldberg C: Clinical assessment of gestational age in the newborn infant. J Pediatr 77:1, 1970
38. Dorovini-Zis K, Dolman CL: Gestational development of brain. Arch Pathol Lab Med 101:192, 1977
39. Dooling EC, Chi JG, Gilles FH: Telencephalic development: Changing gyral patterns. p. 94. In Gilles FH, Leviton A, Dooling EC (eds): The Developing Brain. Wright, Boston, 1983
40. Scher M, Barmada M: Correlation of electrographic and anatomical findings in the very-low-birth-weight newborn. Ann Neurol 16:404, 1984
41. Volpe JJ: Neonatal seizures. p. 129. In Neurology of the Newborn. Vol. 22. Major Problems in Clinical Pediatrics. Saunders, Philadelphia, 1987
42. Bergman I, Painter MJ, Hirsch RP, et al: Outcome in neonates with convulsions treated in an intensive care unit. Ann Neurol 14:642, 1983
43. Holden KR, Freeman JM: Neonatal seizures and their treatment. Clin Perinatol 2:3, 1975
44. Rose AL, Lombroso CT: Neonatal seizure states: A study of clinical, pathological and electroencephalographic features in 137 full-term babies with a long-term follow up. Pediatrics 45:404, 1970
45. Seay AR, Bray PF: Significance of seizures in infants weighing less than 2500 grams. Arch Neurol 34:381, 1977
46. Mizrahi EM, Kellaway P: Characterization of seizures in neonates and young infants by time-synchronized electroencephalography/polygraphic/video monitoring. Ann Neurol 16:383, 1984
47. Dreyfus-Brisac C, Monod N: Electroclinical studies of status epilepticus and convulsions in the newborn. p. 250. In Kellaway P, Petersen I (eds): Neurological and Electroencephalographic Correlative Studies in Infancy. Grune and Stratton, New York, 1964
48. Volpe JJ: Neonatal seizures. Clin Perinatol 4:43, 1977
49. Fenichel GM: Neonatal Neurology. Churchill Livingstone, New York, 1985
50. Staudt F, Roth JC, Engel RC: The usefulness of electroencephalography in currarized newborns. Electroencephalogr Clin Neurophysiol 51:205, 1981
51. Goldberg RN, Goldman SL, Ramsay RE, Feller R: Detection of seizure activity in the paralyzed neonate using continuous monitoring. Pediatrics 69:583, 1982
52. Eyre JA, Oozen RC, Wilkinson AR: Continuous electroencephalographic recording to detect seizures in paralyzed newborns. Br Med J 286:1017, 1983
53. Tharp BR, Laboyrie PM: The incidence of EEG abnormalities and outcome of infants paralyzed with neuromuscular blocking agents. Crit Care Med 11:926, 1983
54. Scher MS, Morehead LM: Electrographic seizures in the high-risk neonate. Epilepsia 27:609, 1986
55. Burke JB: Prognostic significance of neonatal convulsions. Arch Dis Child 29:342, 1954
56. Brown JK, Cockburn F, Forfan JO: Clinical and chemical correlates in convulsions of the newborn. Lancet 1:135, 1972
57. Scher M: Midline electrographic abnormalities in neonatal EEG. Electroencephalogr Clin Neurophysiol 64:26P, 1986
58. Lombroso CT: A prospective clinical electrophysiological study on intracranial hemorrhages in

the newborn. Reprinted from Fukuyama Y, Arima M, Maekawa K, Yamaguchi K (eds): Child Neurology, International Congress Series No. 579, Proceedings of the IYDP Commemorative International Symposium on Developmental Disabilities. Elsevier Tokyo, p. 251
59. Mannino FL, Trauner DA: Stroke in neonates. J Pediatr 102:605, 1983
60. Watanabe K, Hara K, Miyazaki S, et al: The value of EEG and cerebral evoked potentials in the assessment of neonatal intracranial hemorrhage. Eur J Pediatr 137:177, 1981
61. Clancy R, Malig S, Laragie D, et al: Focal motor seizures heralding stroke in full-term neonates. Am J Dis Child 139:601, 1985
62. Ment LR, Freedman RM, Ehrenkranz RA: Neonates with seizures attributable to perinatal complications. Am J Dis Child 136:548, 1982
63. Levy SR, Abroms IF, Marshall PC, Rosquele EE: Seizures and cerebral infarction in the full-term newborn. Ann Neurol 17:366, 1985
64. Staudt F, Howieson J, Benda GJ, Engel RC: EEG in neonatal intracranial hemorrhage: Comparison with clinical findings and CT scan. Z EEG-EMG 13:143, 1982
65. Fenichel GM, Webster DL, Wong WKT: Intracranial hemorrhage in the term newborn. Arch Neurol 41:30, 1984
66. Allemand F, Monod N, Laroche JCI: An electroencephalographic study of neonatal subdural hemorrhage. Rev EEG Neurophysiol 7:365, 1977
67. Pohowalla P, McIntyre HB, Worthen N: EEG in neonatal intracranial cysts. Electroencephalogr Clin Neurophysiol 28:36P, 1984
68. Lerique-Koechlin A: EEG in neonatal meningitis and cerebral hemorrhages (Section VII). p. 53. In Dreyfus-Brisac C, Ellingson P (eds): Handbook of Electroencephalography and Clinical Neurophysiology, Vol. 15B. Elsevier, Amsterdam, 1972
69. Watanabe K, Hara K, Hakamada S, et al: The prognostic value of EEG in neonatal meningitis. Clin Electroencephalogr 14:67, 1983
70. Prian GW, Wright GB, Rumack CM, O'Meara OP: Apparent cerebral embolization after temporal artery catheterization. J Pediatr 93:115, 1978
71. Korobkin R: Congenital hemiplegia. p. 183. In Korobkin R, Guilleminault C (eds): Progress in Perinatal Neurology, Vol. 1. Williams and Wilkins, Baltimore, 1981
72. Billard C, Dulac O, Diebler C: Cerebral infarction in neonates. A possible etiology of neonatal seizure state. Eight case reports. Arch Fr Pediatr 82:677, 1982
73. Goutieres F, Challamel MJ, Aicardi J, Gilly R: Les hemiplegies congenitaies: Semiologie, etiologie et pronostic. Arch Fr Pediatr 29:839, 1972
74. Challamel M, Isnard H, Brunon A, Revol M: Asymmetric EEG transitoire al'entrée dans le sommeil calme chez le nouveau-ne: Étude sur 75 observations. Rev EEG Neurophysiol 14:17, 1984
75. Scher M, Tharp B: Significance of focal abnormalities in neonatal EEG-radiologic correlation and outcome. Ann Neurol 12:217, 1982
76. Cukier F, Andre M, Monod N, Dreyfus-Brisac C: Apport de l'EEG au diagnostic des hémorragies intraventriculaires du prémature. Rev EEG 2:318, 1972
77. Clancy RR, Tharp BR: Positive rolandic sharp waves in the electroencephalograms of premature neonates with intraventricular hemorrhage. Electroencephalogr Clin Neurophysiol 57:395, 1984
78. Novotny EJ, Tharp BR, Enzmann DR, et al: The significance of positive sharp waves in the electroencephalogram of premature infants. Neurology, suppl., 36:279, 1986
79. Clancy RR, Fischer RA: Midline sagittal epileptogenic foci in children. Epilepsia 25:652, 1984
80. Mizrahi EM: Electroencephalographic/polygraphic/video monitoring in childhood epilepsy. J Pediatr 105:1, 1984
81. Donn SM, Grasela TH, Pharm D, Goldstein GW: Safety of a higher loading dose of phenobarbital in the term newborn. Pediatrics 75:1061, 1985
82. Van Orman CB, Darwish HZ: Efficacy of phenobarbital in neonatal seizures. Can J Neurol Sci 12:95, 1985
83. Coen RW, McCutchen CB, Wermer D, et al: Continuous monitoring of the electroencephalogram following perinatal asphyxia. J Pediatr 100:628, 1982
84. Schulte FJ, Hinze G, Schrempf G: Maternal toxemia, fetal malnutrition and bioelectric brain activity of the newborn. Neuropaediatrie 2:439, 1971
85. Harris R, Tizard JPM: The electroencephalogram in neonatal convulsions. J Pediatr 57:501, 1970
86. Watanabe K, Miyazaki S, Hara K, Hakamada S: Behavioral state cycles, background EEGs and prognosis of newborns with perinatal hypoxia. Electroencephalogr Clin Neurophysiol 49:618, 1980
87. Monod N, Pajot N, Guidasci S: The neonatal EEG: Statistical studies and prognostic value in fullterm and preterm babies. Electroencephalogr Clin Neurophysiol 32:529, 1972
88. Lombroso CT: Neurophysiological observations in diseased newborns. Biol Psychiatry 10:527, 1975

89. Ellingson RJ, Peters JF: Development of EEG and daytime sleep patterns in trisomy-21 infants during the first year of life: Longitudinal observations. Electroencephalogr Clin Neurophysiol 50:457, 1980
90. Lombroso CT, Matsumiya Y: Stability in waking-sleep states in neonates as a predictor of long-term neurological outcome. Pediatrics 76:52, 1985
91. Dunn HG, Auckland NL, Low MD: Electroencephalograms. p. 219. In Dunn HG (ed): Sequelae of Low Birthweight: The Vancouver Study. Mac Keith Press, Philadelphia, 1986
92. Ellingson RJ, Dutch SJ, McIntire MS: EEGs of prematures: 3–8 years follow-up study. Dev Psychobiol 7:529, 1974
93. Kellaway P: Ontogenic evolution of the electrical activity of the brain in man and in animals. p. 141. In: Proceedings of the 1st Int. International Congress of Neurological Sciences, Brussels, 1957
94. Dreyfus-Brisac C, Fischgold H, Samson-Dollfus D, et al: Reactivité sensorielle chez le premature, le nouveau-ne et le, ourrisson. Electroenceph Clin Neurophysiol, suppl., 6:417–440, 1957
95. Engel R: Abnormal Electroencephalograms in the Neonatal Period. Thomas, Springfield, 1975
96. Parmelee AH, Akiyama Y, Stern E, Harris MA: A periodic cerebral rhythm in newborn infants. Exp Neurol 25:575, 1969
97. Eisengart M, Gluck L, Glaser GH: Maturation of the EEG of infants of short gestation. Dev Med Child Neurol 12:49, 1970
98. Joseph JP, Lesevse N, Dreyfus-Brisac C: Spatio-temporal organization of EEG in premature infants and full-term newborns. Electroencephalogr Clin Neurophysiol 40:153, 1976
99. Ellingson RJ, Peters JF: Development of EEG and daytime sleep patterns in low risk premature infants during the first year of life: Longitudinal observations. Electroencephalogr Clin Neurophysiol 50:165, 1980
100. Anderson CM, Torres F, Faoro A: The EEG of the early premature. Electroencephalogr Clin Neurophysiol 60:95, 1985
101. Watt J, Strongman K: The organization and stability of sleep states in full-term, pre-term and small-for-gestational-age infants: A comparative study. Dev Psychobiol 18:151, 1985
102. Guilleminault C, Baker RL: Sleep and electroencephalography: Points of interest and points of controversy. J Clin Neurophysiol 1:275, 1984
103. Ellingson RJ: EEGs of premature and full-term newborns. p. 149. In Klass DW, Daly DD (eds): Current Practice of Clinical Electroencephalography. Raven Press, New York, 1979
104. Mizrahi EM, Dorfman LJ: Sensory evoked potentials: Clinical application in pediatrics. J Pediatr 97:1, 1980
105. Jewett DL, Romano MN: Human auditory development potential averaged from the scalp of rat and cat. Brain Res 36:101, 1972
106. Despland PA: Maturational changes in the auditory system as reflected in human brainstem evoked responses. Dev Neurosci 7:73, 1985
107. Despland PA, Galambos R: Use of the auditory brainstem responses by premature and newborn infants. Neuropadiatrie 11:99, 1980
108. Starr A, Amlie RN, Martin WH, Sanders S: Development of auditory function in newborn infants revealed by auditory brainstem potentials. Pediatrics 60:831, 1977
109. Hecox K: Electrophysiological correlates of human auditory development. p. 151. In Infant Perception: From Sensation to Cognition, Vol. 1. Academic Press, New York, 1975
110. Salamy A, McKean CM, Pettett G, Mendelson T: Auditory brainstem recovery processes from birth to adulthood. Psychophysiology 15:214, 1978
111. Scher MS, Ahdab-Barmada M, Fria T: Neurophysiological and anatomical correlations in neonatal nonketotic hyperglycinemia. Neuropediatrics 17:137, 1986
112. Miranda SB, Hack M, Fantz RL, et al: Neonatal pattern vision: A predictor of future mental performance. J Pediatr 91:642, 1977
113. Brazelton TB: Neonatal Behavioural Assessment Scale. Clinics in Developmental Medicine. No. 50. London SIMP with Heinemann, J.B. Lippincott, Philadelphia, 1973
114. Fantz RL: Pattern vision in newborn infants. Science 140:296, 1963
115. Sokol S: Measurement of infant visual acuity from pattern reversal evoked potentials. Vision Res 18:33, 1978
116. Hrbek A, Karlberg P, Olsson T: Development of visual and somatosensory evoked responses in pre-term newborn infants. Electroencephalogr Clin Neurophysiol 34:225, 1973
117. Umezaki H, Morell F: Developmental study of photic evoked responses in premature infants. Electroencephalogr Clin Neurophysiol 28:55, 1970
118. Watanabe K, Iwase K, Hara K: Maturation of visual evoked responses in low-birthweight infants. Dev Med Child Neurol 14:425, 1972
119. Harden A: Maturation of the visual evoked potentials. p. 41. In Chiarenza GA, Papakostopoulos

(eds): Clinical Application of Cerebral Evoked Potentials in Pediatric Medicine. Excerpta Medica, Amsterdam, 1982

120. Harden A, Pampiglione G: Visual evoked potentials, electroretinogram, and electroencephalogram studies in progressive neurometabolic "storage" diseases of childhood. p. 470. In Desmedt JE (ed): Visual Evoked Potentials in Man. Clarendon Press, Oxford, 1977
121. deVries LS, Connell JA, Dubowitz LMS, et al: Correlation of the pattern of cerebral palsy with the distribution of multicystic brain lesions in preterm infants. International Child Neurology Congress, Jerusalem, 1986
122. Graziani LJ, Weitzman ED, Pineda G: Visual evoked responses during neonatal respiratory disorders in low weight infants. Pediatr Res 6:203, 1972
123. Hrbek A, Karlberg P, Kyellmer I, et al: Clinical application of evoked electroencephalographic responses in newborn infants. I. Perinatal asphyxia. Dev Med Child Neurol 19:34, 1977
124. Cracco JB, Cracco RQ, Graziani LJ: The spinal evoked response in infants and children. Neurology 25:31, 1975
125. Willis J, Seales D, Frazier E: Short latency somatosensory evoked potentials in infants. Electroencephalogr Clin Neurophysiol 59:366, 1984
126. Laget P, Salbreux R, Raimbault J, et al: Relationship between changes in somesthetic evoked responses and electroencephalographic findings in the child with hemiplegia. Dev Med Child Neurol 18:620, 1976
127. Duckworth T, Yamashita T, Franks CI, et al: Somatosensory evoked cortical responses in children with spina bifida. Dev Med Child Neurol 18:19, 1976
128. Dorfman LJ, Perkash I, Bosley TM, et al: Use of cerebral evoked potentials to evaluate spinal somatosensory function in patients with traumatic and surgical myelopathies. J Neurosurg 52:654, 1980
129. Dorfman LJ, Pedley TA, Tharp BR, et al: Juvenile neuroaxonal dystrophy: Clinical, electrophysiological and neuropathological features. Ann Neurol 3:419, 1978
130. Duffy FH: Topographic Mapping of Brain Electrical Activity. Butterworth Publishers, Boston, 1986
131. Duffy FH, Als H: Neurophysiological assessment of the neonate; an approach combining brain electrical activity mapping (BEAM) with behavioral assessment (APIB). In Brazelton TB, Lester BM (eds): New Approaches to Development Screening of Infants. Elsevier-North Holland, New York, 1983
132. Watanabe K, Inokuma K, Takeuchi T, Aso K: Neurophysiology of neonates and sequelae of early brain damage. In Arima M, Suzuki Y, Yabuuchi H (eds): The Developing Brain and Its Disorders. S. Karger, Basel, 1985
133. Havlicek V, Childiaeva R, Chernick V: EEG frequency spectrum characteristics of sleep states in full-term and pre-term infants. Neuropaediatrie 6:24, 1975
134. Dittrichova' J, Brichacek V, Paul K, Tautermannoua M: The structure of infant behavior: An analysis of sleep and waking in the first months of life. p. 73. In Hartup WW (ed): Review of Child Development Research, Vol. 6. University of Chicago Press, Chicago, 1982
135. Harper RM, Leake B, Miyahara, et al: Development of ultradian periodicity and coalescence at 1 cycle per hour in electroencephalographic activity. Exp Neurol 73:127, 1981
136. Willekens H, Dumeruth G, Duc G, et al: EEG spectral powers and coherence analysis in healthy full-term neonates. Neuropediatrics 15:180, 1984
137. Dreyfus-Brisac C, Monod N: Sleeping behavior in abnormal newborn infants. Neuropaediatrie 1:354, 1970
138. Parmelee AH: EEG power spectral analysis of newborn infants' sleep states. Electroencephalogr Clin Neurophysiol 27:690, 1969
139. Scholten CA, Vos JE, Prechtl HFR: Compiled profile of respiration, heart beat and motility in newborn infants: A methodological approach. Med Biol Eng Comput 23:15, 1985
140. Stratton P: Rhythmic functions in the human newborn. In Stratton P (ed): Psychobiology of the Human Newborn. John Wiley & Sons, New York, 1982
141. Hellbrugge T: The development of circadian rhythms in infants. Cold Spring Harbor Symp Quant Biol 25:311, 1960
142. Hellbrugge T: Ontogenese des rhythmes circadaires chez l'enfant. p. 159. In Ajuriaquerra J de (ed): Cycle Biologiques et Psychiatrie. Masson, Geneva and Paris, 1968
143. Prechtl HFR, Lenard HG: A study of eye movements in sleeping newborn infants. Brain Res 5:477, 1967
144. Dittrichova' J, Paul K, Pavlikova' E: Rapid eye movements in paradoxical sleep in infants. Neuropaediatrie 3:248, 1972
145. Petre-Quadens O, de Lee C: Eye movements during sleep: A common criterion of learning capacities and endocrine activity. Dev Med Child Neurol 12:730, 1970

146. Prechtl HFR, Nijhuis JG: Eye movements in the human fetus and newborn. Behav Brain Res 10:119, 1983
147. Ersyukova II: Oculomotor activity and autonomic indices of newborn infants during paradoxical sleep. Hum Physiol 6:57, 1980
148. Fukumoto M, Mochizuki N, Takeishi M, et al: Studies of body movements during night sleep in infancy. Brain Dev 3:37, 1981
149. Prechtl HFR, Fargel JW, Weinmann HM, Backter HH: Postures, motility and respiration of low-risk pre-term infants. Dev Med Child Neurol 21:3, 1979
150. Hakamada S, Watanabe K, Hara K, Miyazaki S: Development of the motor behavior during sleep in newborn infants. Brain Dev 3:345, 1981
151. deVries JIP, Visser GHA, Prechtl HFR: The emergence of fetal behaviour. II. Quantitative Aspects. Early Hum Dev 12:99, 1985
152. Korner AF: Neonatal startles, smiles, erections, and reflex sucks as related to state, sex, and individuality. Child Dev 40:1039, 1969
153. Erkinjuntti M, Kero P: Heart rate response related to body movements in healthy and neurologically damaged infants during sleep. Early Hum Dev 12:31, 1985
154. Roffwarg HP, Muzio JN, Dement WC: Ontogenetic development of the human sleep-dream cycle. Science 152:604, 1966
155. Robertson SS: Intrinsic temporal patterning in the spontaneous movement of awake neonates. Child Dev 53:1016, 1982
156. Visser GHA, Laurini RN, deVries JIP, et al: Abnormal motor behaviour in anencephalic fetuses. Early Hum Dev 12:173, 1985
157. Hakamada S, Watanabe K, Hara K, Miyazaki S: Hydranencephaly: Sleep and movement characteristics. Brain Dev 4:45, 1982
158. Coons S, Guilleminault C: Motility and arousal in near miss sudden infant death syndrome. J Pediatr 107:728, 1985
159. Lombroso CT: Neonatal polygraphy in full-term and premature infants: A review of normal and abnormal findings. J Clin Neurophysiol 2:105, 1985
160. Beckwith L, Parmelee AH, Jr: EEG patterns of preterm infants, home environment, and later IQ. Child Dev 57:777, 1986
161. Scher MS, Richardson GA, Day NL: The effects of prenatal alcohol exposure on sleep cycling and arousal. Pediatric Research, part 2 20:165A, 1986
162. Scher MS, Richardson GA, Day NL, Guthrie R: Sleep cycle and arousal abnormalities in neonates with bronchopulmonary dysplasia. Child Neurology Society (abstract by title), Boston, 1980

9

Neurodevelopmental Outcome in Low-Birthweight Infants: The Role of Developmental Intervention

Forrest C. Bennett

Approximately 200,000 preterm infants are born annually in the United States. Considering birthweight alone, about 6 percent of all live births in the white population are of infants 2,500 g or less (low birthweight), and about 1 percent are of infants 1,500 g or less (very low birthweight); these birthweight statistics are at least doubled (i.e., 12 percent and 2 to 3 percent, respectively) in nonwhite populations.[1] Since these prematurity and low-birthweight incidence estimates have remained surprisingly stable over the past 25 years, reductions in neonatal mortality are steadily increasing the prevalence of biologically vulnerable infants in the overall population. While much debate and large differences of opinion persist when considering the effects of neonatal intensive care on the long-term neurodevelopmental morbidity encountered in low-birthweight infants, most investigators are in current agreement that the single, clearest outcome result of this technically enhanced care has been a dramatic and continuing reduction in neonatal mortality since the early 1960s, particularly for very low birthweight infants since the mid-1970s.[2,3] Simply stated, with the present standards of practice in neonatal intensive care units (NICUs), many more very premature, very low birthweight infants are surviving to be discharged home than was the case even 5 to 10 years ago. Table 9-1 illustrates expected survival in the 1980s, as averaged from reporting NICUs, for individual birthweight groups of low-birthweight infants. As can be seen, the survival with tertiary care exceeds 50 percent even at 800 grams, and does not become more infrequent until one goes below this birthweight. A 1983 report from a large San Francisco, California, NICU extends this striking trend by describing a 40 percent survival rate for infants between 500 and 750 grams birthweight.[4] Figure 9-1 graphically shows that while survival continues to increase in all low birthweight categories, the greatest impact of neonatal intensive care technology in recent years has clearly been on the smallest (and sickest) infants.

With continued reductions in the neonatal mortality of preterm/low-birthweight infants, serious concerns persist that this improved survival may be accompanied by increased neurodevelopmental morbidity, specifically in the number of permanently handicapped and brain-damaged children that result from it. The major central nervous system/sensory handicapping conditions associated with prema-

Table 9-1. 1980s NICU Survival Rate by Birthweight

Birthweight (g)	Survival (%)
500–600	15
601–800	35
801–1000	55
1001–1200	75
1201–1400	85
1401–1600	87
1601–1800	90
1801–2000	92
2001–2500	95
Total ≤2500 g	85

turity are: cerebral palsy (particularly the spastic diplegia type, with the legs more neurologically affected than the arms), mental or developmental retardation (Intelligence Quotient or Developmental Quotient below 70), sensorineural hearing loss, and visual impairment (primarily the consequences of retinopathy of prematurity, formerly termed retrolental fibroplasia). These handicaps frequently occur together in the same child, and are occasionally complicated by a chronic seizure disorder. They are usually clinically apparent by 2 years of age, and vary in severity from mild to profound. As a group, their incidence increases with decreasing birthweight and gestational age; the handicap rate in males consistently exceeds that in females.[5–7] Table 9-2 provides current, combined incidence figures by birthweight group for these major handicapping conditions. Such major morbidity statistics may be viewed both optimistically and pessimistically. On the one

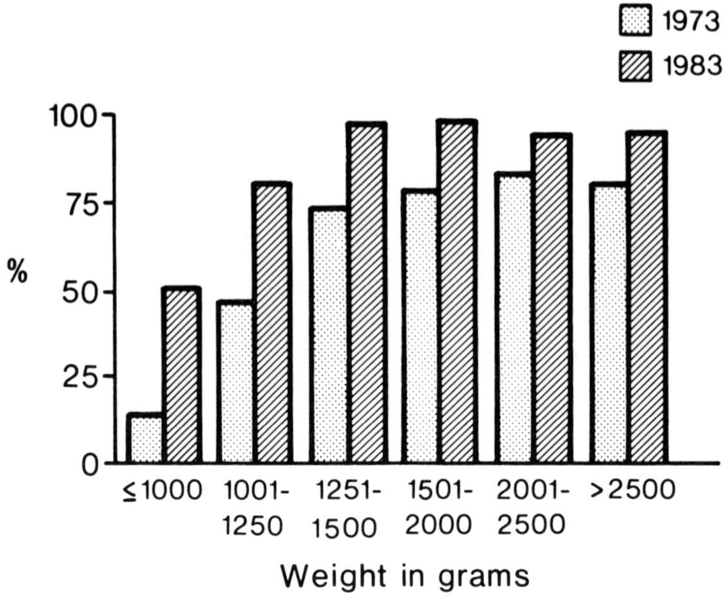

Fig. 9-1. Comparison of NICU survival for mid-1970s and mid-1980s.

Table 9-2. Surviving Low-Birthweight Infants with One or More Major Handicaps

Birthweight (g)	Major Handicapping Conditions (%)
1501–2500	8 (5–20)
1001–1500	15 (5–30)
≤1000	25 (8–40)

hand, the occurrence of these major sequelae is far less frequent than initially predicted at the beginning of the NICU era, and many more nonhandicapped than handicapped (about 15 to 1) survivors are being added to the population. Conversely, the major handicap rate has changed little over the past 10 to 15 years in spite of ongoing decreases in mortality, and very recent data from Sweden,[8] Australia,[9] and the United States[10] strongly suggest an actual current increase in major handicaps among the smallest and sickest survivors.

THE "NEW MORBIDITY"

While major handicapping sequelae are the easiest for NICUs to quantify and report, numerous current long-term follow-up studies are clearly indicating that so-called minor neurodevelopmental and neurobehavioral sequelae are at least, if not more, prevalent in surviving preterm/low-birthweight infants, and become increasingly apparent in a variety of clinical manifestations with increasing age during the first 6 years of life.[11,12] These early, often subtle, developmental and behavioral delays and differences are not necessarily outgrown, but frequently portend future school dysfunction, and may therefore become major impediments to normal academic and social progress. Collectively, these problems, which typically manifest themselves during the preschool and early school years, have been termed the "new morbidity" of prematurity.

Specific types of minor developmental handicap include borderline intelligence (IQ 70 to 84), minor persistent neuromotor abnormalities on the same continuum but of less severity than cerebral palsy (gross- and fine-motor milestone delays, immature balance and coordination), and communication disorders (receptive or expressive language milestone delays, or both, and speech dysfunctions such as malarticulation and dysfluency). Specific areas of observed preterm versus full-term behavioral difference include: (1) neonatal behavior (poorer and more variable performance in most assessed areas, particularly visual and auditory orienting, habituation, and behavioral state organization and modulation), (2) infant and child temperament (more "difficult" with less adaptability to change, less attentive, less motivation for mastery, less smiling, more negative mood, and more irritability), and (3) socioemotional competence (less social perception and more emotional immaturity).[13,14] As with major handicaps, the overall incidence of these "minor" handicapping conditions increases with decreasing birthweight and gestational age, and is also greater in male survivors. Current estimates of their incidence in very low birthweight infants vary between 15 and 25 percent. Accordingly, when the 15 to 20 percent major handicap rate is also considered, between 35 and 45 percent of very low birthweight survivors demonstrate a residual, neurodevelopmental problem that compromises their age-expected function.[15]

Most of the major and minor neurodevelopmental sequelae associated with prematurity and low birthweight are also related to the severity of perinatal/neonatal illness, (i.e., low birthweight infants experiencing a prolonged course of early support with many medical complications have an increased likelihood of developing some type of developmental dysfunction). Specific events highly associated with suboptimal outcomes include: intrauterine growth retardation, severe perinatal asphyxia, neonatal meningitis/encephalitis, symptomatic intracranial hemorrhage (particularly extensive intraventricular or intraparenchymal hemorrage or both), refractory neonatal seizures, and severe chronic lung disease with prolonged mechanical ventilation and oxygen requirements. Typical neonatal complications not so strongly linked to adverse outcomes include respiratory distress syndrome (RDS) and milder forms of chronic bronchopulmonary dysplasia (BPD), apnea of prematurity, and transient metabolic abnormalities (e.g., hypoglycemia, hypocalcemia). However, it must be emphasized that despite the large number of positive group associations in follow-up studies, individual neurodevelopmental outcome remains very difficult to accurately predict prospectively in the NICU, and infants with apparently similar neonatal courses may develop remarkably differently. This repeated observation should be a source of caution and humility to those making critical neonatal care decisions, and also to those providing follow-up evaluations.

This chapter will examine and review recent investigations pertaining to the various "minor" neurodevelopmental morbidities and school function of preterm NICU graduates. This expanded awareness of more subtle central nervous system sequelae is necessary to adequately address and consider the many contemporary medical, legal, ethical, and economic issues related to neonatal intensive care. The unique environment of the NICU will be objectively analyzed in terms of its potential impact on neonatal development and behavior. Finally, the effectiveness of several types of early behavioral interventions in preventing or ameliorating the developmental consequences of prematurity will be historically reviewed and critically evaluated.

NEURODEVELOPMENTAL AND NEUROBEHAVIORAL SEQUELAE

Neurobehavioral, State, and Temperament Development

Numerous studies have compared the neonatal neurobehavioral performance of preterm infants to that of term infants. These studies typically compare preterm infants at their corrected or conceptional age (i.e., chronologic age minus weeks of prematurity), and also tend to employ preterm infants who have relatively uncomplicated neonatal courses. Nevertheless, despite these sampling features that might obscure group differences, preterm infants consistently perform less optimally than healthy term infants on these early measures.

Kurtzberg and colleagues,[14] in one of the largest and most comprehensive neonatal studies to date, compared the neurobehavioral status of 118 low birthweight infants tested at 40 weeks conceptional age with that of 76 nonrisk term infants. A neonatal neurobehavioral examination comprising 21 test items was used. Of

Table 9-3. Comparison of Neonatal Neurobehavioral Performance of Full-term (FT) and Low Birthweight (LBW) Infants

Examination Item	% Adequate FT Infants	% Deviant LBW Infants
Auditory orienting total	100	64
Visual following total	100	66
Head extension	100	19
Traction	100	19
Head lag	99	19
Extremity movement	>95	7
Ventral suspension	100	3
Optic blink	100	1
Rooting, right	>95	33
Sucking	100	0
Rotation	100	1
Moro	100	1
Tonic Neck Reflex	100	0
Grasp	99	10
Popliteal angle	100	24
Arm recoil	100	21
Spontaneous Movement (summary)	100	0
Tonus summary	98	41
Cuddliness	>95	20

(Modified from Kurtzberg D, Vaughan HG, Daum C: Neurobehavioral performance of low birthweight infants at 40 weeks conceptional age: Comparison with normal full-term infants. Dev Med Child Neurol 21:604, 1979.)

these 21 items, 19 could be assigned cutoff scores, below which infants were considered deviant on the specific items. Table 9-3 illustrates both the percentage of term infants with adequate scores and also the percentage of low-birthweight infants with deviant scores on each individual item. As can be seen, the most striking differences between the groups were found in visual and auditory orienting, with approximately two-thirds of the low-birthweight infants falling below the range of performance of the term group. Items testing motor performance (e.g., head extension, traction, head lag, extremity movement) showed a lower, but still apparent, incidence of suboptimal performance among the low-birthweight infants.

Ferrari et al.[16] replicated and amplified these early preterm versus term differences in their investigation comparing 20 low-risk preterm infants to 20 healthy term infants utilizing the Brazelton Neonatal Behavioral Assessment Scale. They found the preterm infants to be significantly inferior in sensory orientation, motor performance, regulation of behavioral state (i.e., quiet–active status), and autonomic regulation. Additionally, the clustering of neurobehavioral items was more heterogeneous among the preterm group. The authors concluded that prematurity, even following relatively normal pre-, peri-, and neonatal experiences, is associated with a behavioral repertoire which is different, more variable, and on the average poorer than that of term infants. Friedman et al.[17] also compared low-risk preterm neonates to healthy term neonates, and found that the preterm infants fussed and cried more, were less soothable, and tended to change state more frequently. They suggested that these neurobehavioral differences are potential contributors to non-optimal interaction between preterms and their caregivers. Aylward and co-workers,[18] in a report from the NIH Collaborative Study on Antenatal Steroid Therapy, analyzed specific factors affecting the neurobehavioral responses of preterm infants. These investigators reported significant effects of gestational age, severity of illness, and race. Specifically, at 40 weeks conceptional age, preterm infants born at younger gestational ages and with greater medical complications demonstrated altered central nervous system development in terms of diminished spontaneous activity and vigor, inability to maintain and modulate responses, and poorer visual orientation capabilities. Thus, these authors cautioned that observed early neurobehavioral differences in preterm versus term infants may be influenced excessively by babies born at the lower end of the gestational age scale. They also described race differences in certain responses, with black infants generally having stronger, more active and coordinated motor performance and better muscle tone than white infants or those of other racial groups (e.g., Hispanic, Native American). Several minor gender differences were found, but overall this variable did not seem to have a strong impact on neurobehavioral responses at term conceptional age.

A number of recent investigations employing a wide variety of electrophysiologic techniques have supported the results of these behavioral measures. As compared to term infants, preterm infants have been shown to have delayed maturation of both cortical and brainstem auditory evoked potentials (EPs), more variable and labile sleep–wake state organization as measured by time-lapse video somnography, and decreased resting heart rate variability and vagal tone (i.e., an indirect measure of overall autonomic nervous system activity).[19–22] Several of these functions, particularly sleep organization and autonomic regulation, have been related to longer-term developmental outcome.[23,24] (see also Ch. 8).

Developmental differences between preterm and term infants throughout infancy and in many areas besides those described above have also been extensively explored. Rose[25] investigated the effect of increasing familiarization time on the visual recognition memory of 6- and 12-month-old preterm and term infants. The infants were given trials in which they viewed a shape for 10-, 15-, 20-, or 30-second familiarization periods and were then tested for specific visual memory. While the older infants showed evidence of recognition memory after less familiarization time than the younger ones, at both ages preterms required considerably longer familiarization times than did term infants. These results suggest that there are persistent differences between preterm and term infants throughout at least the first year of life in visual information processing—a very fundamental aspect of cognition.

Because manipulative exploration of objects may be important to the infant's perception and conceptualization of objects, Ruff et al.[26] studied this developmental function in both preterm and term 9-month-old infants by means of coded and scored videotapes. The videotapes were scored for behaviors such as looking, handling, mouthing, turning the object around, transferring the object from hand to hand, and banging. In this case there were no differences between a "low-risk" subgroup (based on neonatal complications) of preterms and the term infants. However, a "high-risk" subgroup of preterms manipulated the objects significantly less than either the low-risk preterms or the term infants. There was a relationship between manipulative exploration at 9 months and later cognitive functioning at 24 months.

Several studies have probed the related developmental areas of temperament,

Table 9-4. Mean Frequency of Affective Behaviors, Contingent Behaviors, and Expressivity Ratings of Infants and Their Mothers

	Term Infant Ratings (n = 20)	Preterm Infant Ratings (n = 20)
Infant's behavior		
Happy	7.8	2.0
Sad	0.4	4.1
Interested	5.8	4.3
Vocalization	4.9	2.4
Crying	0	3.0
Contingent		
Vocalization	1.8	0.9
Smile	4.3	0.5
Smile and vocalization	1.1	0.8
Expressivity rating	3.3	1.5
Mother's behavior		
Happy	8.5	6.5
Sad	0	0.5
Vocalization	5.1	8.8
Expressivity rating	3.1	2.4

(Modified from Field TM: High-risk infants "have less fun" during early interactions. Topics in Early Childhood Special Education 3(1):83, 1983.)

social interaction and competence, and emotional expression and affect. Most of these studies have considered mother–infant interactions, and there is a consensus of findings that indicates an imbalance in preterm dyads, with infants typically unresponsive and low in communicative signaling levels, and mothers compensating for their infant's inactivity by showing high levels of stimulating and engaging activity. This is in contrast to term dyads, in which mothers are typically observed to respond to their infant's overtures. Investigations of preterm infants who have suffered complicated neonatal courses have shown that these infants exhibit high levels of gaze aversion, avoidance of interaction, and low levels of vocalizing and playing.[27–29] These studies all reported high levels of maternal anxiety and activity in interaction in comparison with the mothers of term infants. Field[13] has reported these interactional differences in depth, and succinctly summarizes the problem: "High-risk (i.e., preterm) infants and their parents 'have less fun' than normal (i.e., term) infants and their parents during their early interactions together." In a study comparing 20 preterm–mother dyads with 20 term–mother dyads at approximately 4 months conceptional age, Field (see Table 9-4) found the preterm infants to be less alert and attentive, less responsive, less interested in game playing, less contingent, less smiling and content, and more affectively negative and irritable than the term infants. Correspondingly, preterm mothers exhibited fewer happy expressions than term mothers, but were more vocal as they attempted to elicit social and communicative responses from their infants.

Crnic et al.[30] and Malatesta et al.[31] have replicated and extended these observations throughout the entire first year of life. Preterm–term differences in expressive behavior and affect were persistent, and continued to affect maternal behavior. Malatesta and co-workers emphasized that in their primarily middle-to upper-middle-social class population, these differences were seen even in the absence of confounding neonatal medical complications. They speculated that the differences are probably even more pronounced with less advantaged, more stressed, or sicker preterm infants. Of long term importance and concern is the increasing evidence of continuity between early interactional disturbances and later developmental dysfunctions.

Motor Development

Numerous studies from several continents have repeatedly documented that the neuromotor development of preterm/low birthweight infants during the first 2 years of life is different, more deviant, more delayed, and generally more worrisome than that of healthy term infants. Not only are preterm developmental scores (utilizing such measures as the Bayley Scales of Infant Development) consistently and significantly below those of term infants at 12 months conceptional age, but preterm motor scores are also usually 10 to 15 points (i.e., practically one standard deviation) below preterm mental scores at this age.[32]

This phenomenon of transiently abnormal neuromotor signs in the first years of life was initially described by Drillien,[33] in a 1972 report from Scotland, as "transient dystonia of low birthweight infants." Drillien reported that its prevalence during the first half of infancy varied inversely with birthweight, involving approximately 35 percent of infants weighing 1,501 to 2,000 g at birth and 60 to 70 percent of infants weighing 1,500 g or less at birth, and that its prevalence also varied directly with neonatal complications (i.e., with it more frequently occurring among sick preterm infants). Transient dystonia includes such neurologic findings as increased or decreased muscle tone, diminished volitional movement, retention and accentuation of primitive reflex patterns, delayed appearance of normal infantile automatic reactions, and asymmetric neuromotor development. Because these neuromotor signs are also the very signs seen in infants who are developing cerebral palsy, it is not surprising that a reliable diagnosis of cerebral palsy is quite difficult in most preterm infants throughout early infancy. However, as detailed by Amiel-Tison,[34] by 8 to 10 months conceptional age the great majority of low-birthweight infants with transient dystonia are gradually and spontaneously becoming normal upon examination, and making motor developmental gains, whereas those relatively few infants developing permanent cerebral palsy appear increasingly abnormal. With the knowledge of this common evolution of neuromotor signs, every very low birthweight infant can theoretically be assigned to one of three diagnostic and prognostic groups at 12 months of age: (1) those who are always normal in a neurologic examination (25 to 30 percent), (2) those who show transient dystonia with subsequent normalization (65 to 70 percent), and (3) those with cerebral palsy (5 to 10 percent). Such categorization might provide more rapid and meaningful morbidity information for both intra-NICU and inter-NICU comparisons than what is currently available from traditional follow-up reports.

Coolman et al.[35] and others have extended these observations to 24 months of age, albeit that most neuromotor changes occur in the first year of life. They also found that some infants with transient dystonia retained subtle, persistent neuromotor differences that would not be labeled as cerebral palsy but which represented qualitative deviations from the norm. Longitudinal studies indicate that infants who have experienced transient dystonia are far more likely to develop language, learning, and(or) behavioral problems (i.e., minimal brain dysfunction) in later childhood than are infants who never demonstrated these abnormalities.[36–38] This would indicate that even though transient dystonia largely resolves, this suspicious neuromotor sign in early infancy may be a predictive marker for other, later manifestations of central nervous system disorganization.

Two recent investigations have addressed the effectiveness of very early physical therapeutic intervention (i.e., so-called neurodevelopmental therapy, as described by the Bobaths[39]) in preventing or ameliorating neurologic dysfunction in preterm/low birthweight infants.[40–41] Both of these controlled studies involved regular, individual physical therapeutic intervention of varying intensity, including home instructions for daily parental follow-through, prior to 4 months conceptional age and prior to the age at which any definitive neurologic diagnosis could be made. Both studies continued this motor intervention program until 12 months of age. Both studies were entirely negative, in that the early physical therapeutic programs employed were not efficacious in altering the pattern of motor development in participating preterm infants. These findings fail to support the notion that very early physical therapy either prevents neuromotor dysfunction or promotes motor development in infants at risk for such dysfunction. This conclusion supports Drillien's original concern that some children reported as having cerebral palsy in the first year of life, and supposedly demonstrating a favorable response to early physical therapy, may in fact represent cases of transient neuromotor abnormalities in which the same good results could have occurred without such therapy.

Preterm-versus-term differences in motor development have been reported throughout the preschool years as well. Burns and Bullock[42] compared the motor abilities of 105 preterm children to those of 102 term children at 5 years of age. No children with cerebral palsy were included in either subject group, thus allowing an accurate comparison of detailed gross- and fine-motor function. Factors significantly distinguishing the preterm children from their term peers included small, tremulous involuntary hand movements, less competent gross motor ability, and difficulties in postural control and balance. Motor performance was unrelated to socioeconomic and environmental factors. The authors note that the variables that differentiated the preterm children from the maturely born children were similar to those often associated with central nervous system dysfunction and school learning problems.

Language Development

Communication skills involving auditory and visual perception, the learning and conceptualizing of a verbal symbol system (language), and the actual production of speech are critical to academic learning and social adjustment. While the overall development of children born as preterm infants has been studied extensively by means of developmental and intelligence testing, language development has been relatively underinvestigated in this population. Nevertheless, several key investigations have focused exclusively on this important area of development.

Zarin-Ackerman and colleagues[43] noted both receptive and expressive language deficiencies at 2 years of age in a group of children born as at-risk (predominately preterm) infants as compared to others born as healthy term infants. They emphasized that these deficits could not be a function of social class (a major factor influencing language development), since this variable was controlled. In Switzerland, Largo et al.,[44] in the most comprehensive language investigation to date, compared 114 preterm children to 97 healthy term children throughout the first 5 years of life. Most stages of language development occurred at slightly later ages among the preterm children than among those born at term. Birthweight and gestational age were negatively correlated with language development at all ages. Perinatal/neonatal complications were also significantly negatively correlated with the ages at which the stages of language development were reached, and also with final language performance at 5 years of age. A permanent hearing deficit as a cause of the mild language delay in the preterm children was excluded by repeated hearing examinations; neurologically impaired children were also excluded from the basic analyses. In addition, there were no significant differences in socioeconomic status between the preterm and term groups, because of the relative homogeneity of the Swiss population. This is in contrast to many reports from other countries, including the United States and England, in which preterm babies are born more frequently to teen-age mothers of lower social class, who have a high caretaking risk. Thus, the particular demographics of this unique study allowed the authors to conclude that biomedical factors exert a considerable effect on the early language development of preterm children, and that this effect is greater than has previously been recognized.

Several smaller studies have confirmed the existence of linguistic dysfunctions among preterm children, particularly those with complicated neonatal courses.[11,45,46] Utilizing a wide variety of measures, inferior performance has been consistently reported in receptive language or comprehension, expressive language parameters such as vocabulary and word-finding, and speech qualities such as articulation and fluency.

Cognitive and Perceptual Development

Consistent differences in performance on intelligence measures have been repeatedly observed and reported in preterm/low birthweight versus term/normal birthweight children.[47,48] Furthermore, these differences in the preschool and early school years appear to persist even when the single most powerful predictor of IQ (i.e., socioeconomic status) is adequately controlled. In other words, significant deficits in cognitive and perceptual function occur frequently even in middle- to upper-middle-social class children born before term, particularly in comparison to their full-term siblings.

Wiener et al.,[49] reporting on a very large sample of low-birthweight children who had been tested with the Wechsler Intelligence Scale for Children, found that the Verbal IQ (predominantly language and cognitive items), Performance IQ (predominantly motor-perceptual items), and Full-Scale IQ (a combination of the Verbal and Performance Scales) scores showed increasing impairment with decreasing birthweight even though all subgroup means remained within the "average" range of intelligence (IQ 85 to 115). Moreover, approximately twice as great a proportion of low birthweight children as of control children fell into the borderline IQ category (70 to 84), which is invariably associated with special educational needs. Visual-motor-perceptual skills, as measured independently by the Bender Gestalt Test, also varied directly with birthweight. Klein and colleagues,[12] in a recent investigation of the preschool performance of very low birthweight children with "average" intelligence, described significant deficiencies on specific visual-motor-perceptual measures as compared to term/normal birthweight children. These authors emphasize the importance of continuing the follow-up of high-risk neonates until school age or later, in order to facilitate the early identification of such dysfunctions, which may be associated with eventual school learning problems, and the potential intervention to ameliorate these dysfunctions. By school age, many prematurely born children may exhibit subtle problems that are often very difficult to define clinically but which are likely to adversely affect their ability to cope with the demands of life both at school and at home.

Among any population of low birthweight children, a frequently asked question concerns the relative performance of those who experienced retarded intrauterine growth, and small for their gestational age (SGA), as compared to that of appropriately grown (AGA) preterm children. Most studies, including several longitudinal investigations into the early school years, have found significantly inferior cognitive, perceptual, and school educational readiness performance among SGA children, particularly those who were also born before term.[50–52] This is in contrast to the gross motor deficits that are highly correlated with decreasing gestational age. It would clearly appear that while the lowest developmental risk is associated with appropriate growth and term birth, in terms of overall intellectual and behavioral function "it is better to be born too soon than too small."

School Function

Finally, as increasing numbers of studies have longitudinally followed preterm/low birthweight infants into the school years, the full spectrum of these children's learning and behavioral performance is emerging and becoming clearer. While prevalence estimates of school problems vary between reports, almost all investigators currently agree that low-birthweight survivors have a distinctly increased risk of school dysfunction in some form.[36,53] There is also general agreement that while this substantial risk certainly exists independently of socioeconomic status, the combination and interaction of biologic and environmental risks produces an especially worrisome "double vulnerable" milieu, and a highly appropriate target population for early developmental intervention efforts. Expectedly, as with antecedent major and minor handicapping conditions, school learning or behavioral problems or both also occur with greatest frequency in the smallest and sickest NICU graduates.

Dunn et al.,[53] in one of the most extensive longitudinal follow-up studies published, reported minimal brain dysfunction (MBD) to be the single most prevalent (20 percent) handicapping syndrome at school age in a population of over 300 preterm children who weighed less than 2,000 g at birth. The authors describe these children, most of whom had IQ scores in the average range, as clinically presenting with language disorders, reading disability, attentional deficits plus overactivity, clumsiness, and various other developmental and behavioral problems. Furthermore, they stress the difficulty in adequately predicting or identifying such minor forms of cerebral dysfunction prior to school entry at age 5. This important group of neurodevelopmental sequelae is consequently liable to be missed when the outcome of preterm/low birthweight children is assessed before

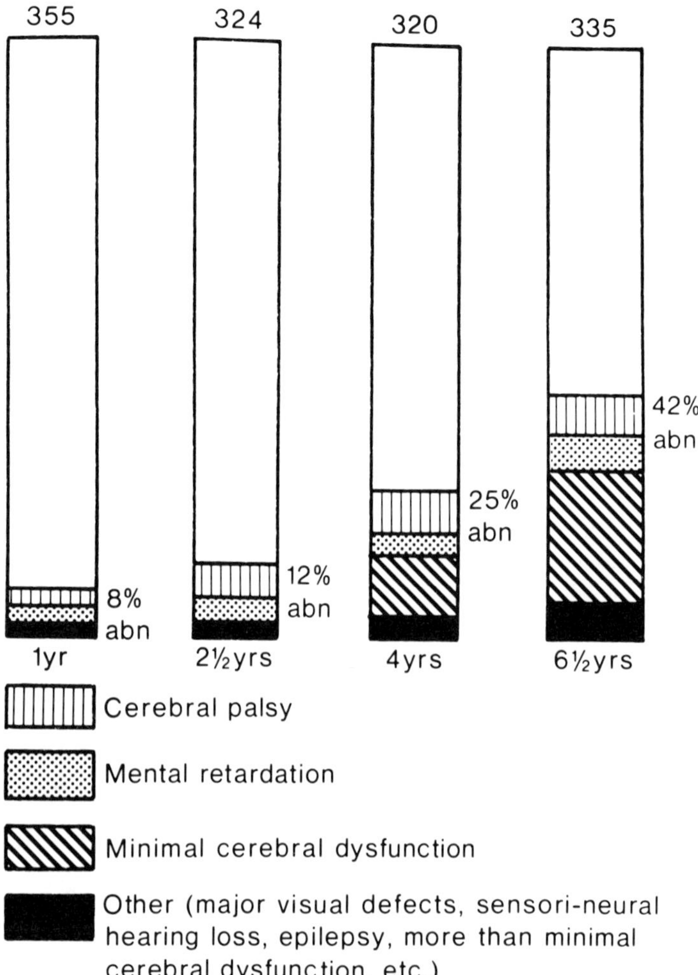

Fig. 9-2. Evolution of developmental dysfunction in preterm/low birthweight children. (Modified from Dunn HG, Krichton JU, Grunau RVE.: Neurological, psychological and educational sequelae of low birthweight. Brain Dev 2:62, 1980.)

that age. Figure 9-2 illustrates this diagnostic evolution and increase in developmental/behavioral problems over time; the authors reported a total prevalence of abnormality (i.e., all degrees of handicap) in their population of 42 percent at early school age. The disproportionate number of male children in this study who experienced school dysfunction and required remedial assistance is shown in Table 9-5. This descriptive investigation has recently been continued into adolescence.[54] While several of the low-birthweight children with earlier problems were no longer demonstrating MBD symptomatology, an almost equal number of previously unrecognized children had developed academic and social problems, thus resulting in a relatively stable number of such problems over time. Additionally, while behaviors such as hyperactivity, temper tantrums, and perservation had greatly subsided, symptoms of neuropsychiatric disturbance, including distractibility, ir-

Table 9-5. School Placement of Preterm/Low-Birthweight Children

	n	School Placement		
		At Grade Level	Regular Class With Problems	Special Class, School, or Institution
Male	150	83 (55%)	36 (24%)	31 (21%)
Female	162	115 (71%)	32 (20%)	15 (9%)
Total	312	198 (63%)	68 (22%)	46 (15%)

(Modified from Dunn HG, Krichton JU, Grunau RVE: Neurological, psychological and educational sequelae of low birthweight. Brain Dev 1:65, 1980.)

ritability, unhappiness, low frustration tolerance, fears, disobedience, poor motivation, and sleep difficulties, persisted or increased.

Other studies have confirmed these observations in very low birthweight children at 8 to 15 years of age, and have documented, in such areas as verbal expression, academic achievement, social competence, and emotional maturity, continued problems that cannot be attributed to social class or differences in the quality of parenting.[49,55,56] Nickel et al.[57] evaluated the school performance at a mean age of 10 years of 25 extremely low birthweight (1,000 g or less) children who were cared for at a time (1960 to 1972) when only very preterm infants who had little or no neonatal illness survived. Despite an overall mean IQ of 90 (range 50 to 141), 16 (64 percent) of these children had been or currently were in special educational programs. Only 7 (28 percent) were rated by their teachers to be achieving at or above grade level. Arithmetic reasoning, mathematics achievement, reading comprehension, balance, fine-motor coordination, and perceptual function were specific and common weaknesses for these children. With the marked increase in survival of extremely small and sick infants at the present time, it would seem reasonable to anticipate at least a continued, and possibly an increased, occurrence of these "new" long-term neurodevelopmental morbidities.

In summary, even though most preterm/low birthweight children are not functionally impaired, they perform and score lower on most measures of mental development, language proficiency, and scholastic achievement throughout childhood when compared on a group basis to term/normal birthweight children, and particularly in the case of very low birthweight children, should be considered at higher risk developmentally and behaviorally. Complete "catch-up" may never actually occur in terms of group differences. Because the severity of neonatal illness by itself is an unreliable predictor of neurodevelopmental outcome, all preterm/low birthweight infants merit sensitive, continuous developmental screening, and developmental assessment and management, if indicated, throughout infancy, childhood, and adolescence. However, while the need for regular developmental surveillance in this "high-risk" population is stressed, an attitude of supportive, cautious optimism, rather than presumption of handicap, is usually appropriate and reinforced by current follow-up information. Most infants and children do not develop the conditions for which they are at increased risk. Counseling and intervention directed at those infants who are also at increased risk environmentally and with regard to parenting would seem to demand high priority because of the documented importance of psychosocial variables in the ultimate prognosis for preterm/low birthweight infants.[58]

NEONATAL DEVELOPMENTAL INTERVENTION

Environment of the Preterm Infant

Before describing the rationale for and specific forms of early developmental intervention, it is worthwhile to briefly picture the NICU environment in which the sick, preterm infant first experiences extrauterine life. Hopefully, such a portrayal will explain the great interest and concern surrounding developmental interventions for preterm/low birthweight newborns, and will also provide the appropriate background setting for the remainder of this chapter.

The contemporary NICU is a highly unique, lifesaving, intensive-medical-care world experienced by the preterm newborn for an average duration of 1 to 3 months, and occasionally longer, depending on the degree of prematurity and the extent of complications. Proper care of the many neonatal complications of prematurity requires marked invasiveness and disruption of diurnal sleep/wake patterns through the use of isolettes with continuous bright lights, by loud noises, mechanical respirators with oral or nasal intubation, indwelling catheters for the administration of fluid and calories and for blood sampling, gastric and intestinal tubes for feeding, prolonged phototherapy with eye patching, multiple needle punctures for blood, urine, and spinal fluid collection, multiple radiologic and ultrasound procedures, countless different examiners and nurses with repetitive, disruptive handling, and, at best, significantly restricted opportunities for normal parent–infant interaction.[59] Dr. Jerold Lucey,[60] a prominent neonatalogist, recently questioned whether intensive care was becoming too intensive. He vividly contrasted the sleeping, quiescent intrauterine fetus with the vastly different extrauterine world of the sick, preterm newborn. He painted a stark but quite realistic picture of the NICU resident:

> Picture yourself in a brightly lit room, nude, defenseless, and your eyes hurting from silver nitrate. You are blindfolded, chilly, and surrounded by a tepid fog. You are gasping for air, fighting to breathe, and choking and gagging every so often on mucus. You are unable to clear your throat or cough. A mask is placed over your face, and blasts of air are forced into your lungs. Somebody sticks a catheter into your mouth, occasionally too far, causing you to retch or vomit. You are startled and frightened by loud, strange noises (beepers, voices, roaring respirators, telephones, radios, incubator noise). Some giant is pouring food into a tube which has been forced through your nose or throat into your stomach. It is uncomfortable and obstructs your nasal airway. You are probably nauseated; you are certainly not hungry, but you are expected to eat—and soon.
>
> "You have a headache, probably the worst one of your life. You are sleep deprived. Every time you doze off, somebody gets worried about you. They think you are in a coma. You have to be very careful to breathe very regularly. You are not allowed the multiple long pauses (15 seconds or more) of a sleeping, dreaming adult. If you do pause, a bell goes off, waking you up, and somebody slaps your feet or pulls your hair to see if you will or can cry. If you are exhausted or unresponsive, you are in trouble. If you have any jerky movements, you are suspected of having a convulsion.
>
> "Every few hours somebody cuts your foot or sticks a needle into your scalp

or one of your arteries. Your arms and legs are taped down to boards. Electrodes are attached to your chest. You are immobilized, You may even have an itch, but you can't scratch. Cool, rude hands probe your abdomen ever so often, feeling for your liver, kidneys, or bladder. After a few days of this 'intensive' care you are exhausted and you may need assistance to continue breathing just because you are too tired to do it on your own." (pp. 1064–1065).

Considering all this, the increasingly prevalent suggestion that the contemporary management of newborns receiving intensive care may be responsible for newly recognized iatrogenic complications, and may contribute to the developmental deficits associated with prematurity, is certainly not surprising.

Neonatal Intervention Rationale

Two major, incompletely resolved debates have markedly influenced the rationale and direction of neonatal developmental intervention.[61] The first issue concerns the appropriate developmental perspective and theoretical construct of a preterm newborn. Specifically, one school of thought argues that the preterm infant should be viewed essentially as an extrauterine fetus, with neonatal intervention efforts therefore aimed primarily at simulating the intrauterine environment. Proponents of this view emphasize the importance of peaceful, restful, womb-like experiences, and attempt to artificially recreate this lost "natural" milieu. Conversely, the other school vigorously asserts that since most body systems undergo profound physiologic changes at birth, it is quite reasonable to presume that the central nervous and sensory systems also change, and that the preterm infant therefore differs substantially from the fetus and requires neonatal interventions simulating the extrauterine environment experienced by term infants. Advocates of this position tend to encourage more active, supplemental sensory stimulations with the infant awake, similar to what is done in the normal newborn nursery and the home. Als et al.,[62] in attempting to provide a realistic view of life for the preterm infant immediately following birth, state the following:

> The 32-week old organism is adapted to an intrauterine environment of a regulated temperature, contained movement pattern, suspension of gravity, muted and regular sensory inputs, and physiological supports which have evolved to ensure normal intrauterine development for a large percentage of fetuses. Should a premature delivery ensue, one could predict that most fetuses would die, since their organismic adaptations do not fit the environment they find themselves in. Modern technology and medicine have changed this but are still searching for how best to provide for such organisms after birth, given the incongruence of the situation. Artificial recreation of the intrauterine environment for the preterm infant is inappropriate since the transitions at birth automatically trigger independent functioning of organ systems necessary for survival, such as the respiratory, cardiac, and digestive systems." (pp. 14–15).

Nevertheless, these writers go on to caution that "when one realizes the current organizational issues for the preterm infant, one becomes aware of the flaws and possible dangers of intervention programs which consider preterm infants to be deficient full-term infants and which, therefore, are intended to 'train' infants in behavior appropriate for full-term babies." (p. 17).

The second, and closely related, key issue concerns the appropriate developmental interpretation of the NICU environment. Does this unusual medical setting constitute a source of: (1) sensory deprivation, requiring a variety of added stimulations; (2) constant overstimulation, requiring less handling and less intervention of all types, and more time for protected, uninterrupted sleep; or (3) an inappropriate pattern of interactions rather than simply too much or too little stimulation, and including aspects of both deprivation and overstimulation? Most recent ecologic investigations of the NICU support this third view. Pertaining strictly to physical stimulation, these careful observational studies indicate that preterm newborns are not sensorily deprived, but in fact receive large amounts of ongoing stimulation.[63,64] Newborns monitored in these studies were continuously exposed to cool-white fluorescent lighting with illumination not varying across day and night. Likewise, recording of the acoustic environment revealed continuously high sound levels, higher than in a home or even a busy office. Mean characteristic sound levels were in the range of 70 to 80 decibels (dB); conversational speech ranges predominantly between 30 and 60 dB. For extended periods, the sound levels in the NICU were potentially hazardous, with upper levels reaching 120 dB. These noise levels are comparable to automobile traffic, and at times the noise reached levels of large machinery. Isolettes provided little to no sheltering from this collection of visual and auditory insults, since recordings of light and sound were virtually identical both outside and inside the incubator. The data also indicated that preterm newborns have extensive contact with caregivers. However, almost all contacts were with staff members. In spite of open visiting policies, a minimal percentage of contacts involved family members. This is of particular concern, since mothers have been found to provide an important source of stimulation to their newborns, as compared with nursing personnel. The average frequency of daily contacts ranged from 40 to 70, with some newborns receiving as many as 100 contacts. Virtually all of the contacts involved medical or nursing care with some form of handling. The contacts were brief (2 to 5 minutes in duration) and occurred on the average of every 18 to 30 minutes. In a given day, sick newborns received a total of 2.5 to 3.5 hours of contact with caregivers.

In contrast to the high magnitude of visual, auditory, and tactile stimulation, these time-motion studies found that preterm newborns had infrequent social experiences. Despite the fact that they were in contact with other persons, they seldom received social types of stimulation. The preponderance of contacts between caregivers and newborns could appropriately be described as nonsocial. If social stimulation occurred, it was embedded within routine medical or nursing care. Approaching an infant for the sole aim of providing social stimulation was a rare event. In more than half the instances in which newborns cried during contacts, caregivers did not attempt to soothe them. Additionally, the integration of social sensory experiences was not impressively high. It was not uncommon for newborns to be handled and not talked to, or to be positioned in such a way that they could not see caregivers. Quite often, social stimulation was given independently of the newborns' behavioral states. For example, in no more than approximately half the situations in which social events occurred did the newborns have their eyes opened. Surprisingly, even in the intermediate care (i.e., for infants growing and gaining weight, with less acute needs) nurseries assessed, the large majority of contacts with newborns were devoid of social events. Social touching of, rocking of, or talking to newborns, all of which are felt to be developmentally advantageous, occurred during less than one-third of all contacts.

In summary, with respect to social stimulation, many preterm newborns may indeed be sensorily deprived throughout their course of hospitalization. Despite the constant bombardment by visual, auditory, and tactile physical stimuli that it provides, the NICU appears to be a startlingly nonsocial environment for newborns. Unfortunately, there is also frequently little or no organization, rhythmicity, or developmentally appropriate pattern of physical or social stimulation incorporated into the plan of newborn intensive care.

In light of the foregoing controversial issues, it is no surprise that the specific rationale (i.e., the philosophical goals and objectives) guiding neonatal developmental intervention programs is also not widely consensual and in fact continues to evolve over time. This ongoing theoretical evolution of purpose has dramatically altered the focus and form of current neonatal intervention strategies. Through the end of the 1970s, three prominent rationales variously influenced the types and emphases of initial neonatal interventional efforts.[61] The determination of which of these three rationales was functionally dominant at a given NICU was, of course, predicated on personal, local interpretations of the developmental debates discussed previously. Succinctly, the three neonatal interventional rationales predominating during the decade from 1970 to 1979 may be stated as follows: (1) to attempt to normalize and humanize the disruptive effects of the NICU environment so that it more closely resembled the environment of term newborns; (2) to correct for presumed sensory deprivation endured by the preterm newborn treated in the NICU, and to thereby optimize subsequent development and decrease the likelihood of long-term neurodevelopmental sequelae; and (3) to compensate for intrauterine experiences lost as a result of premature birth.

However, because of continued dispute and the lack of a consensus about the necessity, nature, and effectiveness of neonatal developmental interventions based solely on these early, initial principles, there has been a clear shift in focus and orientation since approximately 1980 away from exclusively newborn- and infant-directed measures toward more family-centered interventions emphasizing and facilitating parent–preterm infant interactions. This recent redirection and alteration in the guiding rationale of neonatal intensive care should not be viewed as a total departure from past approaches nor as a scientific repudiation of earlier efforts, but rather as a very reasonable, practical, and necessary outgrowth of the expanded awareness of the developmental importance of early parent–infant interaction and communication.[65]

Types of Intervention

While one finds great interstudy variability in terms of the specific neonatal interventions (independent variables) utilized, practically all reporting centers in the 1970s employed early supplemental stimulation, environmental modification, or both in basically one or more of four major sensory areas.[66] In fact, the majority of published investigations are of multimodal (i.e., combined) sensory manipulations in more than one circumscribed area.

The four major sensory modalities recommended for neonatal developmental intervention include: (1) visual stimulation (decoration of the surroundings, mobiles with brightly colored objects), (2) auditory stimulation (talking, singing, music boxes, recordings of the mother's voice, recordings of the mother's heartbeat), (3) tactile stimulation (non-nutritive sucking, stroking, flexing, massaging, rubbing, handling, positioning), and (4) vestibular-kinesthetic stimulation (rocking and the use of oscillating beds such as waterbeds). Many different combinations of these infant-focused interventions have been described and analyzed (e.g., stroking, handling, and rocking; specific cephalocaudal message treatment and rocking administered by the mother; use of a rocking bed and heartbeat recording; visual decoration and body rubbing; use of a rocking waterbed, with simulated heartbeats and tapes of the mother's voice played during rocking; and bright mobiles, rubbing, rocking, talking, singing, and music boxes—thus representing all four sensory modalities in this case). As can immediately be appreciated, the number of individual protocols is almost limitless, and intervention programs further vary in terms of their specificity (or lack thereof) within a given sensory area. For example, one program may utilize a variety of vestibular stimulations in differing degrees and sequences, while another may have chosen to assess the effects of vestibular stimulation as specifically provided by a motorized hammock or, alternatively, by an oscillating waterbed. Such marked variability between individual intervention programs seriously impairs both the interpretation of and ability to generalize the outcome from each.

A relatively unique type of physical stimulation, recently advocated by some, is neonatal hydrotherapy.[67] This approach is generally used as an adjunct to the more traditional intervention modalities, particularly in conjunction with tactile stimulations such as rubbing, handling, and positioning. The equipment required for this intervention technique includes a standard infant bassinet or other suitable tub, warm water in which the preterm newborn is immersed, and an overhead radiant heater placed above the tub.

As previously mentioned, there has been an entirely new dimension and direction to the field of developmental intervention for biologically vulnerable infants in the 1980s.[61,68] This more recent type of intervention focuses primarily on the enhancement of the parent–preterm infant relationship by means of both the facilitation of optimal social functioning on the part of the preterm infant, and correspondingly by direct parent-training strategies. The type of neonatal intervention in this current, parent-focused approach closely resembles and parallels the goals and objectives of early developmental intervention for infants at increased environmental risk. In fact, recommendations and protocols regarding intervention for the two risk populations will frequently appear quite similar, with many overlaps and a shared rationale; it is not unusual at individual sites for the preterm/low-birthweight intervention protocol to have been adapted directly from existing intervention programs for infants and families who are impoverished or of low socioeconomic status.

Interventions aimed at improving parent–preterm infant interaction have taken various forms, usually including a component of infant preparation and readiness for such intimate contact and also a component of parent instruction in initiating dialogue and responding to the fragile infant's communicative overtures. The preterm newborn and infant should, when it is medically appropriate, be assisted through environmental structuring, support, and facilitation in interacting with his or her immediate environment in such a way that he or she confirms expectations for elicited social behavior with and feedback to the parents. For example, when the preterm infant becomes overloaded with stimuli, he or she may withdraw, become rigid, or even demonstrate signs of autonomic nervous system stress and dysfunction, including gagging, vomiting, apnea, bradycardia, and cyanosis. In each of these cases the infant becomes unavailable to its environment in terms of obtaining information or giving positive feedback, and in turn may cause the parents and other caregivers to feel less competent and effective. Thus, to the extent that reciprocal social interactions are contingent upon the "readability" and "predictability" of the infant's signals, in addition to the caregiver's ability to respond appropriately to these signals, it becomes critical for infants at risk to engage in interactions without experiencing great physiologic, motor, and homeostatic regulatory costs.

Likewise and concurrently, contemporary neonatal intervention programs emphasize the need for parents to understand preterm newborn and infant behavior. Parmelee[69] has stressed the importance of carefully interpreting the individual infant's different behaviors to the parent as a key first step in this. He states that it is also helpful to very specifically model techniques of dealing with the infant for the parent, and to positively reinforce the parent's successful spontaneous interactions with the infant. Ideally, parents should be assisted in correctly modifying their perceptions of their infant's medical status, should become more successful in implementing programs of brief behavioral intervention, and should be aided in constructing a positive and enhancing psychological environment for themselves and their vulnerable infant. Additionally, since the coexistence of both biologic and environmental risks constitutes a particularly common background for developmental failure, efforts at comprehensive, broad-based intervention must often include both an intensive home visitation component and also an understanding of the parents' (especially the mother's) coping abilities, support services for the parents' physical and mental health, and economic support for the family, including adequate, stable daycare for the infant and siblings when required.

Intervention Parameters and Settings

As with the specific combinations of sensory stimulations, great variability also exists in the reported onset, frequency, and duration of interventions. The timing of initial developmental intervention varies from immediately after birth, to some relatively arbitrary starting point such as 14 days of age, to the time when the preterm newborn is deemed clinically and physiologically stable. Likewise, even though most studies have provided an intervention program taking place at least several times daily, marked interstudy variability in intervention frequency is again the norm. Some stimulations were given only during feedings, some were prescribed every 15 minutes regardless of the infant's readiness or state of alertness, and others were continuous, discontinuous, or contingent upon the infant's own activity and responsiveness. The greatest variation of all is in the duration of reported intervention programs. For example, typical intervention endpoints include term gestational age, attainment of normal birthweight, or nursery discharge. Thus, the overall length of sensory stimulation might be 1 week or 8 weeks. Furthermore, while most interventions with preterm infants have focused exclusively on manipulating the environment during the infant's initial hospitalization, in recent years an increasing number of programs also provide interventional protocols for parents that continue after hospital discharge of the infant to its home. These home follow-through programs also vary in duration from several months to the entire first year of life.

Nurses in the NICU have been the principal agents of neonatal intervention in most reports of the various forms of sensory stimulation described earlier. Other agents are physical therapists, occupational therapists, and early childhood special educators. With the previously discussed evolution from solely infant-focused programs to more parent-focused strategies, parents and other family members are, naturally, increasingly involved in the active intervention plans.

Intervention Subject Selection

The study of comparability of experiments involving neonatal developmental interventions is further hampered by the inconsistent reporting of and limited information given about sample characteristics. This too constitutes a source of great interstudy and intrastudy variability. Many studies have involved families of low socioeconomic status with predominantly black, young, unmarried mothers. Unfortunately, most have also involved relatively healthy preterm infants without early signs and symptoms of neurologic dysfunction; infants who may theoretically benefit from intervention the most—such as those of extremely low birthweight (less than 1,000 g at birth) and experiencing numerous neonatal complications—are quite underrepresented in most published investigations. Thus, the bulk of experimental evidence has been accumulated from infants who, biologically and medically, are at relatively lower risk and environmentally are at higher risk. Additionally, study differences abound in such basic infant characteristics as birthweight mean and range (700 to 2,400 g), gestational age mean and range (24 to 37 weeks), inborn–outborn status, severity of neonatal illness, types of medical intervention, and duration of hospitalization. These are important sources of variability in interpreting intervention results, since all have been associated to some degree with neurodevelopmental outcome in preterm infants. Other sources of variation that prevent direct comparison of the results of intervention protocols include socioeconomic status, race, and maternal age and parity.

Intervention Outcome Measures

Adding to the variability of the study populations and intervention methodologies used is the extensive variability in the types of dependent outcome measures that have been employed. Assessed outcome parameters of neonatal intervention can be grouped into three broad categories: developmental, medical, and parental. The various developmental outcome measures employed include performance on standardized neurodevelopmental and neurobehavioral evaluations (e.g., Brazelton Neonatal Behavioral Assessment Scale, Bayley Scales of Infant Development, Cattell Infant Intelligence Scale), performance on specific cognitive–sensory tasks (e.g., visual orienting, auditory responsivity, recognition memory), sleep-wake state organization and stabilization, temperament characteristics such as activity level and irritability, and neuromotor criteria such as muscle tone and volitional movement. The dependent medical variables that are typically assessed are weight gain, head growth, change in vital signs such as heart or respiratory rate or both, frequency of apnea, frequency of emesis, and length of hospitalization. Parental outcome measures have included the frequency of parental visitation and attempted evaluation of the quality of the parent–infant interaction.

Interventional studies have varied considerably in both the number and types of intervention outcome measures utilized. For example, one study may examine only a single medical outcome, such as the frequency of apnea, using different sensory stimulations, while another will evaluate a combination of developmental, medical, and parental results for very similar interventions. In sum, the critical appraisal of neonatal intervention involves a difficult, confusing search for effects amid a complex mixture of structural, methodologic, sampling, and outcome variables.

Results of Neonatal Developmental Intervention

As might be anticipated, the reported results of intervention studies are as various as the methodologies employed, and the outcome patterns reveal great variability in terms of their exact nature, extent, significance, and duration. The positive developmental outcomes most frequently reported include improved neonatal neurobehavioral performance (particularly in visual and auditory orienting and general maturation items), increased state stabilization, higher performance on infant developmental (both mental and motor) assessment scales, normalized muscle tone, and more manageable temperament, with decreased irritability and increased positive affect. Encouraging medical outcomes typically cited include improved weight gain with better feeding, decreased incidence of apnea, and more mature heart-rate responses. Reported positive parental outcomes primarily involve an increased frequency of parental visitation and enhanced parent–infant interaction. However, while most studies report at least some measured benefit attributable to the specific intervention employed, many of these benefits are not replicated in other investigations which, in contrast, report essentially negative findings. Because of these frequently contradictory results, only limited generalizations can be made from most of the individual, isolated outcomes.

Nineteen scientifically credible neonatal developmental intervention studies reported since 1970 could be categorized into three groups according to the basic intervention philosophy employed: (1) 13 were investigations of infant-focused, sensory stimulation interventions, (2) 3 were investigations of parent-focused, training interventions and (3) 3 were investigations of a combination of both infant-focused and parent-focused interventions. The 13 infant-focused studies were further subdivided on the basis of the specific sensory modalities utilized: two reports[70,71] of auditory stimulation alone, one report[72] of tactile stimulation alone, one report[73] of vestibular-kinesthetic stimulation alone, three reports[74–76] of combined auditory and vestibular-kinesthetic stimulation, four reports[77–80] of combined tactile and vestibular-kinesthetic stimulation, and two reports[81,82] of multimodal sensory stimulation combining all four principal modalities (visual, auditory, tactile, and vestibular-kinesthetic). As expected, the majority of acceptable studies, particularly prior to 1980, primarily examined infant-focused interventions, while more recent studies have often included a parent-training component. However, in only 3 of the 13 infant-focused programs[72,78,82] were parents directly involved in administering the sensory stimulations. In most of the 19 studies, regardless of focus, the actual interventions occurred exclusively while the infant was hospitalized in the intensive care or intermediate care nursery. Only five of the studies[78,82–85] investigated interventions that were partially or entirely home-based—by far the most extensive being the Bromwich and Parmelee study,[84] which provided parent-focused home intervention to 2 years of age. The comprehensive nature and complex requirements of these home programs generally make them more difficult to adequately perform as individual, clinical research projects.

All 13 infant-focused studies reported at least one statistically significant group difference favoring the experimental, intervention group over a randomly or sequentially chosen control group. All of the 13 studies also found an absence of significant intergroup differences in numerous assessed outcome measures. However, beyond these superficial similarities, the results diverge dramatically, with the positive findings of one study often being the negative findings of another. Interpretation is rendered even more difficult, as previously discussed, by the great interstudy variability, which makes each investigation seem almost anecdotal. For example, rapidity of weight gain is a desired medical outcome easily measured in many of the 13 infant-focused studies. Kramer and Pierpont,[76] using a combination of auditory and vestibular-kinesthetic stimulations, reported improved growth parameters, particularly weight gain, as their only significant group difference attributable to their intervention program. In contrast, both Barnard[74] and Burns et al.,[75] employing virtually the same intervention modalities 10 years apart, found no experimental-versus-control group differences in weight gain: an outcome that was their major negative result. To complete this total disparity, Kramer and Pierpont found no significant group differences in newborn neurologic status or in standardized neonatal behavioral assessment, while again, almost the exact opposite was reported by Barnard and Burns and colleagues, both of whom found very significant improvements for experimental group infants in these same developmental areas—specifically, an increased state stabilization and greater neuromotor maturation. Korner et al.[73] reported no weight gain or other physiologic group differences following a study of purely vestibular-kinesthetic stimulation via oscillating waterbeds, with the single exception of a significant reduction of apnea in the experimental group. Even though this potentially important finding has not been reliably corroborated by other investigators, it has altered practices in a number of neonatal intensive care units (see Ch. 5).

Even the two studies utilizing similar multimodal sensory stimulations reported conflicting results. Scarr-Salapatek and Williams,[82] in a frequently cited study, found significantly greater weight gain and significantly superior performance in measures of neonatal behavior for experimental group infants receiving interventions in all four major sensory modalities. However, Leib et al.,[81] using the same modalities, reported no significant group differences in the identical outcome measures. The two studies did both report significantly higher scores on assessments of mental and motor development during the first year of life for experimental infants. But even this general agreement in findings must be cautiously interpreted because of its short-term nature (i.e., 1 year of age or less), and also because of other studies[86] showing essentially no infant performance differences. It is particularly striking that two reviews of neonatal developmental interventions reached conclusions as disparate as the individual studies themselves. Cornell and Gottfried[87] argued that the accumulated literature failed to substantiate convincing effects of intervention on most outcome measures, including weight gain, neonatal behavior, and mental development; only in the area of motor development could they detect a trend of positive influence. Nevertheless, Campbell,[88] referring to many of the same studies, summarized the effects of neonatal intervention programs as positively influencing weight gain and mental development during the first year of life, but having no demonstrable influence on early motor development.

The most consistent finding of the six studies[83–86,89,90] that were partially or completely parent-focused involved the positive facilitation of parent–infant interactions. Five of these six studies reported at least some significant, objective enhancement of the mother–infant relationship, with only Brown et al.[86] failing to detect any group differences in interactional quantity or quality. However, clear documentation of other benefits of this practical, parent-training approach cannot be obtained from the results of these studies. The postulated parental outcome of an increased frequency of hospital visitation was reported only by Minde et al.[89]; Brown and co-workers[86] found that experimental group mothers, during their own hospitalizations, visited their infants in the NICU significantly more often than control group mothers, but that this encouraging group difference rapidly disappeared once the mothers were discharged from the hospital and returned to their homes. No consistent group differences in weight gain, neonatal behavioral performance, or mental or motor development were apparent across the six studies.

Analysis of the three most rigorous, long-term parent-focused studies, all of which were conducted primarily in the infant's home following nursery discharge, and which utilized structured, educational home visitation as the principal intervention modality, highlights this dilemma. Field et al.[85] reported numerous optimistic results from a 8-month home intervention program combining both parent-focused and infant-focused strategies. Significantly better outcomes were realized for their experimental group preterm infant/teenage mother dyads in practically all of the dependent variables assessed (i.e., infant temperament ratings, mother-infant interaction ratings, weight gain, and mental development scores). Unique to this study was that the authors expanded their investigation to include other demographic types of infant/mother pairs, and remarkably found that the preterm infant/teenage mother experimental-control group differences were greater than the preterm infant–term infant, teenage mother–adult mother, or preterm infant/teenage mother–preterm infant/adult mother group differences. Barrera et al.,[83] employing a year-long home intervention program, found that a parent-focused intervention group scored somewhat higher in terms of mental but not motor development than did either an infant-focused intervention or a control group. However, the finding of greatest statistical significance in this investigation was the consistently superior performance of a term control group to all three preterm groups on measures of both mental and motor development. In contrast, Bromwich and Parmelee[84] reported far more modest, almost discouraging, results from their highly individualized home intervention program for preterm infants between 10 and 24 months of age. This study was unique in that free, regular health care and supervision from birth to 2 years of age was provided to all participating families, while only the experimental group received the education component of the combined intervention effort. The only significant group difference discovered was enhanced mother-child interaction at 2 years of age for experimental group pairs.

No group differences were apparent on any child-developmental measures at the study conclusion. The authors suggested that among possible interpretations for the failure to find cognitive group differences were the extensive health care component available to both the experimental and control groups, and the temporal proximity of outcome measures to the intervention experience, since there is evidence that parent-focused, educational interventions may be expected to show greater effects over a period of time rather than immediately after program termination.[91]

Conclusions and Recommendations

How can one sort out and respond to these mixed effects that occur within a framework of incredible interstudy variability? Following a thorough review of infant-focused, primarily hospital-based neonatal sensory stimulation interventions, one is almost forced to conclude that practically any early intervention protocol can be expected to yield at least some benefits in some measured area of performance. However, reported positive effects are generally of very short duration, with significant developmental differences highly unusual even at 1 year of age, and virtually no studies providing post-infancy data. Thus, the accumulated evidence hardly provides a convincing rationale on which to base specific recommendations for nursery developmental intervention protocols, nor does it seem, at this time, to justify the routine employment of such programs in multiple sites to normalize or facilitate the development of biologically vulnerable infants in the NICU environment.

There are several important reasons for this cautious, conservative interpretation. Too little evidence now exists on how to achieve maximal and optimal effects from these types of intervention programs; the key variables responsible for success have not as yet been defined. There has been insufficient consideration and discussion of potentially adverse side effects of neonatal developmental intervention in most individual studies or reviews of the field. The link between repeated, intrusive handling and disturbance of the physiologically fragile preterm/low birthweight infant and such deleterious neonatal complications as hypoxia, acidosis, apnea, and bradycardia has recently been documented.[92] Increasing numbers of detailed investigations into the typical "life" and ecology of the NICU emphasize both the instability of the autonomic nervous system of the immature newborn and the surprising ease of exacerbating this instability by continual and unpredictable disruptions of quiet sleep.[93,94] These observations confirm and partially explain longstanding anecdotal nursing descriptions of the seemingly paradoxical association between decreased physical examination and sensory stimulation of the neonate and its increased neurophysiologic stability and readiness for nursery discharge.

Some of the most sustained neonatal interventional effects were best demonstrated in those relatively few programs[82,85] that continued their stimulation protocol after hospital discharge into the infant's home, with close and considerable parental involvement. Unfortunately, these very comprehensive programs would be prohibitively costly in many centers, but more importantly, may actually owe the bulk of their apparent success to the extensive period of support given the mother, rather than to the various infant stimulation modalities themselves. Another reason for cautious conclusions about exclusively infant-focused interventional approaches is the lack of evidence for the effectiveness or safety of intervention for those preterm/low birthweight infants at greatest risk for developmental deviance, since most reported studies have dealt predominantly with relatively healthy preterm newborns.

Finally, original theoretical bases for neonatal developmental intervention, as described earlier in this chapter, have been found wanting in terms of appropriately conceptualizing the preterm infant and the NICU environment. The majority of early studies were designed around a model of the preterm infant as an isolated, sensorily deprived organism in serious need of supplemental stimulation. This inadequate model led quite naturally to attempts to "train" immature, unready, disorganized preterm infants in behavior appropriate for mature, term infants. More recent, complex models of the preterm infant and its parents and unique surroundings have suggested new interventional directions.

As has been discussed, the shift to more parent-focused, parent-training-oriented neonatal interventions, based primarily on the "new" rationale of enhancement of the quality of parent–infant interactions, also cannot be clearly and convincingly supported by the accumulated research evidence. Nevertheless, contemporary neonatal intervention programs that attempt to facilitate effective parenting strategies for immature, often unresponsive infants, and which incorporate some type of extended home visitation plan, appear to best fit current child-development models, to be most acceptable and useful to families, and to have the greatest likelihood of achieving functional, meaningful results. Sufficient clinical interventional experience with preterm/low birthweight infants has been gathered to permit generating suggested practical guidelines for neonatal intervention programs. These include: (1) recognizing the unusual physiological stresses being endured by the preterm infant, (2) modifying the environment to decrease overstimulation and protect the fragile infant; specifically, screening out strongly noxious and unnecessary sensory stimuli such as handling during periods of quiet sleep, (3) introducing diurnal rhythms to promote behavioral organization, (4) gradually facilitating reciprocal visual, auditory, tactile, vestibular-kinesthetic, and social feedback during alert periods, (5) immediately terminating or altering approaches that produce avoidance responses, and (6) educating and assisting parents in "reading," anticipating, and appropriately responding to their own infant's cues and signals.[88]

This final programmatic recommendation is particularly important. Klaus and Kennell[95] have emphasized the developmental utility of infant imitation, which is frequently observed in mother–term infant interactions, rather than simple infant stimulation, which tends to predominate in mother–preterm infant interactions. Several investigators have reported the unexpected observation that decreasing the maternal activity level and substituting imitation for stimulation results in increased infant responsiveness and gaze time.[96,97] Thus, early intervention programs should strive to help parents by interpreting the infant's behavior for them, by demonstrating how to handle the preterm infant, and by fostering and reinforcing parental feelings of competence. The specific intervention plan chosen must be individualized, flexible, modifiable, and always sensitive to the changing, dynamic neurodevelopmental status of the particular infant.

The lack of definitive conclusions about the effectiveness of early intervention on the behavior and development of the preterm human infant should not be overly discouraging, but instead should be a strong, urgent stimulus to the planning, financing, and completion of new comprehensive, prospective, longitudinal investigations. Such a national collaborative early intervention project, the Infant Health and Development Program, is currently in progress, with results still several years away. With the increasing survival of ever smaller and sicker infants, early intervention studies must include these most vulnerable survivors as well as those infants with less complicated neonatal courses. New studies must attempt to differentiate the effectiveness of intervention and its need by preterm infants of middle and high socioeconomic status in comparison to preterm infants of low socioeconomic status. Children "graduating" from intervention programs must be followed and assessed developmentally beyond 1 or even 2 years of age, to seek long-term effects that might initially be obscured and inapparent.

Lastly, essentially negative studies should be critically analyzed in order to ascertain mitigating variables leading to program ineffectiveness. Brown et al.,[86] discussing their failure with a combined infant- and parent-focused approach to involve socially disadvantaged mothers with their babies and thereby enhance mother–infant interactions, enumerated such interventional impediments as mothers' lack of transportation to and from the hospital, mothers' need to care for older children at home, mothers' inability to leave the home because of cultural concerns of their own mothers, and crises of daily living (e.g., inadequate or no housing, lack of financial support). Brown and co-workers succinctly summarized this unfortunate reality, saying that "Most of the mothers seemed so overwhelmed by the inadequacies of their social environments that no intervention short of massive environmental alteration was likely to have any lasting consequences." This sobering conclusion should serve both to keep individual, limited neonatal interventions in perspective and also to challenge us to develop innovative, broad-based approaches to the enormously complex task of optimizing the developmental and behavioral outcome of preterm/low birthweight infants.

REFERENCES

1. McCormick MC: The contribution of low birthweight to infant mortality and childhood morbidity. N Engl J Med 312:82, 1985
2. Paneth N, Kiely JL, Wallenstein S, et al: Newborn intensive care and neonatal mortality in low birthweight infants. N Engl J Med 307:149, 1982
3. Philip AGS, Little GA, Polivy DR, Lucey, JF: Neonatal mortality risk for the '80s: The importance of birthweight/gestational age groups. Pediatrics 68:122, 1981
4. Hirata T, Epcar JT, Walsh A, et al: Survival and outcome of infants 501 to 750 grams: A six year experience. J Pediatr 102:741, 1983
5. Brothwood M, Wolke D, Gamsu H, et al: Prognosis of the very low birthweight baby in relation to gender. Arch Dis Child 61:559, 1986
6. Fitzhardinge PM: Early growth and development in low birthweight infants following treatment in an intensive care nursery. Pediatrics 56:162, 1975
7. Hack M, Fanaroff AA, Merkatz IR: The low birthweight infant—evolution of a changing outlook. N Engl J Med 301:1162, 1979
8. Hagberg B, Hagberg G, Olow I: The changing panorama of cerebral palsy in Sweden. Acta Pediatr Scand 73:433, 1984
9. Stanley FJ: An epidemiological study of cerebral palsy in western Australia, 1956–1975. I. Changes in total cerebral palsy incidence and associated factors. Dev Med Child Neurol 21:701, 1979

10. Paneth N, Kiely JL, Stein Z, Susser M: Cerebral palsy and newborn care. III. Estimated prevalence rates of cerebral palsy under differing rates of mortality and impairment of low birthweight infants. Dev Med Child Neurol 23:801, 1981
11. Ehrlich CH, Shapiro E, Kimball BD, Huttner M: Communication skills in five-year-old children with high-risk neonatal histories. J Speech Hearing Res 16:522, 1973
12. Klein N, Hack M, Gallagher J, Fanaroff AA: Preschool performance of children with normal intelligence who were very low birthweight infants. Pediatrics 75:531, 1985
13. Field TM: High risk infants "have less fun" during early interactions. Topics in Early Childhood Special Education 3(1):77, 1983
14. Kurtzberg D, Vaughan HG, Daum C, et al: Neurobehavioral performance of low birthweight infants at 40 weeks conceptional age: Comparison with normal full-term infants. Dev Med Child Neurol 21:590, 1979
15. Saigal S, Rosenbaum P, Stoskopf B, Milner R: Follow-up of infants 501 to 1500 grams birthweight delivered to residents of a geographically defined region with perinatal intensive care facilities. J Pediatr 100:606, 1982
16. Ferrari F, Grosoli MV, Fontana G, Cavazzuti GB: Neurobehavioral comparison of low-risk preterm and fullterm infants at term conceptual age. Dev Med Child Neurol 25:450, 1983
17. Friedman SL, Jacobs BS, Werthmann MW: Preterms of low medical risk: Spontaneous behaviors and soothability at expected date of birth. Infant Behav and Dev 5:3, 1982
18. Aylward GP, Hatcher RP, Leavitt LA, et al: Factors affecting neurobehavioral responses of preterm infants at term conceptional age. Child Dev 55:1155, 1984
19. Kurtzberg D, Hilpert PL, Kreuzer JA, Vaughan HG: Differential maturation of cortical auditory evoked potentials to speech sounds in normal fullterm and very low birthweight infants. Dev Med Child Neurol 26:466, 1984
20. Kaga K, Hashira S, Marsh RR: Auditory brainstem responses and behavioral responses in preterm infants. Br J Audiol 20:121, 1986
21. Anders TF, Keener M: Developmental course of nightime sleep-wake patterns in full-term and premature infants during the first year of life. I. Sleep 8(3):173, 1985
22. Fox NA, Porges SW: The relation between neonatal heart period patterns and developmental outcome. Child Dev 56:28, 1985
23. Anders TF, Keener MA, Kraemer H: Sleep-wake state organization, neonatal assessment and development in premature infants during the first year of life. II. Sleep 8(3):193, 1985
24. Cohen SE, Parmelee AH, Beckwith L, Sigman M: Cognitive development in preterm infants: Birth to 8 years. Dev Behav Pediatr 7:102, 1986
25. Rose SA: Differential rates of visual information processing in full-term and preterm infants. Child Dev 54:1189, 1983
26. Ruff HA, McCarton C, Kurtzberg D, Vaughan HG: Preterm infants' manipulative exploration of objects. Child Dev 55:1166, 1984
27. DiVitto B, Goldberg S: The effects of newborn medical status on early parent-infant interactions. p. 311. In Field TM (ed): Infants Born at Risk. Spectrum, New York, 1979
28. Field TM: Interaction patterns of preterm and term infants. p. 333. In Field TM (ed): Infants Born at Risk. Spectrum, New York, 1979
29. Watt J: Interaction and development in the first year. I. The effects of prematurity. Early Hum Dev 13:195, 1986
30. Crnic KA, Ragozin AS, Greenberg MT, et al: Social interaction and developmental competence of preterm and full-term infants during the first year of life. Child Dev 54:1199, 1983
31. Malatesta CZ, Grigoryev P, Lamb C, et al: Emotion socialization and expressive development in preterm and full-term infants. Child Dev 57:316, 1986
32. Bennett FC, Robinson NM, Sells CJ: Hyaline membrane disease, birthweight, and gestational age: Effects on development in the first two years. Am J Dis Child 136:888, 1982
33. Drillien CM: Abnormal neurologic signs in the first year of life in low birthweight infants: Possible prognostic significance. Dev Med Child Neurol 14:575, 1972
34. Amiel-Tison C: A method for neurologic evaluation within the first year of life. Curr Probl Pediatr 7:1, 1976
35. Coolman RB, Bennett FC, Sells CJ, et al: Neuromotor development of graduates of the neonatal intensive care unit: Patterns encountered in the first two years of life. Dev Behav Pediatr 6:327, 1985
36. Drillien CM, Thomson AJM, Burgoyne K: Low birthweight children at early school age: A longitudinal study. Dev Med Child Neurol 22:26, 1980
37. Ross G, Lipper EG, Auld PAM: Consistency and change in the development of premature infants weighing less than 1501 grams at birth. Pediatrics 76:885, 1985

38. Vohr BR, Coll CTG: Neurodevelopmental and school performance of very low birthweight infants: A seven-year longitudinal study. Pediatrics 76:345, 1985
39. Bobath K, Bobath B: The diagnosis of cerebral palsy in infancy. Arch Dis Child 31:408, 1956
40. Goodman M, Rothberg AD, Houston-McMillan JE, et al: Effect of early neurodevelopmental therapy in normal and at-risk survivors of neonatal intensive care. Lancet 2:1327, 1985
41. Piper MC, Kunos VI, Willis DM, et al: Early physical therapy effects on the high-risk infant. A randomized controlled trial. Pediatrics 78:216, 1986
42. Burns YR, Bullock MI: Comparison of abilities of preterm and mature born children at 5 years of age. Aust Pediatr J 21:31, 1985
43. Zarin-Ackerman J, Lewis M, Driscoll JM: Language development in 2-year-old normal and risk infants. Pediatrics 59:982, 1977
44. Largo RH, Molinari L, Comenale-Pinto L, et al: Language development of term and preterm children during the first five years of life. Dev Med Child Neurol 28:333, 1986
45. Hubatch LM, Johnson CJ, Kistler DJ, et al: Early language abilities of high-risk infants. J Speech Hearing Dis 50:195, 1985
46. Michelsson K, Noronen M: Neurological, psychological and articulatory impairment in five-year-old children with a birthweight of 2000 g or less. Eur J Pediatr 137:96, 1983
47. Rubin RA, Rosenblatt C, Balow B: Psychological and educational sequelae of prematurity. Pediatrics 52:352, 1973
48. Ungerer JA, Sigman M: Developmental lags in preterm infants from one to three years of age. Child Dev 54:1217, 1983
49. Wiener G, Rider RV, Oppel, WC, Harper PA: Correlates of low birthweight. Psychological status at eight to ten years of age. Pediatr Res 2:110, 1968
50. Neligan GA, Kolvin I, Scott D, Garside RF: Born Too Soon or Born Too Small. Clinics in Developmental Medicine, Vol. 61 J. B. Lippincott, Philadelphia, 1976
51. Eaves LC, Nuttall JC, Klonoff H, Dunn HG: Developmental and psychological test scores in children of low birthweight. Pediatrics 45:9, 1970
52. Silva PA, McGee R, Williams S: A longitudinal study of the intelligence and behavior of preterm and small for gestational age children. Dev Behav Pediatr 5:1, 1984
53. Dunn HG, Krichton JU, Grunau RVE, et al: Neurological, psychological and educational sequalae of low birthweight, Brain Dev 2:57, 1980
54. Dunn HG (ed): Sequaelae of Low Birthweight: The Vancouver Study Clinics in Developmental Medicine no. 95/96. J.B. Lippincott, Philadelphia, 1986
55. Wright FH, Blough RR, Chamberlin A, et al: A controlled follow-up study of small prematures born from 1952 through 1956. Am J Dis Child 124:506, 1972
56. Caputo DV, Goldstein KM, Taub HB: The development of prematurely born children through middle childhood. p. 219. In Field TM (ed): Infants Born at Risk. Spectrum, New York, 1979
57. Nickel RE, Bennett FC, Lamson FN: School performance of children with birthweights of 1000 g or less. Am J Dis Child 136:105, 1982
58. Kopp CB: Risk factors in development. p. 1081. In Haith MM, Campos JJ (eds): Handbook of Child Psychology: Vol. 2. Infancy and Developmental Psychobiology. John Wiley & Sons, New York, 1983
59. Gottfried AW, Hodgman JE, Brown KW: How intensive is newborn intensive care? An environmental analysis. Pediatrics 74:292, 1984
60. Lucey JF: Is intensive care becoming too intensive? Pediatrics 59:1064, 1977
61. Meisels SJ, Jones SN, Stiefel, GS: Neonatal intervention: Problem, purpose, and prospects. Topics in Early Childhood Special Education 3(1):1, 1983
62. Als H, Lester BM, Tronick EC, Brazelton TB: Towards a research instrument for the Assessment of Preterm Infants' Behavior (APIB). p. 1. In Fitzgerald HE, Lester BM, Yogman MW (eds): Theory and Research in Behavioral Pediatrics, Vol 1. Plenum Press, New York, 1982
63. Gottfried AW, Gaiter JL (eds): Infant Stress under Intensive Care: Environmental Neonatology. University Park Press, Baltimore, 1984
64. Gottfried AW, Wallace-Lande P, Sherman-Brown S: Physical and social environment of newborn infants in special care units. Science 214:637, 1981
65. Bee HL, Barnard KE, Eyres SJ, et al: Prediction of IQ and language skill from perinatal status, child performance, family characteristics, and mother-infant interaction. Child Dev 53:1134, 1982
66. Field TM: Supplemental stimulation of preterm neonates. Early Hum Dev 4:301, 1980
67. Sweeney JK: Neonatal hydrotherapy: An adjunct to developmental intervention in an intensive care setting. Phys Occup Ther Pediatr 3:1, 1983
68. Ramey CT, Bryant DM, Sparling JJ, Wasik BH: A biosocial systems perspective on environmental interventions for low birthweight infants. Clin Obstet Gynecol 27:672, 1984

69. Parmelee AH: Early intervention for preterm infants. p. 82. In Brown CC (ed): Infants at Risk: Assessment and Intervention. Johnson and Johnson Baby Products Company, Skillman, NJ, 1981
70. Katz V: Auditory stimulation and developmental behavior of the premature infant. Nurs Res 20:196, 1971
71. Segall ME: Cardiac responsivity to auditory stimulation in premature infants. Nurs Res 21:15, 1972
72. Powell LF: The effect of extra stimulation and maternal involvement on the development of low birthweight infants and on maternal behavior. Child Dev 45:106, 1974
73. Korner AF, Kraemer HC, Haffner ME, Cosper LM: Effects of waterbed flotation on premature infants: A pilot study. Pediatrics 56:361, 1975
74. Barnard KE: The effect of stimulation on the sleep behavior of the premature infant. Commun Nurs Res 6:12, 1973
75. Burns KA, Deddish RB, Burns WJ, Hatcher RP: Use of oscillating waterbeds and rhythmic sounds for premature infant stimulation. Dev Psychol 19:746, 1983
76. Kramer LI, Pierpont ME: Rocking waterbeds and auditory stimuli to enhance growth of preterm infants. J Pediatr 88:297, 1976
77. Field TM, Schanberg SM, Scafidi F, et al: Tactile/kinesthetic stimulation effects on preterm neonates. Pediatrics 77:654, 1986
78. Rice RD: Neurophysiological development in premature infants following stimulation. Dev Psychol 13:69, 1977
79. Rosenfield AG: Visiting in the intensive care nursery. Child Dev 51:939, 1980
80. White JL, Labarba RC: The effects of tactile and kinesthetic stimulation on neonatal developmental in the premature infant. Dev Psychobiol 9:569, 1976
81. Leib SA, Benfield DG, Guidubaldi J: Effects of early intervention and stimulation on the preterm infant. Pediatrics 66:83, 1980
82. Scarr-Salapatek S, Williams ML: The effects of early stimulation on low birthweight infants. Child Dev 44:94, 1973
83. Barrera ME, Rosenbaum PL, Cunningham CE: Early home intervention with low birthweight infants and their parents. Child Dev 57:20, 1986
84. Bromwich RM, Parmelee AH: An intervention program for preterm infants. p. 389. In Field TM (ed): Infants Born at Risk. Spectrum, New York, 1979
85. Field TM, Widmayer SM, Stringer S, Ignatoff E: Teenage, lower class, black mothers and their preterm infants: An intervention and developmental follow-up. Child Dev 51:426, 1980
86. Brown JV, LaRossa MM, Aylward GP, et al: Nursery-based intervention with prematurely born babies and their mothers: Are there effects? J Pediatr 97:487, 1980
87. Cornell EH, Gottfried AW: Intervention with premature human infants. Child Dev 47:32, 1976
88. Campbell SK: Effects of developmental intervention in the special care nursery. p. 165. In Wolraich M, Routh DK (eds): Advances in Developmental and Behavioral Pediatrics, Vol. 4. JAI Press, Greenwich, CT, 1983
89. Minde K, Shosenberg N, Marton P, et al: Self-help groups in a premature nursery–A controlled evaluation. J Pediatr 96:933, 1980
90. Widmayer SM, Field TM: Effects of Brazelton demonstrations for mothers on the development of preterm infants. Pediatrics 67:711, 1981
91. Bronfenbrenner U: Is early intervention effective? p. 449. In Friedlander BZ, Sterritt GM, Kirk GE (eds): Exceptional Infant, Vol. 3. Bruner-Mazel, New York, 1975
92. Long JG, Philip AGS, Lucey JF: Excessive handling as a cause of hypoxemia. Pediatrics 65:203, 1980
93. Gorski PA, Hole WT, Leonard CH, Martin JA: Direct computer recording of premature infants and nursery care: Distress following two interventions. Pediatrics 72:198, 1983
94. Lawson K, Daum C, Turkewitz G: Environmental characteristics of a neonatal intensive care unit. Child Dev 48:1633, 1977
95. Klaus M, Kennell J: Interventions in the premature nursery: Impact on development. Pediatr Clin North Am 29:1263, 1982
96. Field TM: Effects of early separation, interactive deficits and experimental manipulations on infant-mother face-to-face interaction. Child Dev 48:763, 1977
97. Trevarthen C: Descriptive analysis of infant communicative behavior. p. 227. In Schaffer HR (ed): Studies in Mother-Infant Interaction. Academic Press, New York, 1977

10
Neonatal Sepsis: A Review of New Treatment Methods

Harry R. Hill
Robert D. Christensen

MORBIDITY AND MORTALITY DUE TO NEONATAL SEPSIS

Bacterial sepsis is a major contributor to morbidity and mortality during the neonatal period.[1–7] The incidence of sepsis in the first month of life ranges from one to as high as ten cases per thousand live births.[1–5] Recent studies have suggested that the rate may even be significantly higher.[8,9] In one series, 41 percent of infants who died within the first month of life had positive bacterial cultures from blood or cerebrospinal fluid. While these cultures were often obtained postmortem, the results do suggest that bacterial infection contributes to the death of neonates in a high percentage of cases. Infants who are the products of complicated pregnancies are clearly even at higher risk for developing bacterial sepsis than are normal, term neonates. Thus, sepsis occurs much more frequently in preterm infants and in infants with whom there have been maternal complications, such as premature rupture of the membranes or intrapartum infections.[1–5] While recent developments in neonatal intensive care have clearly decreased morbidity and mortality in the preterm infant, prolonged hospitalization and invasive procedures have contributed to a high incidence of infection.[10,11] This is especially true for infants with birthweights of less than 1,000 grams.[12]

In spite of the development of potent new antimicrobial agents and the use of "state-of-the-art" support techniques, the mortality rate in neonatal sepsis still ranges from 30 to 70 percent.[1–4] Furthermore, the compromised nature of the neonate's host defense system often allows the widespread dissemination of microorganisms from the bloodstream to a variety of local sites.[13] These defects contribute to the seeding of organisms to the meninges, lungs, bones, and other sites. The morbidity from these secondary infections is high. For instance, it has been estimated that up to 50 percent of neonates who develop meningitis have significant residual neurologic sequelae.[1–3]

In the present chapter, we will review new treatment methods that seek to reduce the high morbidity and mortality due to bacterial sepsis in the neonate. Some of these methods include conventional therapies, such as the use of new antimicrobial agents or combinations of agents. Others, most of which are still experimental, are aimed at correcting host-defense abnormalities in the neonate. Hopefully, a combination of these two approaches may, in the future, be capable of further lowering infant mortality from bacterial infection.

Changing Etiology of Neonatal Sepsis

Group A streptococci and other gram-positive organisms were often the etiologic agents in sepsis of the newborn prior to the introduction of antibiotics. Later, after penicillins and sulfonamides were introduced, gram-negative organisms such as *Escherichia coli, Klebsiella pneumoniae*, and *Pseudomonas aeruginosa* became common.[5] Since the mid-1960s, we have observed a high incidence of group B streptococcal infections throughout the United States and other developed countries.[4] Interestingly, this organism has not played a major role in neonatal sepsis in developing countries such as Mexico, where *Klebsiella* and *E. coli* are still the predominant pathogens. The reasons for this are not understood.

More recently, coagulase-negative staphylococci have been isolated from a large number of blood cultures from neonates, especially in intensive care nurseries.[5,14] Noel and Edelson[14] found 23 instances of what appeared to be clinically significant *Staphylococcus epidermidis* bacteremia during a 17-month period in a neonatal intensive care unit (NICU) at a New York city hospital. Ten of these episodes were associated with colonized indwelling vascular catheters, while 4 episodes were in infants with necrotizing enterocolitis (NEC). Six cases occurred in infants without colonized vascular catheters or NEC; three were in full-term infants. Ten patients had focal *S. epidermidis* infections including omphalitis, a wound abscess, mastitis, and cervical abscesses. All 23 episodes were considered true infections by the clinicians caring for the patients. Scherer and co-workers,[15] in reviewing 60 cases of *S. epidermidis* sepsis in children, found 4 sepsis-related deaths in preterm infants. Thus, this organism appears to be capable of producing clinical illness, focal infection, and even death in compromised neonates, especially in those requiring indwelling vascular catheters.

While Group B streptococci and *E. coli* together still account for over 70 percent of serious infections in the neonates,[1–3] other infections, such as those due to *Listeria monocytogenes, Haemophilus influenzae, Neisseria meningitidis*, and groups C, D, and G streptococci can also produce serious neonatal infection.[1,2,10,17] Anaerobic organisms may additionally be isolated alone or in combination with aerobes from septic neonates. *Campylobacter fetus, jejuni*, and *coli* have also recently been implicated in premature delivery associated with fetal or neonatal infection and mortality.[18] This wide diversity of potential pathogens, all of which can produce similar clinical syndromes, makes the appropriate choice of antimicrobial agents for neonatal bacterial sepsis a difficult one.

NEW DEVELOPMENTS IN ANTIMICROBIAL THERAPY

In a recent review of neonatal sepsis, Siegel[17] indicated that approximately 10 percent of all neonates are treated for suspected sepsis. Only 1 to 10 percent of these are documented to be cases of sepsis, however.[17,19] In a study reported from two Boston hospitals, the ratio of treated to infected neonates was even higher.[20] In one hospital, the ratio was 15:1 while in the other it was 28:1. Thus, antimicrobial use in neonates is exceedingly high throughout the United States and the world.

Are there well-documented advances in the antibiotic therapy of neonatal infections over the past 5 years? In spite of the development of several potent new antimicrobial agents, one would have to say that these have not yet proved to be of significant benefit in terms of morbidity or mortality. In fact, the combination of ampicillin and an aminoglycoside has remained the preferred initial regimen for suspected sepsis during the first month of life.[17] Group B and D streptococci as well as *Listeria* are susceptible to ampicillin alone. Several studies, however, have documented synergism and more rapid killing kinetics with these organisms when an aminoglycoside is also utilized.[1,3,4,17] This combination is also effective against *E. coli*. Such a combination is not optimal for sepsis due to staphylococci, however. While most *S. aureus* strains are sensitive to aminoglycosides, these agents certainly are not the drugs of choice for this type of infection. A penicillinase-resistant penicillin such as methicillin or a cephalosporin should probably be combined with the aminoglycoside in place of ampicillin in older infants with nosocomial infections acquired in intensive care units.[5,17] However, *S. epidermidis* is often resistant to these agents. Methicillin-resistant strains accounted for 63 to 75 percent of clinically significant infections due to *S. epidermidis* in two series.[14,21] Cephalosporin resistance among *S. epidermidis*, as well as the unreliability of disk-diffusion techniques with cephalosporins, make these agents unsuitable for treating such infections in neonates.[14] These organisms demonstrate hetero-resistance in culture and in vivo, which probably accounts for the emergence of resistant strains during therapy. The only agent that has consistently been found to be effective against clinically infectious *S. epidermidis* is vancomycin.[14,22,23] While this drug may have significant nephrotoxic and ototoxic effects, these can usually be prevented by keeping the serum level below 30 μg/ml.[14,23] Doses of 30 to 60 mg/kg/day, given in 2 to 4 divided doses (depending on the age), have been recommended in neonates, with close monitoring of the serum concentration of the drug.[14,22,23] While many of the susceptible *S. epidermidis* strains may also be sensitive to rifampin, there are no current data indicating that the addition of rifampin to vancomycin offers a significant advantage. The use of rifampin alone usually leads to the development of resistance, and is therefore discouraged. Removing the colonized vascular catheter is critical to the successful treatment of *S. epidermidis* infection, although there have been a few reports of successful therapy through an infected line. In general, therapy must be continued for 10 to 14 days.[17]

Multiply resistant gram-negative organisms have made the selection of appropriate antimicrobial agents for treating neonatal sepsis more difficult. It was hoped that the advent of the third-generation cephalosporins would greatly simplify and improve the therapy of neonatal sepsis and meningitis. These drugs offer a truly broad spectrum of activity and are relatively nontoxic, allowing higher serum and tissue levels to be reached. While moxalactam and cefotaxime have been employed in the successful treatment of neonatal infections,[24,25] control trials, such as that conducted by the Neonatal Meningitis Cooperative Study Group, found no significant benefit of moxalactam over a combination of ampicillin and amikacin.[26] In addition, the third-generation cephalosporins have poor activity against *S. aureua* and *S. epidermidis*, while enterococci and *Listeria* are generally resistant to these drugs.[5] Moxalactam has also been associated with undue bleeding caused by decreased synthesis of prothrombin, a problem not shared by cefotaxime.

When *Pseudomonas aeruginosa* or aminoglycoside-resistant *Klebsiella* are identified as the etiologic agents in neonatal sepsis, the acylamino-penicillins may be of value. These agents, which include piperacillin, mezlocillin, and azlocillin, have increased activity against such strains, but their superiority to carbenicillin or ticarcillin has not yet been clinically documented.[5] A number of common strains causing neonatal infection are unaffected by the third-generation cephalosporins or the acylamino-penicillins, making them poor choices as initial or single drugs in the treatment of neonatal sepsis.

Two additional drugs, aztreonam and imipenem, may be beneficial in the future for therapy of neonatal sepsis.[5] Aztreonam has excellent activity against most gram-negative organisms including *Pseudomonas*, while imipenem has activity against gram-positives, gram-negatives, and anaerobes. Studies are currently in progress with these agents in infants.

THE USE OF BLOOD AND BLOOD PRODUCTS IN TREATING NEONATAL SEPSIS

Whole-Blood Transfusion

Exchange transfusion has been attempted for some time as an adjunct in the treatment of neonatal sepsis in Europe.[27–29] Initial isolated reports date back almost 20 years. The rationale for using exchange transfusion includes the removal of endotoxins, other bacterial toxins, and live organisms, as well as better tissue perfusion and a decrease in hemorrhagic manifestations. Belohradsky and coworkers[29] reported one of the largest series in which exchange transfusions were used to treat septic neonates. They noted a modest reduction in mortality from 55 percent (72 of 132) to 42 percent (14 of 33) in infants with sepsis who were transfused. Increases in serum IgG, IgA, IgM, and complement were noted after transfusion.

In 1978, we reported that the transfusion of fresh whole blood from walking donors was effective in raising opsonic antibody levels against one common pathogen, the group B streptococcus in human neonates.[30] In previous studies, we[31] and others[32] had shown that infants, or mothers of infants, who developed group B streptococcal sepsis often lacked type-specific antibody to their infecting strain. As shown in Figure 10-1, the transfusion of blood from a donor who possessed serum antibody to the infecting strain resulted in an increase in opsonic activity as measured by neutrophil chemiluminescence production.[30] When the donor lacked antibody or had a lower level than that in the neonate, transfusion either had no effect or actually resulted in a decrease in serum opsonic activity. Another important observation made in this study was that most donors had relatively low levels of serum opsonic activity against the various types of group B streptococci. Thus, it was necessary to employ a relatively large transfusion volume, equal to or greater than 40 percent of the patient's blood volume, in order to effect a significant rise in neonatal serum opsonic activity. In this initial study, performed in association with Dr. Robert Hall of Children's Mercy Hospital in Kansas City,

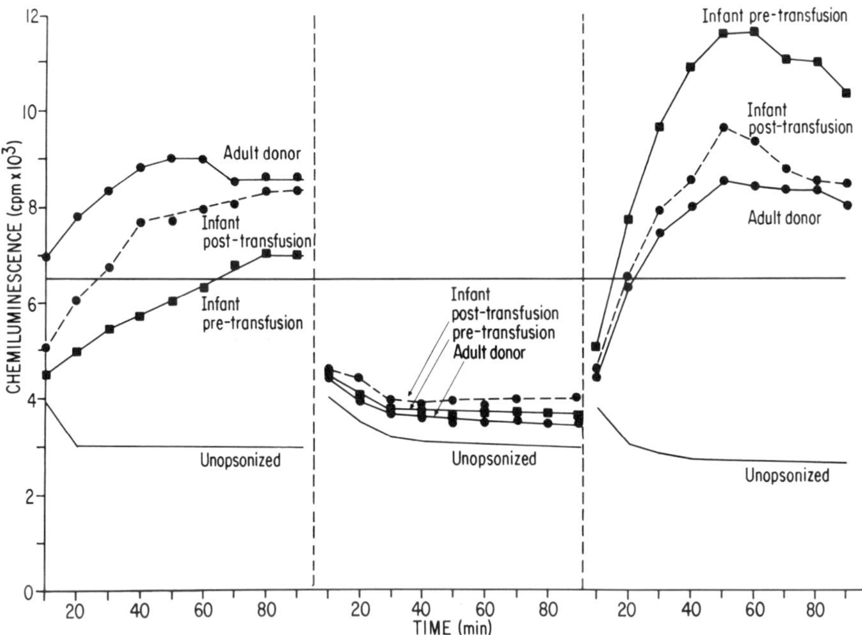

Fig. 10.1. Effect of fresh whole blood transfusion on group B streptococcal opsonins in neonatal serum, as measured by neutrophil chemiluminescence. (Shigeoka AO, Hall RT, Hill HR: Transfusion in group B streptococcal sepsis. Lancet 1:636, 1978.)

we found that infants who received transfusions of whole blood and had an increase in opsonic activity against their infecting strain of organism were more likely to survive than those who did not.[30] All 9 patients who demonstrated post-transfusion increases in type-specific antibody levels survived, versus only 3 of 6 infants who had no such increase. The differences in survival between the two groups in this small pilot study were significant, however ($P = 0.04$).

Courtney and co-workers,[33] in an uncontrolled larger trial, examined the effect of exchange transfusion with fresh blood (less than 1 hour old) on the survival rate in infants with group B streptococcal sepsis. Infants were selected for exchange transfusion (40 to 100 ml/kg) based on the choice of the attending physician, the availability of a blood donor, and the condition of the infant. There was, however, a significant difference in survival among those who underwent transfusion (23 of 27) versus those who did not (11 of 22) ($P < 0.05$). Although there were clearly problems inherent in the method used for determining who would and who would not receive exchange transfusion, survival was still significantly greater among those receiving transfusion as an independent variable.

In 1980, Vain et al.[34] reported that 7 of 10 severely ill infants with sclerema and sepsis survived following exchange transfusion with up to 160 ml/kg of citrated blood. These authors reported that acidosis, hypotension, urine output, platelet counts, and prothrombin times improved following transfusion.

White Blood Cell Transfusions

We and a number of other authors have shown that human neonates often develop a profound neutropenia and depletion of marrow granulocyte stores during bacterial sepsis.[35–40] For this reason, we initially sought to determine, in experimental animals, if leukocyte administration might provide protection against group B streptococcal infection. In a study published in 1980, we found that the administration of functional polymorphonuclear leukocytes (PMNs) from adults protected newborn rats from intraperitoneal infection with group B streptococci.[41] In fact, the degree of protection afforded by the leukocytes (50 percent survival) was equivalent to that observed with the administration of type-specific antibody (51 percent). When PMNs were administered along with antibody, protection approached the 75 percent level in this animal model. Of interest was the fact that PMNs obtained from human neonates, which have inherent abnormalities in movement, resulted in only an intermediate level of protection.[41]

Subsequent studies have indicated that the myeloid response of neonatal rats to group B streptococcal infection is profoundly depressed when compared to that of adult animals.[42] As shown in Figure 10-2, adult animals inoculated with group B streptococci develop a significant neutrophilia within 5 hours, which peaks at 24 hours and then returns to normal as the animal recovers. The adult rats also developed a significant left shift to more immature cells at 2 hours which had disappeared by 24 hours. In contrast, the newborn animal develops a profound and irreversible neutropenia with a marked left shift (Fig. 10-3). The adult animal's bone marrow response to infection is also strikingly different from that of the neonate. The adult animal's neutrophil storage pool (NSP), which consists of mature PMNs, bands, metamyelocytes decreases slightly at 2, 5, and 15 hours after

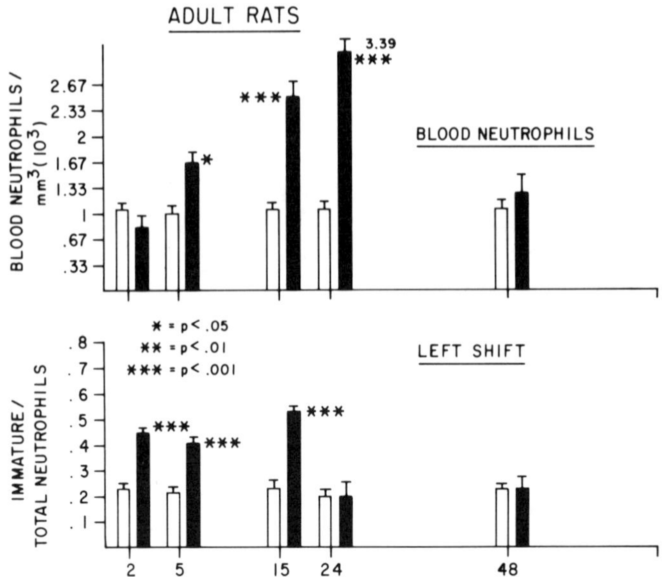

Fig. 10.2. Absolute blood neutrophil counts in group B streptococcus-infected (solid bars) versus uninfected adult rats (clear bars). (Christensen RD, Macfarlane JL, Taylor NL, et al: Blood and marrow neutrophils during experimental group B streptococcal infection: Quantification of the stem cell, proliferative, storage, and circulating pools. Pediatr Res 15:549, 1982.)

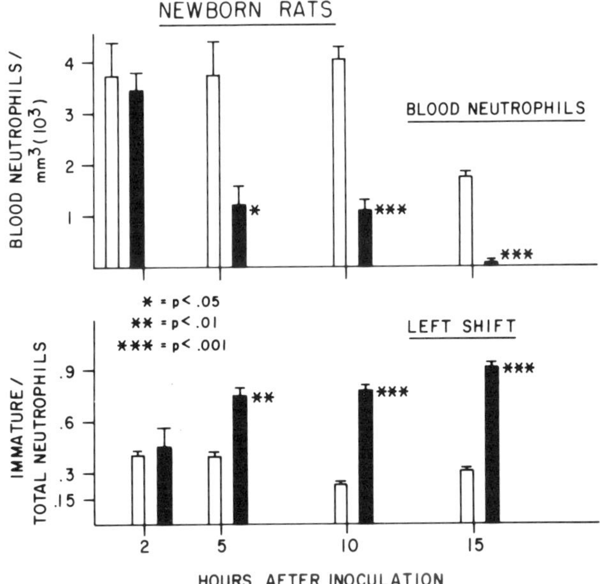

Fig. 10.3. Absolute blood neutrophil counts in group B streptococcus-infected (solid bars) versus uninfected neonatal rats (clear bars). (Christensen RD, Macfarlane JL, Taylor NL, et al: Blood and marrow neutrophils during experimental group B streptococcal infection: Quantification of the stem cell, proliferative, storage, and circulating pools. Pediatr Res 15:549, 1982.

infection, as the more mature cells are released into the peripheral circulation (Fig. 10-4). The animals proliferative pool of myeloblasts, promyelocytes, and myelocytes remains essentially the same in the 48 hours after infection. In order to maintain the proliferative pool and prevent severe depletion of the marrow, the adult animal markedly increases the number of marrow colony forming units (CFUc). This response is detectable at 5 hours and peaks at 48 hours (Fig. 10-4). The infant's marrow following infection rapidly develops a severe depletion of its NSP and a significant decrease in the proliferative pool (Fig. 10-5). In contrast to the marrow of infected adult rats, the neonatal marrow cannot develop an increase in colony-forming cells during infection.[42] The exact reason for this is not completely understood, but subsequent studies have suggested that this is most likely due to the fact that the proliferative rate is already maximal in neonates.[43]

In January of 1981, Laurenti and co-workers,[44] in Rome, reported their initial experiences employing granulocyte transfusions to treat neonates with bacterial sepsis. In their study, 20 infected infants received from 2 to 15 leukocyte transfusions which contained from 0.5 to 1 $\times$ 10^9 leukocytes each. Only 2 of these infants died, as opposed to 13 of 18 infected infants who received only conventional therapy. While the study was not well controlled, the results were still impressive, and prompted one of us to write an accompanying editorial.[45] It was hoped that the question mark at the end of the title of this editorial would be emphasized.

Subsequently, Christensen and co-workers[46] examined a total of 26 neonates with bacterial infection and peripheral neutropenia. Ten of the patients with neutropenia did not demonstrate severe depletion of their marrow NSP (neutrophils + bands + metamyelocytes totaling 7 percent or more), and all lived. When

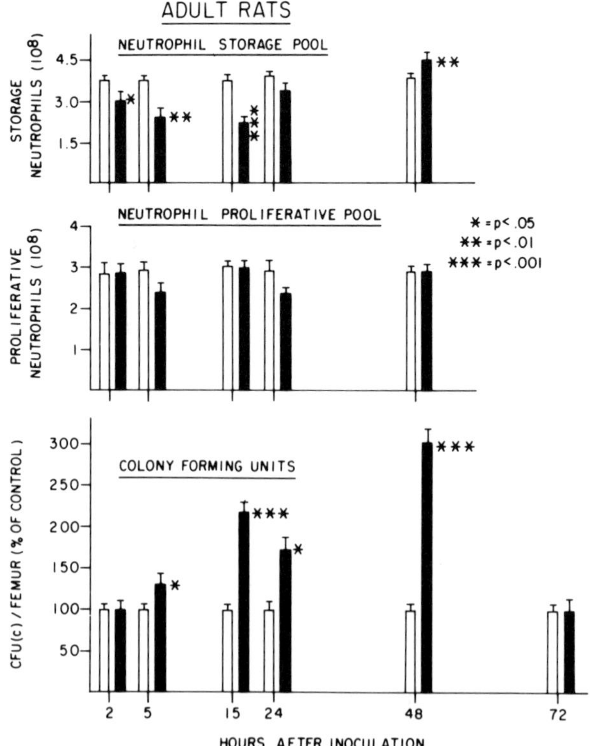

Fig. 10.4. Neutrophil storage pools, proliferative pools, and unipotent stem cells (CFUc) in infected (solid bars) and uninfected (clear bars) adult rats. (Christensen RD, Macfarlane JL, Taylor NL, et al: Blood and marrow neutrophils during experimental group B streptococcal infection: Quantification of the stem cell, proliferative, storage, and circulating pools. Pediatr Res 15:549, 1982.)

neutropenia was associated with NSP depletion (a total of 7 percent or less), however, 8 or 9 infected infants died. Seven additional patients had neutropenia and NSP depletion associated with sepsis, but each was given a single leukocyte transfusion containing from 0.2 to 1.0 $\times$ 10^9 PMNs. All 7 patients survived; the difference in survival between those transfused and not transfused was statistically significant (P <0.01). Limited follow-up failed to reveal adverse effects of the transfusions on PAO_2, PCO_2, pH, or chest x-rays, and there was no evidence of acquired cytomegalovirus, hepatitis, or Epstein-Barr virus infection.

Additional reports appeared in the literature, suggesting that the transfusion of leukocytes had been beneficial in an infant with necrotizing enterocolitis,[47] and in 3 of 6 infants with refractory sepsis.[48] Obviously, no attempt was made to control these studies. In 1984, Cairo and colleagues[49] described a second randomized trial of granulocyte transfusions in infected neonates. The infants he studied were not necessarily neutropenic or marrow depleted, and all were over 1,000 g body weight. The transfused infants received 0.5 to 1.0 $\times$ 10^9 granulocytes collected by continuous-flow centrifugation. Thirteen of the patients were transfused and all survived. In contrast, 6 of 10 infants who were not transfused died (P <0.02). When only those infants with positive cultures were examined, however, the difference in survival between those receiving transfusion (7 of 7) versus those without transfusion (4 of 7) was not statistically significant.[49]

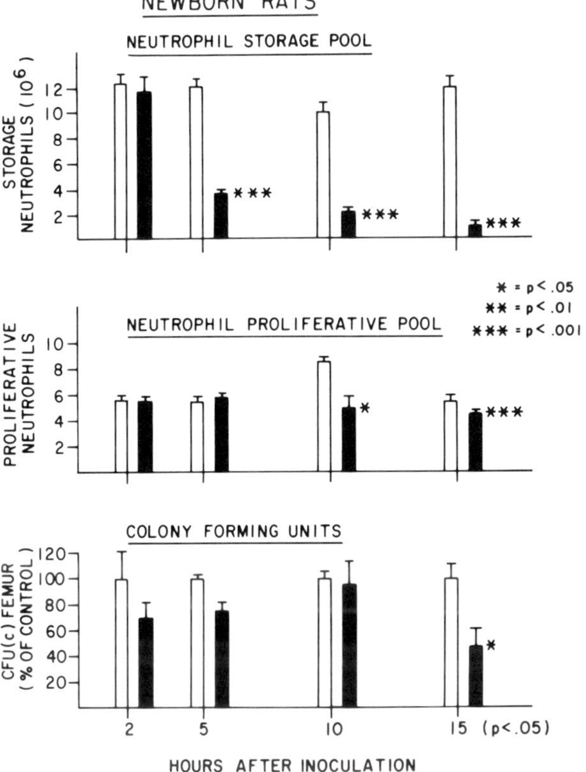

Fig. 10.5. Neutrophil storage pools, proliferative pools, and unipotent stem cells (CFUc) in infected (solid bars) and uninfected (clear bars) neonatal rats. (Christensen RD, Macfarlane JL, Taylor NL, et al: Blood and marrow neutrophils during experimental group B streptococcal infection: Quantification of the stem cell, proliferative, storage, and circulating pools. Pediatr Res 15:549, 1982.)

Stork and co-workers[50] subsequently reported on a controlled trial of granulocyte transfusions in septic neutropenic neonates. A total of 23 neutropenic infants with necrotizing enterocolitis or suspected sepsis were included in the study. The infants were randomized to receive conventional therapy alone or conventional therapy plus transfusions of 0.1 to 0.9×10^9 leukocytes (PMNs + lymphocytes + monocytes) from buffy coat preparations. Seven of 12 (58 percent) of the patients who received transfusions survived, versus 9 of 13 (69 percent) who did not. The presence of an elevated ratio of immature to mature cells (more than 0.8) or a depleted neutrophil storage pool (7 percent or less) in a limited number of patients had no effect on the efficacy of leukocyte transfusion in this study. Of patients with positive cultures, 50 percent (6 of 12) survived in the transfused group, versus 71 percent (7 of 13) in the nontransfused group.

Wheeler and colleagues[51] studied 13 neonates who were neutropenic with proven bacterial sepsis by examining their peripheral PMN counts and marrow NSPs when possible. Seven patients had NSPs of greater than 7 percent, while 3 had NSP depletion. Three patients did not have marrow aspirates because of their condition or because of the unavailability of a hematologist. (These three individuals survived, and their PMN counts rose spontaneously.) Five of the seven septic patients who did not have NSP depletion on marrow examination survived with conventional therapy. In contrast, only one of three of the NSP-depleted infants survived (33 percent). Two of these three infants were given granulocyte transfusions, and one survived. Obviously, the number of cases included in this study was far too few to make any firm conclusions about the role of NSP depletion or granulocyte transfusion in mortality from neonatal sepsis.

An expanded study by Wheeler and associates[52] included 28 infants with less than 1,500 PMN/mm^3 on two samples. Twenty-four patients had sepsis as documented by culture or antigen detection tests. Among septic infants with NSP depletion (7 percent or less), 5 of 9, or 56 percent, died. This compared to 1 of 11 (9 percent) of septic infants without NSP depletion who died. Marrow-depleted infants were randomized to receive either 15 ml/kg of buffy coat PMNs (approximately 0.3×10^9 cells) or 15 ml/kg of packed red blood cells. The mortality rate in the NSP-depleted, septic infants who received transfusion (2 of 4; 50 percent) was not different from those who were not transfused (3 or 5; 60 percent).

These studies obviously do not provide an answer to the question of how effective leukocyte transfusions are in neonatal sepsis. They serve only to raise additional critical issues, including: (1) the means of collection, number of cells, and number of doses of granulocytes needed; (2) the suitability of the patient for transfusion, including the degree of neutropenia, the immature-to-total PMN ratio, and whether there is NSP depletion; (3) the type of infection (early versus late) being considered, etiologic agent, and presence or absence of NEC; and (4) the need for antibody, complement, and other factors along with granulocytes.

The Use of Immunoglobulins

The full-term newborn infant receives a considerable quantity of immunoglobulin G from its mother. Unfortunately, the maternal immunoglobulin usually does not contain functional opsonic antibody directed against the etiologic agent causing sepsis in the offspring.[1–4,31,32] Furthermore, some of the IgG subclasses (notably IgG2 and IgG4) have been reported to pass the placenta poorly, and IgM and IgA do not cross at all in most circumstances.[13] The problem is even more severe in the preterm infant, since active transport of maternal IgG is minimal until 30 to 32 weeks of gestation. Thus, there is clear indication that the newborn infant, and especially the preterm one, has a relative antibody deficiency. For this reason, a number of studies have been undertaken in experimental animals, and more recently in human infants, to determine the efficacy of antibody administration in neonatal sepsis.

Initial studies by our group[53] and by Fischer and colleagues[54] showed that human gamma globulin, modified for intravenous use (IGIV), could prevent mortality in neonatal rats inoculated with group B streptococci (Fig. 10-6). The survival rate following antibody therapy only approached 40 to 50 percent in our studies, however, using conventional doses of IGIV (100 to 200 mg/kg). Furthermore, the immunoglobulin preparations had little activity against more resistant strains (R), even when utilized in higher doses (Figs. 10-6 and 10-7). Thus, in our opinion and that of Fischer and colleagues, something additional was needed for the effective antibody treatment of group B sepsis in neonates.

We therefore turned to the development of monoclonal antibodies to group B streptococci. These preparations, made in association with Drs. Seth Pincus and

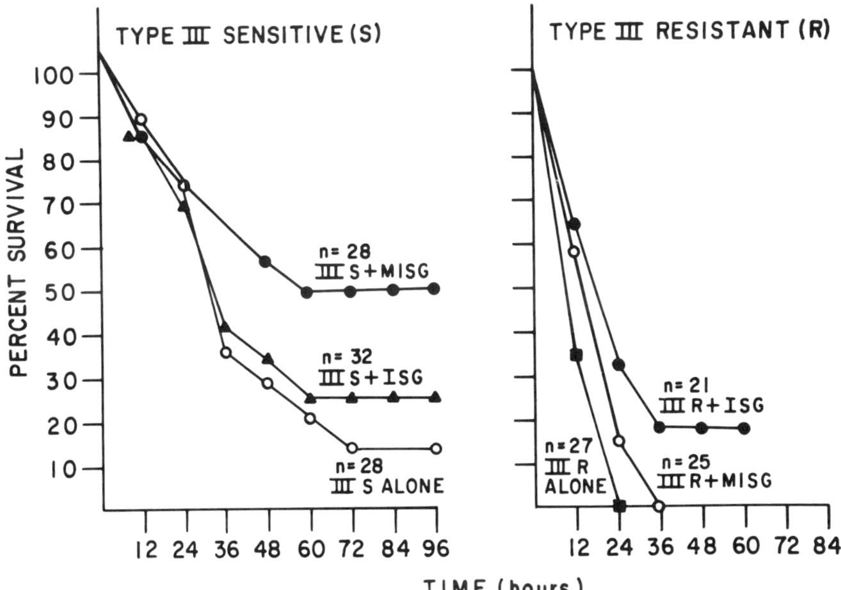

Fig. 10.6. Protective efficacy of modified immune serum globulin (MISG, IGIV) and intramuscular immune serum globulin (ISG) in neonatal rats infected with type III group B streptococci. (Santos JI, Shigeoka AO, Rote NS, Hill HR: Protective efficacy of a modified immune serum globulin in experimental group B streptotoccal infection. J Pediatr 99:875, 1981.)

Ann Shigeoka, were prepared by injecting mice with whole, type III group B streptococci.[55] After 14 days the spleens from these animals were removed and the B cells were fused with a murine myeloma cell line (Fig. 10-8). After screening individual cell lines for type-specific antibody production, clones were selected that produced highly active antibody in opsonic and protective studies. As can be seen in Figure 10-9, the type-specific murine monoclonal IgM antibody was ex-

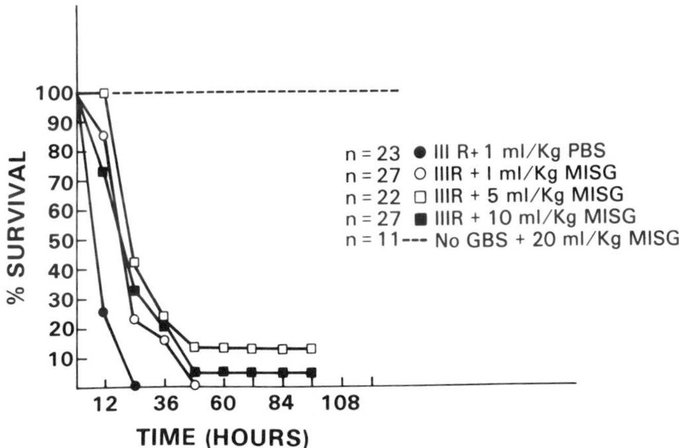

Fig. 10.7. Lack of protection of increasing doses of intravenous immune globulin (MISG, IGIV) against a resistant strain of type III group B streptococci in neonatal rats. (Santos JI, Shigeoka AO, Rote NS, Hill HR: Protective efficacy of a modified immune serum globulin in experimental group B streptococcal infection. J Pediatr 99:875, 1981.)

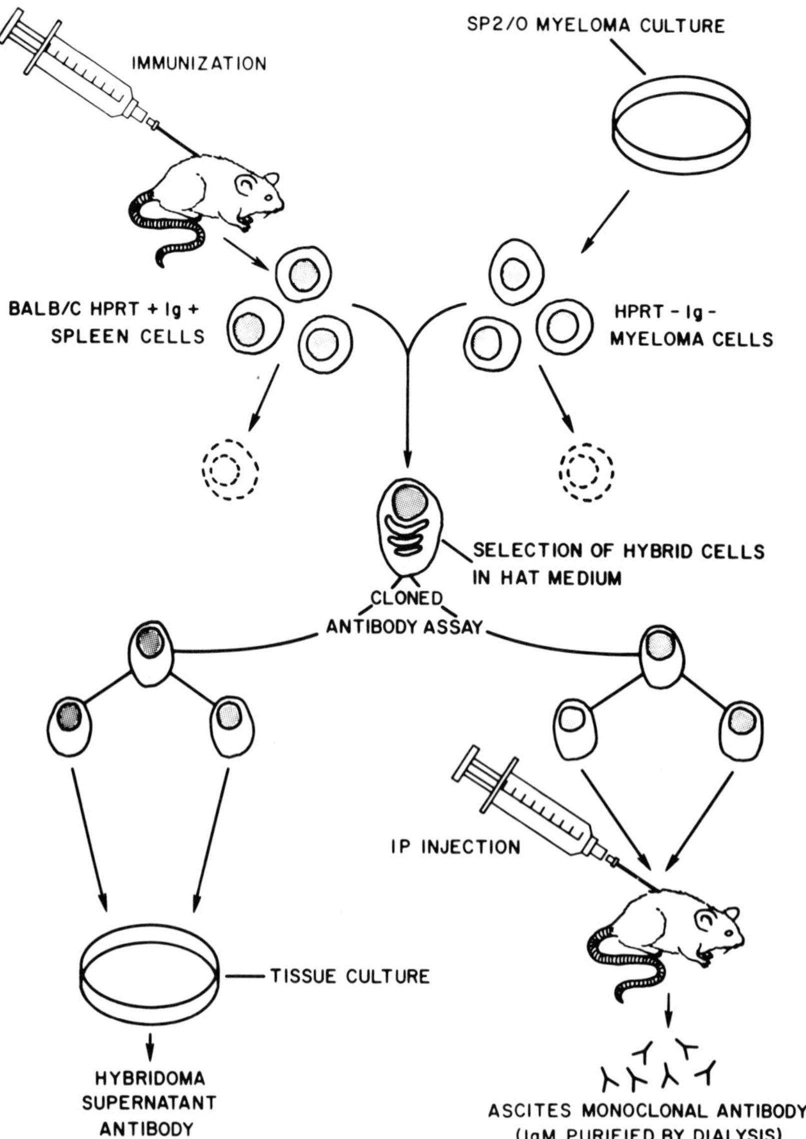

Fig. 10.8. Production of type-specific group B streptococcal monoclonal murine antibody. (Reprinted from Shigeoka AO, Pincus SH, Rote NS, Hill HR: Protective efficacy of hybridoma type-specific antibody against experimental infection with group B streptococcus. J Infect Dis 149:363, 1984 by permission of The University of Chicago Press. © 1984 by the University of Chicago. All rights reserved.)

tremely effective in preventing the death of newborn rats from respiratory (shown here) or peritoneal infection with type III group B streptococci. Moreover, the preparation was effective against even the more resistant strains of group B streptococci.

In additional studies, we have found that the monoclonal antibodies directed against the type-specific polysaccharide antigens of group B streptococci not only

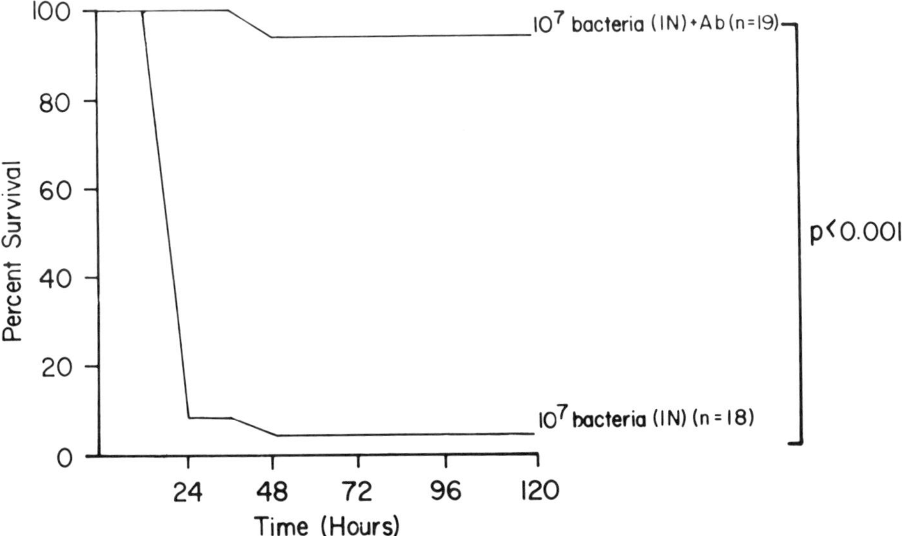

Fig. 10.9. Protection afforded by murine monoclonal antibody against respiratory infection with type III group B streptococci in neonatal rats. (Reprinted from Shigeoka AO, Pincus SH, Rote NS, Hill HR: Protective efficacy of hybridoma type-specific antibody against experimental infection with group B streptococcus. J Infect Dis 149:363, 1984 by permission of The University of Chicago Press. © 1984 by the University of Chicago. All rights reserved.)

act to opsonize bacteria, but also promote the marrow release and localization of PMNs at the site of infection.[56,57] This is most likely due to the release of breakdown products of the third component of complement.[58]

In association with Dr. Robert Hall and colleagues at Children's Mercy Hospital in Kansas City, we have found some evidence that transfusion may promote marrow granulocyte release in septic human neonates. In those studies, a significant post-transfusion increase in immature PMNs was observed in 25 infants who received whole blood transfusions that probably contained antibody. This suggests that such therapy may have actually been acting to "turn on" the infant's marrow by supplying antibody or necessary complement components.

Unfortunately, murine monoclonal antibodies will probably never be approved for use in human neonates, even though they have been employed in the therapy of some leukemias and in transplant patients. Human monoclonal antibodies have been made, but are relatively difficult to produce, and their functional activity has not yet been adequately documented. Dr. Richard Wasserman of the University of Texas Southwestern Medical School in Dallas has prepared a series of human monoclonal antibodies to group B streptococci.[60] While these clearly bind to antigen in an enzyme-linked immunoabsorbent assay (ELISA), we have yet to find, in collaborative efforts with Dr. Wasserman, significant opsonic or protective activity in these preparations.

In spite of the relatively low levels of activity of commercial IGIV preparations against group B streptococci and *E. coli* K1, clinical trials of these agents in neonatal sepsis have been reported from Europe. Sidiropoulos and colleagues[61] randomized 35 infected infants to receive conventional therapy or conventional therapy plus

IGIV (1 g daily in term infants and 0.5 g daily in preterm infants). The mortality rate in the IGIV-treated group was 10 percent (2 of 20), versus 26 percent (4 of 15) in the controls. The differences ($P = 0.16$) were not significant. When only preterm infants were considered, however, there was a significant difference in mortality between those who received antibiotics alone (4 of 9) versus those who received antibiotics plus IGIV (1 of 13; $P = 0.04$).

Studies in this country have demonstrated the safety and kinetics of IGIV administration in human neonates with doses up to 500 mg/kg. At present, efficacy studies are being carried out with these preparations in the United States.

In seeking to circumvent the problem of low levels of specific antibody to bacterial pathogens in regular preparations of IGIV, Gloser and colleagues[62] have made a hyperimmune IGIV against group B streptococci. Human volunteers (30) have been immunized with the type-specific polysaccharides of types Ia, Ib, II, and III group B streptococci. These individuals were then plasmapheresed and a pentavalent (Ia, Ib, Ic, II, and III) hyperimmune IGIV was prepared. Gloser et al.,[62] as well as Fischer and associates,[63] have clearly shown that the antibody titers and protective efficacy of this preparation in an experimental animal model far exceed that of conventional IGIV. Controlled trials of this preparation in human neonates are in the planning stages.

One additional published study warrants mentioning. Adhikari and associates[64] have used a gamma globulin preparation with high antibody levels to Gram-negative endotoxin (lipopolysaccharide; LPS) to treat human neonates with sepsis who also had positive *Limulus amoebocyte* lysate tests for endotoxin. There was no difference between the mortality rate among those treated with the anti-LPS immunoglobulin (6 of 16) and those who received an albumin control (7 of 20). The recovery periods were decreased in survivors, from an average of 310 hours in controls to 120 hours in the treated patients. Whether an immunoglobulin preparation with activity against LPS will have a role in the treatment of neonatal Gram-negative sepsis remains to be determined.

Fibronectin Administration

Fibronectin (FN) is a high-molecular-weight glycoprotein that is present throughout the body. It circulates in plasma and is a major constituent of the intracellular matrix.[65] In the plasma it helps to maintain vascular integrity and promotes the reticuloendothelial clearance of particulate matter. The fibronectin content is often low in the plasma of patients with sepsis, shock, severe trauma, and burns. We[66] and others[67] have found that newborn infants have low levels of plasma FN as compared to adult concentrations. Furthermore, we have found that FN promotes the opsonic and protective activity of monoclonal antibody or IGIV against group B streptococci.[68] As can be seen in Figure 10-10, the protective effect of a low concentration of monoclonal IgG antibody was markedly enhanced by the addition of fibronectin in a neonatal rat model of group B streptococcal disease. While we are unaware of specific studies showing a beneficial effect of fibronectin administration in human neonates with sepsis, such studies may be warranted.

Hazards of Blood Produce Use

There clearly are hazards to the use of blood and blood products in human neonates. These include such obvious hazards as the transmission of hepatitis viruses, cytomegalovirus, Epstein-Barr virus, and the human immunodeficiency virus (HIV

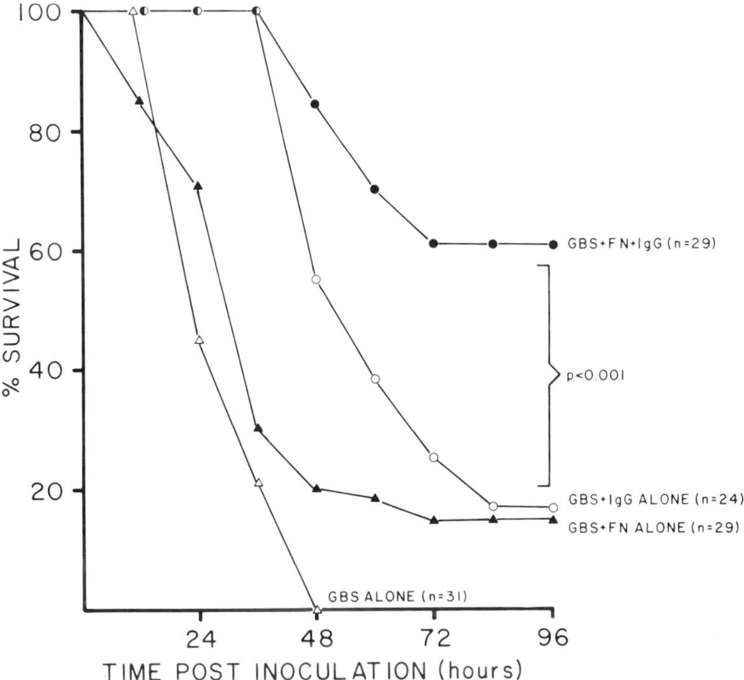

Fig. 10.10. Effect of fibronectin and monoclonal IgG type-specific antibody on the survival of neonatal rats infected with type III group B streptococci. (Hill HR, Shigeoka AO, Augustine NH, et al: Fibronectin enhances the opsonii motective activity of monoclonal polyclonal antibody against group B streptococci. J. Exp Med 159:1618, 1984. By copyright permission of the Rockefeller University Press.)

or HTLV-III). Since the advent of screening for hepatitis B with antigen detection and serologic tests, it is apparent that over 90 percent of cases of transfusion-associated hepatitis are of non-A, non-B hepatitis. Only 2 percent or less are actually hepatitis B, and these are most likely the result of using blood from viremic donors prior to the development of serologic evidence of infection. Non-A, non-B hepatitis, while usually not severe as an acute disease, may lead to persistently elevated liver enzyme activities and chronic liver disease. In one study of post-transfustion non-A, non-B hepatitis, liver biopsy revealed evidence of chronic active hepatitis in 60 percent and cirrhosis in 12 percent of the subjects.[69] Non-A, non-B hepatitis may be transmitted by all untreated blood products. In addition, a few batches of IGIV prepared by other than the standard Cohn fractionation procedure have resulted in non-A, non-B hepatitis in recipients.[70] To our knowledge, this is the only infectious agent that has been transmitted by gamma globulin preparations. Furthermore, no preparation licensed in the United States has ever been documented to transmit non-A, non-B hepatitis, HIV, or other viral agents.[71]

Cytomegalovirus (CMV) has a high prevalence in the general population. Exposure to this virus results in a lifetime of potential infectiousness. Therefore, individuals with serologic evidence of past infection can transmit CMV in their donated blood. Transfusion-acquired CMV can result in serious disease in human neonates, especially those with prematurity or low birthweight. The transmission of CMV to previously unexposed (seronegative) patients can be prevented, however, through the use of seronegative blood.[72] Such antibody screening, even on a "stat" basis, can be done easily, with conventional antibody tests or recently developed latex agglutination procedures.

The problem of transmission of HIV (HTLV-III) in blood or blood products is becoming more widespread daily. A number of transfusion-associated cases of HIV have been reported, including cases involving neonates.[73,74] Tests are now routinely used to screen potential blood donors for anti-HIV antibodies, but these are only 98 to 99 percent sensitive. Thus, there is a slight chance that an individual infected with HIV might not yet have a serologic response to the virus at the time of blood donation, and could transmit the virus.

Other potential problems from the use of blood or blood products may be encountered.[45] These include the sequestration of leukocytes within the lung in an "adult respiratory distress-like picture." In the initial study of Christensen and co-workers,[46] no evidence for this was detected, and no deterioration in blood gas valves or pulmonary function was observed. We must continue to watch for such occurrences, however.

Graft-versus-host disease (GVHD) has also commonly been mentioned as a hazard of the use of whole blood or leukocyte transfusions in human neonates. This can be prevented by irradiation of the blood or leukocytes prior to administration (3,000 rads is believed by most to inactivate T cells while not affecting granulocyte function), and is generally recommended.

Because of the hazards mentioned above, and since there is not yet definitive proof that any of the mentioned experimental regimens actually improves survival or decreases morbidity in human neonatal sepsis, the practicing neonatologist must proceed cautiously. Clearly, well-designed, large clinical trials will be needed to prove the efficacy of immunotherapy for infection in this population. Still, it is our firm belief that further reduction in the still exceedingly high mortality and morbidity rate from neonatal sepsis will come about only if we devise means to replace or enhance those portions of the neonate's host defense system that are clearly deficient.

ACKNOWLEDGMENTS

This work was supported in part by U.S. Public Health Service Grants AI 19094, AI 13150, and HD 14419.

REFERENCES

1. Hill HR: Diagnosis and treatment of sepsis in the neonate. p. 219. In Root RK, Sande MA (eds): Septic Shock: Contempory Topics in Infectious Diseases. Churchill Livingstone, New York, 1985
2. Santos JI, Hill HR: Bacterial infections of the neonate. p. 179. In Wedgwood RJ, Davis, RD, Ray CG, Keley VC (eds): Infections in Children. Harper and Row, Philadelphia, 1982
3. Klein JO: Recent advances in management of bacterial meningitis in neonates. Infection, suppl. 12:S44–S48, 1984
4. Hill HR: Group B streptococcal infections. p. 397. In Holmes KK, Mardh PA, Sparling PF, Wiesner PJ (eds): Sexually Transmitted Diseases. McGraw Hill, New York, 1984
5. Stamm SE: Antimicrobial therapy of bacterial sepsis in the newborn infant. J Pediatr 106:1043, 1985

6. Siegel JD, McCracken GH: Sepsis neonatorum. N Engl J Med 304:642, 1981
7. Klein JO, Dashefsky B, Norton CR, Mayer J: Selection of antimicrobial agents for treatment of neonatal sepsis. Rev Infect Dis, suppl. 5:555, 1983
8. Eisenfeld L, Ermocilla R, Wirtschafter D, Cassidy G: Systemic bacterial infections in neonatal deaths. Am J Dis Child 137:645, 1983
9. Pierce JR, Merenstein GB, Stocker JT: Immediate postmortem cultures in an intensive care nursery. Pediatr Infect Dis 3:510, 1984
10. Hemming VG, Overall JC, Britt MR: Nosocomial infections in a newborn intensive care unit. N Engl J Med 294:1310, 1976
11. Hill HR, Hunt CE, Matsen JM: Nosocomial colonization with *Klebsiella*, type 26, in a neonatal intensive care unit associated with an outbreak of sepsis, meningitis and necrotizing enterocolitis. J Pediatr 85:415, 1974
12. La Gamma EF, Drusin LM, Mackles AW, et al: Neonatal infections: An important determinant of late NICU mortality in infants less than 1,000 g at birth. Am J Dis Child 137:838, 1983
13. Hill HR: Host defense in the neonate: Prospects for enhancement. Semin Perinatol 9:2, 1985
14. Noel GJ, Edelson PJ: *Staphylococcus epidermidis* bacteremia in neonates: Further observations and the occurrence of focal infection. Pediatrics 74:832, 1984
15. Scherer LR, West KW, Weber TR, et al: *Staphylococcus epidermidis* sepsis in pediatric patients: Clinical and therapeutic considerations. J Pediatr Surg 19:358, 1984
16. George P, Singer DB: Respiratory distress and shock in a term neonate. J Pediatr 96:946, 1980
17. Siegel JD: Neonatal sepsis. Semin Perinatol 9:20, 1985
18. Simor AE, Karmal A, Jadavji T, Roscoe M: Abortion and perinatal sepsis associated with *Campylobacter* infection. Rev Infect Dis 8:397, 1986
19. Prober CG: Treatment of bacterial infections in the neonate. Clin Invest Med 8:368, 1986
20. Hammerschlag MR, Klein JO, Herschel M, et al: Patterns of use of antibiotics in two newborn nurseries. N Engl J Med 296:1268, 1977
21. Archer GL: Antimicrobial susceptibility and selection of resistance among *Staphylococcus epidermidis* isolates recovered from patients with infection of indwelling foreign devices. Antimicrob Agents Chemother 14:353, 1978
22. Schaad VB, McCracken GH, Nelson JD: Clinical pharmacology and efficacy of vancomycin in pediatric patients. J Pediatr 96:119, 1980
23. Cook FV, Farrer WF: Vancomycin revisited. Ann Intern Med 88:813, 1978
24. Kafetzis DA, Brater DC, Kapiki AN, et al: Treatment of severe neonatal infections with cefotaxime: Efficiency and pharmacokinetics. J Pediatr 100:483, 1982
25. Schaad VB, McCracken GH, Threlkeld N, Thomas WL: Clinical evaluation of a new broad-spectrum oxa-beta-lactam antibiotic, moxalactam, in neonates and infants. J Pediatr 98:129, 1981
26. McCracken GH, Threlkeld N, Mize S, et al: Moxalactam therapy for neonatal meningitis due to gram-negative enteric bacilli: A prospective controlled evaluation. JAMA 252:1427, 1984
27. Xanthou M, Zypolyta A, Anagnostakis D, et al: Exchange transfusion in severe neonatal infection with sclerema. Arch Dis Child 50:901, 1975
28. Tollner U, Pohlondt F, Heinze F, et al: Treatment of septicemia in the newborn infant: Choice of initial antimicrobial drugs and the role of exchange transfusion. Acta Pediatr Scand 66:605, 1977
29. Belohradsky BH, Roos R, Marget W: Exchange transfusion in neonatal septicemia. Infection, suppl. 6:139, 1978
30. Shigeoka AO, Hall RT, Hill HR: Transfusion in group B streptococcal sepsis. Lancet 1:636, 1978
31. Hemming VG, Hall RT, Rhodes PG, et al: Assessment of group B streptococcal opsonins in human and rabbit serum by neutrophil chemiluminescence. J Clin Invest 48:1379, 1976
32. Baker CJ, Kasper DL: Correlation of maternal antibody deficiency with susceptibility to neonatal group B streptococcal infection. N Engl J Med 294:753, 1976
33. Courtney SE, Hall RT, Harris DJ: Effect of blood transfusion on mortality in early-onset group B streptococcal septicemia. Lancet 2:462, 1979
34. Vain NE, Mazlumian JR, Swarner OW, Cha CC: Role of exchange transfusion in the treatment of severe septicemia. Pediatrics 66:693, 1980
35. Christensen RD, Bradley PP, Rothstein G: The leukocyte left shift in clinical and experimental neonatal sepsis. J Pediatar 98:101, 1981
36. Boyle RJ, Chandler BD, Stonestreet B, Oh W: Early identification of sepsis in infants with respiratory distress. Pediatrics 62:744, 1978
37. Squire E, Favara, Todd J: Diagnosis of neonatal bacterial infection: Hematologic and pathologic findings in fatal and nonfatal cases. Pediatrics 64:60, 1979
38. Christensen RD, Rothstein G: Exhaustion of mature marrow neutrophils in neonates with sepsis. J Pediatr 96:316, 1980

39. Christensen RD, Shigeoka AO, Hill HR, Rothstein G: Circulating and storage neutrophil changes in experimental type II group B streptococcal sepsis. Pediatr Res 14:806, 1980
40. Gregory J, Hey E: Blood neutrophil response to bacterial infection in the first month of life. Arch Dis Child 47:747, 1972
41. Santos JI, Shigeoka AO, Hill HR: Functional leukocyte administration in protection against experimental neonatal infection. Pediatr Res 14:1408, 1980
42. Christensen RD, Macfarlane JL, Taylor NL, et al: Blood and marrow neutrophils during experimental group B streptococcal infection: Quantification of the stem cell, proliferative, storage and circulating pools. Pediatr Res 15:549, 1982
43. Christensen RD, Hill HR, Rothstein G: CFUc proliferation in experimental neonatal and adult group B streptococcal sepsis. Pediatr Res 17:278, 1983
44. Laurenti F, Fero R, Isacchi G, et al: Polymorphonuclear leukocyte transfusion for the treatment of sepsis in the newborn infant. J Pediatr 98:118, 1981
45. Hill HR: Phagocyte transfusion: Ultimate therapy of neonatal infection? J Pediatr 98:59, 1981
46. Christensen RD, Rothstein G, Anstall HB, Bybee B: Granulocyte transfusion in neonates with bacterial infection, neutropenia and depletion of mature marrow neutrophils. Pediatrics 70:1, 1982
47. DeCurtis M, Romano G, Scarpato N, et al: Transfusion of polymorphonuclear leukocytes (PMNs) in an infant with necrotizing enterocolitis (NEC) and a defect of phagocytosis. J Pediatr 99:665, 1981
48. Laing IA, Boulton FE, Hume R: Polymorphonuclear leukocyte transfusion in neonatal septicaemia. Arch Dis Child 58:1003, 1983
49. Cairo MS, Rucker R, Bennetto GA, et al: Improved survival of newborns receiving leukocyte transfusions for sepsis. Pediatrics 74:887, 1984
50. Stork E, Baley J, Shurin S: A controlled trial of granulocyte transfusions in neutropenic neonates. Pediatr Res 19:366A, 1985
51. Wheeler JG, Chauvenet AR, Johnson CA, et al: Neutrophil storage pool depletion in septic neutropenic neonates. Pediatr Infect Dis 3:407, 1984
52. Wheeler JG, Abramson JS, Johnson CA, et al: Preliminary findings of a randomized study of buffy coat transfusions in septic neutropenic neonates. Pediatr Res 20:403A, 1986
53. Santos JI, Shigeoka AO, Rote NS, Hill HR: Protective efficacy of a modified immune serum globulin in experimental group B streptococcal infection. J Pediatr 99:875, 1981
54. Fischer GW, Hunter KW, Wilson SR: Modified human immune serum globulin for intravenous administration: In vitro opsonic activity and in vivo protection against group B streptococcal disease in suckling rats. Acta Paediatr Scand 71:639, 1982
55. Shigeoka AO, Pincus SH, Rote NS, Hill HR: Protective efficacy of hybridoma type-specific antibody against experimental infection with group B streptococcus. J Infect Dis 149:363, 1984
56. Christensen RD, Rothstein G, Hill HR, Pincus SH: The effect of hybridoma antibody administration upon neutrophil kinetics during experimental type III group B streptococcal sepsis. Pediatr Res 17:795, 1983
57. Shigeoka AO, Weber ME, Pincus SH, et al: Type-specific monoclonal antibody enhances the local phagocytic response to group B streptococcal infections. J Infect Dis 153:1170, 1986
58. Shigeoka AO, Bathras J, Janatova J, Hill HR: Neutrophil mobilization responses induced by the purified C3d-k fragment of complement in experimental group B streptococcal infection. Clin Res 34:133A, 1986
59. Hall RT, Shigeoka AO, Hill HR: Serum opsonic activity and peripheral neutrophil counts before and after exchange transfusion in infants with early onset group B streptococcal septicemia. Pediatr Infect Dis 2:356, 1983
60. Wasserman RL, Kuhls TH: In vitro sensitization prior to fusion generates a high frequency of human-human hybridomas binding to group B streptococci (GBS). Pediatr Res 18:266A, 1984
61. Sidiropoulos D, Boehme W, Muralt GV, et al: Immunoglobulin supplementation in prevention or treatment of neonatal sepsis. Pediatr Infect Dis, suppl., 5:S193–S194, 1986
62. Gloser H, Backmayer H, Helm A: Intravenous immunoglobulin with high activity against group B streptococci. Pediatr Infect Dis, suppl., 5:S176–S179, 1986
63. Fischer GW, Hemming VG, Hunter KW, et al: Intravenous immunoglobulin in the treatment of neonatal sepsis: Therapeutic strategies and laboratory studies. Pediatr Infect Dis, suppl., 5:S171–S175, 1986
64. Adhikari M, Coovadia HM, Gaffin SL, et al: Septicaemic low birthweight neonates treated with human antibodies to endotoxin. Arch Dis Child 60:382, 1985
65. Mosesson MW, Amrani DL: The structure and biological function of plasma fibronectin. Blood 56:145, 1980
66. Hill HR, Shigeoka AO, Pincus S, Christensen RD: Intravenous IgG in combination with other modalities in the treatment of neonatal infection. Pediatr Infect Dis, suppl., 5:S180–S184, 1986

67. Barnard DR, Arthur MM: Fibronectin (cold insoluble globulin) in the neonate. J Pediatr 102:453, 1983
68. Hill HR, Shigeoka AO, Augustine NH, et al: Fibronectin enhances the opsonic and protective activity of monoclonal and polyclonal antibody against group B streptococci. J Exp Med 159:1618, 1984
69. Berman M, Alter HJ, Ishak KG, et al: The chronic sequelae of non-A, non-B hepatitis. Ann Intern Med 91:1, 1979
70. Lever AML, Brown D, Webster ADB, Thomas HC: Non-A, non-B hepatitis occurring in agammaglobulinaemic patients after intravenous immunoglobulin. Lancet 2:1062, 1984
71. Bossell J: Safety of therapeutic immune globulin preparations with respect to transmission of human T lymphotropic virus type III/Lymphadenopathy-Associated Virus infection. MMWR 35:231, 1986
72. Yeager AS, Grumet FC, Hafleigh EB, et al: Prevention of transfusion-acquired cytomegalovirus infections in newborn infants. J Pediatr 98:281, 1981
73. Curran JW, Lawrence DN, Jaffe H, et al: Acquired immunodeficiency syndrome (AIDS) associated with transfusion. N Engl J Med 310:69, 1984
74. Oleske J, Minnefor A, Cooper R, et al: Immune deficiency syndrome in children. JAMA 240:2345, 1983

11

Prevention and Reduction of Iatrogenic Disorders in the Newborn

Trevor A. Macpherson
Susan Shen-Schwarz
Marie Valdes-Dapena

> Perinatology was born and has come of age in the last 20 years. When it was very young, its problems were few, but now as it emerges full-grown, the problems have increased in number and magnitude—and as it is with human beings, many of its difficulties are of its own creation.[1]
>
> (Valdes-Dapena)

> Neonatal intensive care relies heavily on mechanical devices and invasive procedures; indeed so much is being done to the desperately ill infant that at times it might be difficult to appreciate that he or she is not just another component in a complex array of mechanical devices.[2]
>
> (Ablow)

In a book on advances neonatal intensive care, it might appear paradoxical to include a chapter on iatrogenic disorders. However, such complications are and always will be the consequence of, and the impetus for, advances in neonatal intensive care. They appear to hold us back, but in fact they drive us forward. Described as "diseases of medical progress,"[3] they might also be designated as "diseases of and for medical progress," particularly in the young discipline of neonatal intensive care.

The term "iatrogenic," given us by O.H. Perry Pepper,[4] combines the Greek words "iatros," meaning physician, with "genesis," signifying origin, and is applied to those diseases induced by physicians in the care of their patients. The term, originally restricted to pyschiatric disorders induced in patients by autosuggestion resulting from misinterpretation of the doctor's attitude, comments, or both, now has broader application, including complications that result from diagnostic and therapeutic interventions. These disorders are so important to the practice and process of health care that Meyers[3] has suggested that the category "iatrogenic disorders" be added to the classic etiologic categories of disease that now include congenital/developmental, traumatic, infectious/inflammatory, metabolic, neoplastic, and degenerative. The adverse effects described in iatrogenic disorders are generally those of commission, those of omission usually being excluded because they are difficult to substantiate with certainty; what might have been is not as accurately determined as that which is.

The term "iatrogenic" or "physician-induced disease" in neonatology should not be interpreted as accusatory, since the majority of iatrogenic complications in the neonate are the result of well-intended and accepted diagnostic and therapeutic procedures. In newborns the risk of iatrogenic disease is often equal to that of the affliction being treated, especially in the very low birthweight/young gestational age group. The smaller the patient, the narrower the gap between "helping" and "hurting," and the more difficult it is to predict with certainty those patients destined for a more favorable outcome. We must be grateful for our successes, while rising to meet the challenge of our failures.

A major hindrance to better recognition, documentation, and communication of iatrogenic diseases is the threat of litigation. This threat is useful insofar as it protects the public from incompetent, inadequately trained, or careless physicians. It has less, if any, value if it prevents concerned physicians from sharing information on their failures with a view to prevention. Specific iatrogenic diseases might be recognized earlier and investigated more widely, their incidence might be reduced sooner, and harmful agents or procedures would be eliminated more readily if individual cases could be collected in some sort of registry without the threat of an increased risk of litigation. This is particularly important in diseases of low incidence, where significant time may pass before the problem is recognized in individual institutions. The lack of such a registry is one reason that the incidence of many such disorders is not known.

The intent of this chapter is to review, in the neonate in the neonatal intensive care unit (NICU), those iatrogenic complications that have their onset after birth. Prenatal and natal events, such as maternal medications, invasive fetal procedures, perinatal asphyxia, birth trauma, iatrogenic respiratory distress syndrome, and complications of cardiac catheterization are excluded; the interested reader is referred to excellent previous reviews of these subjects.[1,5–6] Iatrogenic disorders that become manifest years after the discharge of an infant from the nursery are also excluded, as are the myriad drug complications. We will discuss prevention, the role of the neonatologist in post-discharge follow-up, and the potential for collaborative research in reducing the incidence of iatrogenic complications in the newborn. If total prevention is not possible, our goal should, at the very least, be to commit ourselves to achieve the utmost care and skill, so that iatrogenic complications are brought to an "irreducible minimum."[3]

The authors will have achieved their goal if our readers learn something new or are made aware of the importance of individual and collective efforts in recognizing, documenting, communicating, investigating, educating, and thereby reducing iatrogenic complications in the newborn.

DEFINITION

Iatrogenic complications are defined, as "all unintended adverse outcomes, of diagnostic and/or therapeutic interventions, whether due to lack of physician skill, inherent hazard of the intervention, susceptibility of the host, or extent of affliction being managed (as adapted from Kasser[7]). Adverse outcomes may be of early or late onset. The scope of iatrogenic complications is appreciated when one realizes

Table 11-1. Common Indications for Assisted Ventilation

Respiratory distress syndrome
Aspiration syndromes
Pneumonia
Postoperative support
Pulmonary immaturity
Hypoventilation (drug induced)
Sepsis
Central nervous system disorders
Anomalies of the lung

(Data from Ref. 2.)

that almost every diagnostic or therapeutic intervention carries some potential risk, and every organ is susceptible to damage by one or more of the myriad ways in which physicians may be required to intervene in the neonate, either diagnostically or therapeutically.

COMPLICATIONS OF ASSISTED VENTILATION

Pulmonary complications are among the most common iatrogenic problems seen in the NICU. Among neonates with persistent pulmonary hypertension of the newborn (PPHN), it is estimated that up to 50 percent develop pulmonary air leak complications.[8] The evolution of assisted ventilation is one of the major reasons for improved survival in the neonate; however, its course is strewn with testimony to the hazard of its application—it is both a "boon and a bane for the neonatologist."[9]

The common indications for assisted ventilation are listed in Table 11-1, and the air-leak complications of assisted ventilation in Table 11-2. Almost all of the air-leak syndromes are a consequence of barotrauma, the initial event being leakage of air due to alveolar rupture. They are among the most common iatrogenic complications seen in the neonate, and a list of predisposing factors is shown in Table 11-3.

Table 11-2. Pulmonary Complications—Air Leak Syndromes

Acute pulmonary interstitial emphysema
Intrapulmonary pneumatosis
Intrapleural pneumatosis
Chronic persistent interstitial pulmonary emphysema
Generalized (diffuse)
Localized (persistent and loculated)
Pneumothorax
Pneumomediastinum
Pneumopericardium
Pneumoperitoneum
Subcutaneous emphysema
Retroperitoneal air
Air embolism

(Adapted from Perelman R: Reducing iatrogenic lung disease in the premature newborn. Semin Perinatol 10:217, 1986.)

Table 11-3. Predisposing Factors to Pulmonary Air Leaks in Infants

Pulmonary immaturity
Respiratory distress syndrome
Aspiration syndromes
Pulmonary infection
Pulmonary anomalies
Errors at resuscitation
Overzealous resuscitation at birth
Intubation of bronchus
Needle puncture of lung
Assisted ventilation
Excessive peak inspiratory pressure and tidal volume
Excessive artifical sighing
Nonhomogenicity of surfactant development
Asynchronous breathing
CPAP greater than 10 cmH_2O
PEEP greater than 10 cmH_2O
Inadvertent PEEP
Fast frequency of breathing
Small diameter of intubation tubes
Increased airway resistance
Peribronchial edema
Prolonged time constants
Absent pores of Kohn

(Valdes-Dapena M: Iatrogenic disease in the perinatal period as seen by the pathologist. p. 382. In Naeye RL, Kissane JM, Kaufman N (eds): Perinatal Diseases. © 1981 The Williams & Wilkins Co., Baltimore)

Pulmonary Interstitial Emphysema

Pulmonary interstitial emphysema (PIE) is the initiating event in all air-leak syndromes, and is defined as the presence of air in the intrapulmonary (perivascular-peribronchial-peribronchiolar-intralymphatic) and intrapleural (subpleural) connective tissue compartments. This entity can occur in the absence of assisted ventilation, when a ball-valve effect results from air obstruction due to mucus or meconium. Reid and Rubino consider that the more extensive connective tissue system in preterm infants, makes them more susceptible to PIE.[10] The high mechanical ventilatory pressures required to ventilate the immature, "stiff," surfactant-deficient lung of the preterm neonate predisposes it to PIE and is the reason why this complication continues to be a major problem in the NICU.

Macklin and Macklin[11] were the first to conclude that PIE resulted from the entrapped interstitial air derived from the rupture of alveolar walls, which in turn resulted from the disequilibrium of alveolar and vascular lung compartments. Caldwell[12] has depicted these mechanical stresses, and Thibeault[13] has suggested that high-stress gradients occur at the alveolar base, where it is in opposition to blood vessels. An imbalance of alveolar expansion and alveolar pulmonary blood flow appears to be an important predisposing factor in the development of PIE.

Even though PIE in the preterm infant does not always lead to further air-leak syndromes[14]—possibly because of increased interstitial water[13]—it can cause significant morbidity and mortality. Air dissecting through the interstitium of the lung makes the lung rigid, causing mechanical "splinting" of the lung with sub-

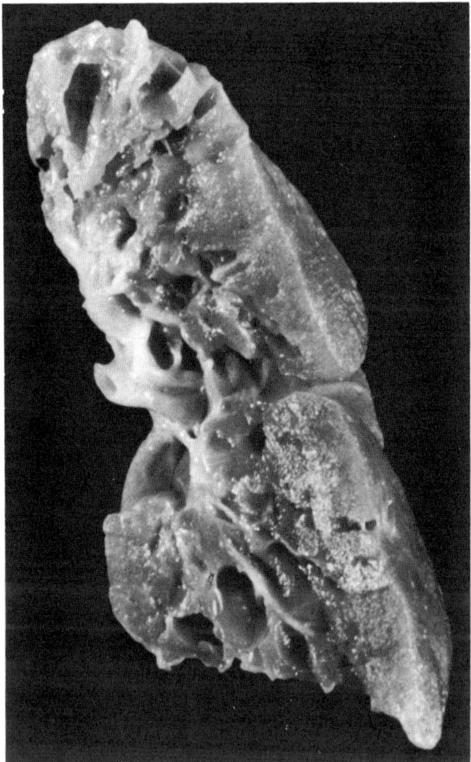

Fig. 11.1. Cut section of lung with PIE. The "air" dissects along interlobular septae and bronchovascular sheaths and is most striking at the hilum of the lung.

sequent "compression" of alveolar and other blood vessels (air block).[1] The ensuing reduced blood flow compounds an already present alveolar air/blood-flow imbalance, further increasing the predisposition to PIE. In addition, adjacent lung parenchyma is compressed. This cycle, once in operation, is difficult to interrupt. From the interstitium, air readily tracks along lymphatics and blood vessels via the path of least resistance to reach the pleura or mediastinum or both, forming large, thin-walled bullae that readily rupture to cause a pneumothorax (Fig. 11-1). From the above discussion, it is not surprising that air-leak syndromes occur most frequently in preterm newborns,[13] and can be attributed directly to the use of mechanical ventilation techniques that apply a continuous, distending pressure.[2,15] Term infants who develop PIE usually have underlying pulmonary disease such as aspiration syndrome, pneumonia, or lung anomalies.

The exact location of the air in the pulmonary interstitium in PIE has been a matter of dispute; some maintain that the air is in the lymphatics,[16,17] whereas others contend that it is in the interstices of the interstitial tissue.[16,18,19] Others have difficulty distinguishing between the two microscopically, and conclude it may be present in both[1] (Fig. 11-2).

Radiographic criteria for the diagnosis of PIE have been reviewed.[2] At autopsy, subpleural blebs are often noted, and in severe cases the lung may show a Swiss-cheese appearance. At autopsy, the extent and distribution of PIE can be dramatically demonstrated by inflating the lungs with formaldehyde.

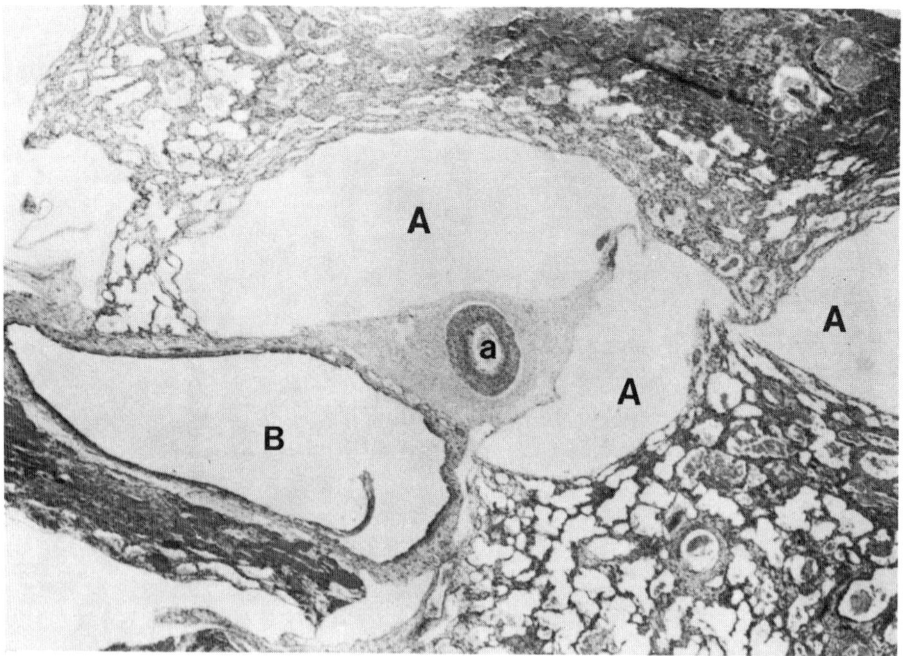

Fig. 11.2. Photomicrograph of pulmonary interstitial emphysema. The "air pockets" (A) are seen in the connective tissue surrounding the bronchiole (B) and artery (a).

Pneumothorax

Air can reach the pleural cavity from rupture of a subpleural or hilar bleb, but air in the cavity is more commonly due to rupture of an anterior mediastinal collection of air.[13] This is probably because interstitial air tracks along the line of least resistance—such resistance becoming progressively weaker in the direction of vessels of increasing caliber.[20] Air is thus more likely to locate finally around large vessels in the mediastinum, rather than in peripheral subpleural sites. In rare instances, pneumothorax may be due to perforation of the lung or bronchus by an endotracheal suction catheter.[21] The radiographic diagnosis of pneumothorax has been reviewed.[2] At autopsy, the diagnosis is made readily by postmortem radiography, by opening the chest under water, or by needle aspiration. The last method may miss small, localized collections of air. In tension pneumothorax, the diaphragm may be everted, the mediastinum displaced, or the ipsilateral lung collapsed. The lung and internal thoracic wall may be bright red.

Pneumopericardium, Pneumoperitoneum, and Subcutaneous Emphysema

Pneumopericardium is usually associated with PIE,[22] although the mechanism of its occurrence is not fully explained.[23] It can result from bronchial perforation secondary to perforation at intubation, or from endotracheal tube suction for lung toilet.[13] When massive, it may have significant hemodynamic consequences[24,25] (Fig. 11-3).

Pneumoperitoneum usually results when mediastinal air tracks along the aorta

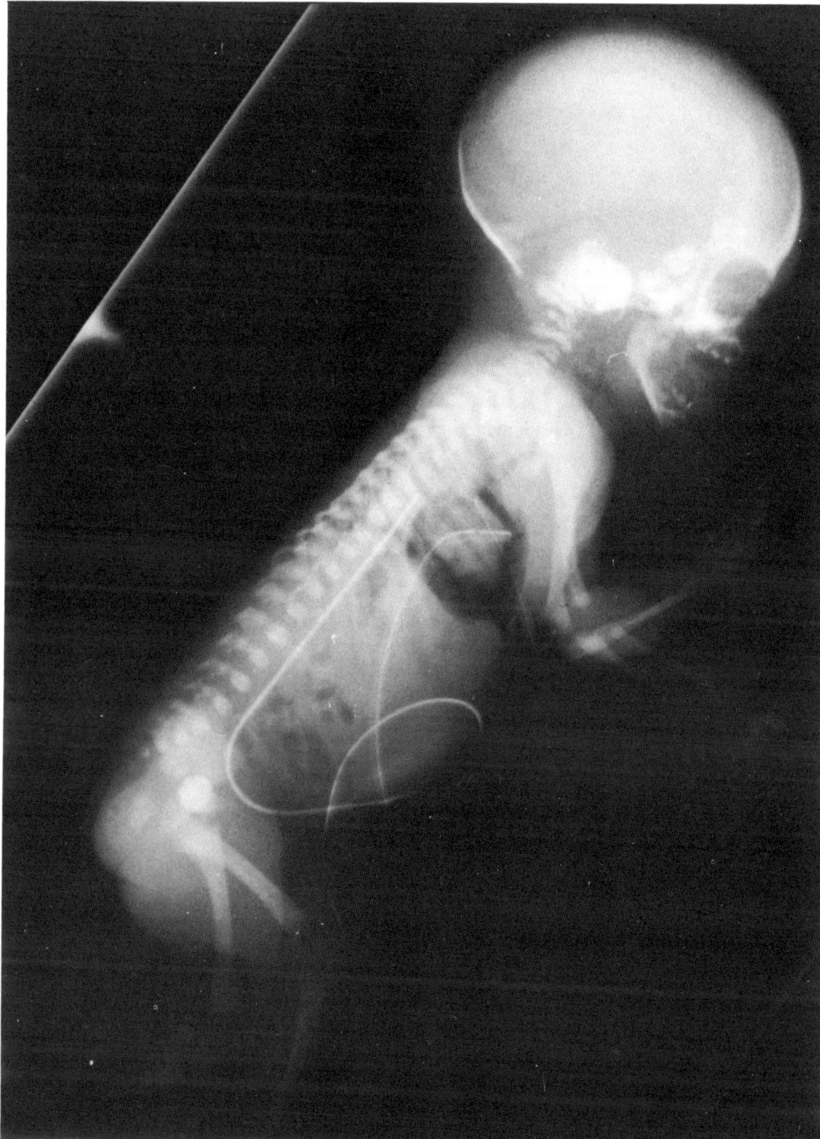

Fig. 11.3. x-Ray showing pneumopericardium. In this lateral-view, whole-body x-ray of a 26-weeks gestation, 920 g infant who lived for 5 hours, the air distends the pericardium and extends along the root of the great vessels.

or inferior vena cava through the diaphragm into the retroperitoneum, and ultimately via mesenteric vessels to form subserosal cysts whose rupture results in pneumoperitoneum. Another iatrogenic cause is bowel perforation due to trauma from a nasogastric tube.[26,27] Except when due to bowel perforation, pneumoperitoneum is of less consequence than other air-leak syndromes.

Subcutaneous emphysema results when air dissects from the mediastinum along the great vessels into the subcutaneous tissues of the neck, and is the least common air-leak syndrome. It can also result from perforation of the trachea by instrumentation.

Persistent Interstitial Pulmonary Emphysema

Persistent interstitial pulmonary emphysema (PIPE) is a complication that occurs almost exclusively in infants who have had assisted ventilation, and can be defined as a localized or diffuse, space-occupying and persistent emphysematous lesion in the lung. It can compromise ventilation. Two varieties have been described by Stocker and Madewell.[28] The localized form, which can be diagnosed during life, involves the left upper lobe of the lung in 50 percent of cases,[29] and often requires surgery. The diffuse form can be established only at autopsy.[28] In both forms there is usually associated bronchopulmonary dysplasia, but this is more severe in the diffuse variety. Foreign-body giant cells surrounding the "emphysematous cysts" are characteristic of PIPE. The disease is probably the result of a localized or diffuse persistent air leak.

A localized area of overinflation may cause sufficient mediastinal shift to necessitate surgical removel of the involved segment of the lung so as to relieve respiratory distress. More recently, selective bronchial intubation has been performed with some success in PIPE, obviating the need for surgery.[30] This technique has, however, been complicated by hypoxia, bradycardia, right-upper-lobe atelectasis, pneumonia, and additional air leaks. Since 1977, 19 cases treated by this method have been reported.[30]

Air Embolism

Air embolism is a rare event, and when noted radiologically is generally fatal.[31,32] It is most readily visualized in the heart, but other sites include the aorta, hepatic vessels, and the liver.[2]

Bronchopulmonary Dysplasia

Bronchopulmonary dysplasia (BPD) is an excellent example of the dilemma neonatologists face in attempting to eliminate iatrogenic complications in the newborn. Originally described in 1967,[33] it is still an important complication. There are no precise or universally accepted diagnostic criteria for BPD, and the overall incidence is uncertain "because published data are variable and the pathogenic relationship between anatomic immaturity, surfactant deficiency, mechanical ventilation, and oxygen exposure are unclear[9] (see also Ch. 4).

Bronchopulmonary dysplasia can be defined as a deviation from normal lung development caused primarily by a combination of increased oxygen exposure and barotrauma over time.[34] All lung tissues can be affected, and the most debilitating stage is one in which areas of "emphysema" alternate with areas showing smooth-muscle and connective-tissue proliferation while still others are atelectatic. At this peak stage, pulmonary hypertension is a frequent complication of BPD; it is characterized in the lung by medial smooth-muscle hypertrophy in medium-sized and small pulmonary arteries.[1] Full recovery is apparently possible but, in many patients, pulmonary function tests remain abnormal for months or years.

Currently, the best hypothesis for the pathogenesis of BPD is that it is caused

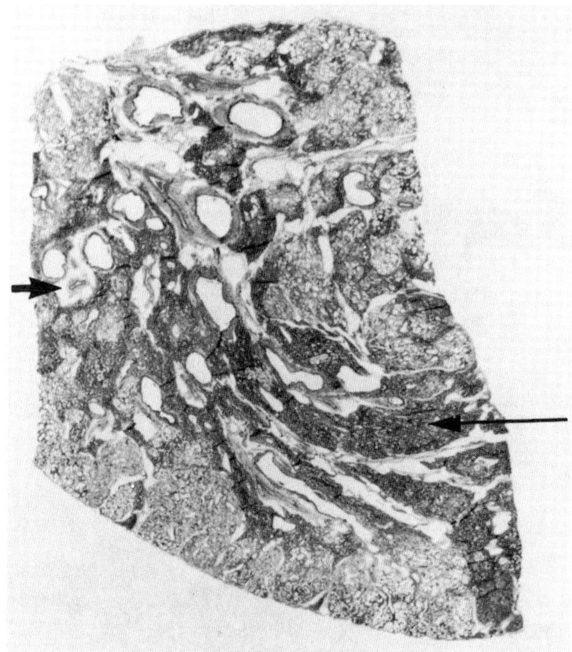

Fig. 11.4. Whole-mount section of lung with early bronchopulmonary dysplasia and pulmonary interstitial emphysema. This 28-weeks gestation, 1,000 g infant lived for 8 days. The lungs show areas of hyperinflation and atelectasia (long arrow) associated with interstitial fibrosis. Pulmonary interstitial emphysema (short arrow) is also present in this section.

by an as yet undefined interaction between increased oxygen exposure and barotrauma over time. The role of endotracheal intubation is less clear, but it is associated with the development of squamous metaplasia and tracheal necrosis.[35] These changes impede normal pulmonary toilet and the function of ciliated epithelium, but the role of these factors in the development of BPD has not yet been established.

The radiographic features of BPD have been reviewed.[2] The histologic changes have been divided into three stages[36]: exudative, proliferative, and recuperative. The initial changes are a deviation from the normal process involved in recovery from respiratory distress syndrome (RDS), including peribronchial interstitial fibroblast proliferation, edema, and persistent hyaline membranes. These features are followed after the first 2 weeks by: (1) progressive proliferation of interstitial fibroblasts, (2) smooth-muscle hypertrophy of bronchiolar walls, and (3) epithelial changes of hyperplasia and squamous metaplasia in larger air-ways.[1] All of these features, together with the organization of mucus secretions, result in obstructive phenomena causing alternating areas of atelectasis and overdistension of the lung[37] (Fig. 11-4). Pulmonary hypertension can also result from vascular smooth-muscle hypertrophy.[1] With all of these pathologic features, it is not suprising that infants with BPD have a significant compromise of respiratory function.

Oxygen[33,38,39] and barotrauma[40,41] contribute to the development of BPD. At least two authors maintain that since high pressure and increased oxygen exposure

Table 11-4. Oxygen Toxicity in Animals

Exudative phase	Proliferative phase (more than 7 to 10 days)
First 6 hours Tracheitis	Proliferation of type II, alveolar cells Thickening of alveolar surface
48 to 72 hours Bronchitis Loss of ciliary function Damage to mucus-secreting cells Fulminant necrotizing bronchiolitis	Interstitial fibrosis Increase in number of Clara cells in airways Subepithelial fibrosis Resolution in short exposures
After 48 to 72 hours Damage to capillary endothelium Extensive interstitial edema Damage to alveolar type I cells Associated atelectasis	Permanent lung scarring in others
Death in the exudative phase Due to respiratory failure from pulmonary edema extensive atelectasis	

(Data compiled from Ref. 43.)

usually occur together, it is difficult to evaluate the contribution of each to the development of BPD.[37,42] The best assessment at present may be that the bronchial epithelial changes and bronchial wall hypertrophy in BPD are due to barotrauma, while those of the interstitium are related to the adverse effects of oxygen.[37]

The spectrum of oxygen-induced damage to the lung has been clearly demonstrated in many animal experiments, and a list of them has been compiled from the review of Hansen and Gest[43] and is presented in Table 11-4. The effects of oxygen in the human are less easily demonstrated, but there have been several reviews detailing its possible effects.[44–47] The cytology of tracheal aspirates has been used to diagnose lung lesions, and wider use of this technique may be helpful in monitoring the effects of oxygen damage.[48,49]

Necrotizing Tracheobronchitis

A "new" lesion called necrotizing tracheobronchitis (NTB), related to assisted ventilation, was described by Metlay et al.[50] and subsequently reported by others.[51] It has also been noted in infants exposed to high-frequency jet ventilation.[52–54] Metlay's group found NTB in 38 newborns who had received assisted ventilation for periods from 3 hours to 13 days. In one case, the patient received assisted ventilation for only 40 minutes, which was the entire length of his life. The lesion showed no preference for gestational age or birthweight. The patients' gestational ages ranged from 25 to 43 weeks (mean 32 weeks), with bimodal distribution peaks at 28 and 38 weeks. Their birthweight ranged from 700 to 4000 g (mean 1740 g). Survival ranged from 40 minutes to 13 days, with a mean survival of 5 days. Necrotizing tracheobronchitis occurred with both the Bird and Seachrist ventilator, and over a range of ventilator rates, pressures, and FIO_2 concentrations. The severity of the lesion (graded as 1 to 4) increased with the duration of assisted ventilation. In severe cases, respiratory obstruction may occur as the result of sloughing of tracheal mucosa; this complication has been treated successfully by tracheal lavage in some cases.[54]

Pathologic changes at autopsy are maximal beyond the tube tip (Fig. 11-5). It

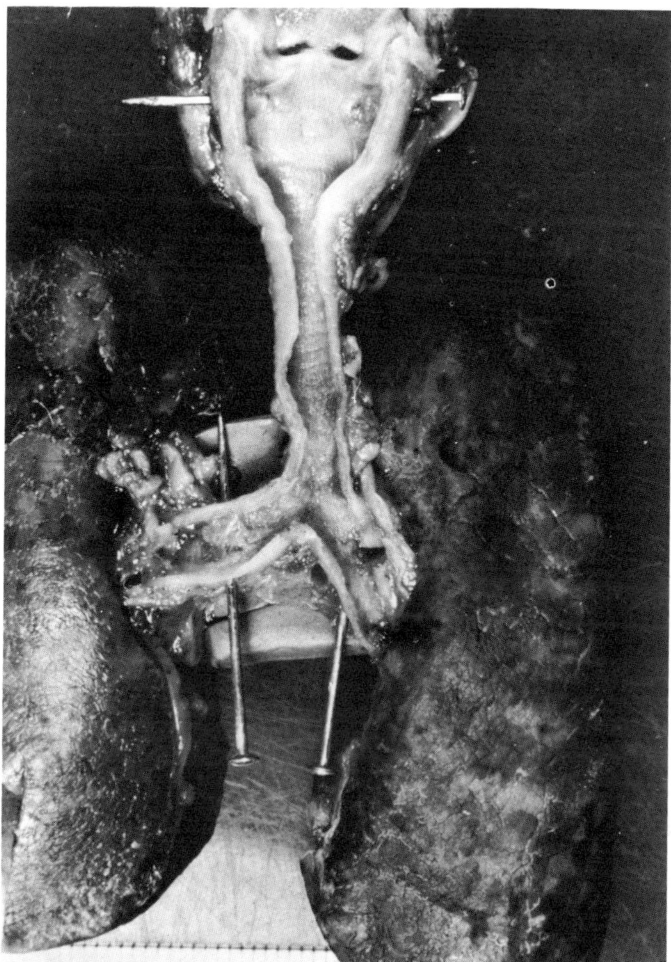

Fig. 11.5. Necrotizing tracheobronchitis: gross. Trachea and lungs of an 8-day-old, 30-weeks gestation infant. The posteriorly opened trachea shows thickening and a cobblestone appearance of the mucosa in the distal portion, involving the bifurcation and extending into the bronchus bilaterally.

is this feature, together with the characteristic basophilic tissue changes on the luminal aspect of the trachea (Fig. 11-6), that makes the lesion in NTB different from previously described lesions produced by, or associated with, endotracheal tubes.[35] Furthermore, the changes extend into both major bronchi—an unlikely effect were the lesion caused by the tube trauma alone. The precise etiology of NTB is not known, but it has been seen only in infants who have received assisted ventilation. Its occurrence with bronchial involvement in an infant who was bagged for only a short time supports the hypotheses that NTB is caused either by airflow or by factors such as inadequate humidification, heat, or toxins derived from the tube itself. The importance of NTB lies in the fact that it may cause obstruction with respiratory compromise. This complication should be suspected when excessive mucus production is noted. Necrotizing tracheobronchitis can be diagnosed

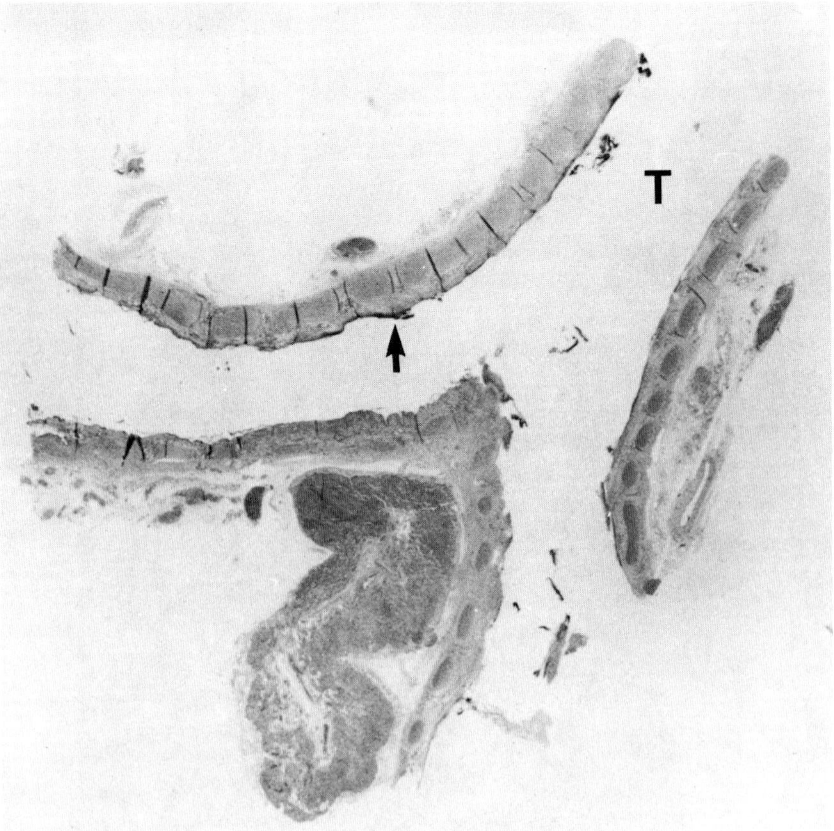

Fig. 11.6. Necrotizing tracheobronchitis: whole mount of longitudinal section of bifurcation of trachea (T) and mainstem bronchus. The mucosa shows complete loss of epithelium, being covered instead by basophilic necrotic material (arrow).

by the cytologic examination of tracheal aspirates when characteristic basophilic material is seen.

Yellow Hyaline Membrane Disease

Yellow hyaline membrane disease (YHMD) is mentioned as an example of a lesion that was a common finding at autopsy at Magee-Womens Hospital, Pittsburgh, Pennsylvania, several years ago but is now rarely encountered.[55] The reason for its decline is uncertain, since several treatment modalities were changed within a short period of time, including a shorter turnaround time for arterial blood gas tension studies as a result of computerization, and the removal of benzyl alcohol as a preservative in infusates. It is likely that several factors are responsible for the virtual elimination of YHMD, but the exact reasons have not yet been determined.

Perforation of the Gastrointestinal Tract

Garland et al.[56] reported 20 cases of gastrointestinal perforation not associated with necrotizing enterocolitis or bowel obstruction (GPNN). All of the infants affected had face masks or nasal prongs used in association with assisted ventilation, as compared with 52 percent of controls. Perforation occurred during the first 5 days in 11 patients and during the first 3 days in 9 instances, and involved the stomach, duodenum, ileum, or jejunum. The authors concluded that GPNN associated with assisted ventilation delivered by face mask or nasal prongs was increased thirtyfold as compared with assisted ventilation delivered by endotracheal tube.

Reducing Complications of Assisted Ventilation

Perelman[9] has suggested that there are three major prerequisites for reducing neonatal respiratory morbidity and mortality: (1) prevention of preterm birth, (2) reduction in the incidence or severity or both of neonatal respiratory disease, and (3) technologic advances toward diminishing complications of mechanical ventilation. The first is beyond the scope of the present discussion. The second can be achieved by accurate assessment of lung maturity prior to elective delivery, via a pulmonary maturity "index or profile" performed according to strict guidelines.[57] More particularly, the incidence and severity of respiratory distress can be reduced if lung maturation can be accelerated in instances in which preterm birth cannot be prevented. The current use of corticosteroids initiated by Liggins[58] and Kotas and Avery[59] is not always effective and is not without side effects.[60] Perelman[9] concludes that "future studies of importance that may increase clinical capabilities (of enhancing lung maturity) include delineation of regulatory mechanisms controlling the metabolism of lung phospholipids, precise elucidation of hormonal influencs on lung maturation, and refined approaches to manipulating surfactant biosynthesis."

Technologic advances required to reduce the complications of mechanical ventilation include: (1) reducing the need for assisted ventilation, (2) developing new methods of ventilation; (3) providing agents that protect the lung from damage, (4) improving nutritional support of the ventilated neonate, and (5) using more accurate monitoring devices that permit a more physiologic management of assisted ventilation.[9] The need for assisted ventilation can be reduced only if lung maturation can be accelerated or stimulated. When ventilation is needed, the lowest pressures possible should be used.[61] Exogenous surfactants are the major hope in this regard, but the definite evidence of their safety and value is still forthcoming,[62,63] although the requirements of an effective agent have been detailed[64] (see Ch. 2). No increase in lung inflammation or activation of the classical pathway of complement has occurred with human-derived surfactant.[65] Advances in mechanical ventilators must reduce the barotrauma and oxygen toxicity caused by conventional ventilatory methods. High-frequency ventilation (HFV) may do that, and is discussed in Chapter 3 of this volume. However, HFV may cause complications such as NTB, with damage ranging from erythema to a severe necrosis with obstruction of the trachea and mainstem bronchus.[52,53] Extracorporeal membrane oxygenation (ECMO) has been associated with intraventricular hemorrhage (IVH) in 8 of 8 infants of less than 35 weeks' gestation, leading Cilley et al.[66] to recommend that ECMO be contraindicated in infants of this gestational age and less. When ECMO is used in older infants, the incidence of IVH can be reduced by avoiding thrombycytopenia, heparin overdose, and rapid changes in blood pressure. Other complications of ECMO are jugular vein injury, equipment failure causing hemolysis, and oxygenation failure due to damaged tubing.[67]

The search for agents to protect the lung from toxic side effects has been un-

Table 11-5. Incidence of Complications of Assisted Ventilation at Magee-Womens Hospital (Data from Autopsy Records)

Lesion	Year 1979–1980 (n = 183)	Year 1984–1985 (n = 157)
Pneumothorax	33.9%	22.2%
PIE	27.5%	19.8%
YHMD	31.6%	3.9%
BPD	14.4%	17.0%
NTB	20.4%	19.0%

successful to date. Antioxidants, steroids, and other agents that have been used produce their own complications, and the benefits of their use do not currently outweigh their potential hazards.[68] The increasing use of computerization in intensive care holds promise for improving monitoring and the real-time adjustment of assisted ventilation.[69] Improvements in the management of other support necessary for the sick neonate are also promising.[70] Computers, however, introduce the possibility of other types of human error.[71]

We determined the incidence of several of the above complications at Magee-Womens Hospital, and compared data from 1979–1980 with that for 1984–1985 (Table 11-5). These data were compiled from a review of neonatal autopsy records. The incidence of BPD and NTB had remained fairly constant, the incidence of YHMD had decreased markedly, and the incidence of pneumothorax and PIE had also declined.

Reduction in neonatal morbidity and mortality due to pulmonary lesions will be a major step in reducing complications in newborns to an irreducible minimum.

Complications Caused by Endotracheal Intubation

The numerous complications of endotracheal tubes are listed in Table 11-6 (Figs. 11-7 and 11-8) and those of suction catheters in Table 11-7 (Fig. 11-9). Acute complications of both can be grouped into (1) mechanical, (2) traumatic, and (3) physiologic categories, while almost all of the chronic lesions are consequences of trauma. Physiologic complications of both endotracheal instillation and suctioning include changes in intracranial, mean arterial, and cerebral perfusion pressures.[72] These complications can be reduced by preoxygenation prior to intubation and suction. Changes in blood pressure increase the risk of intraventricular hemorrhage in these situations. Hypoxia can be induced by excessive handling of neonates.[73]

In general, endotracheal tubes used in the newborn are of the noncuffed variety, making aspiration a potential hazard, as demonstrated by Goodwin et al.[74] These investigators noted that in 80 percent of 20 intubated neonates (birth weight 750 to 2,930 g, gestational age 29 to 36 weeks, mean postnatal age of 14.3 days, and mean duration of intubation 12.5 days), dye put in the mouth was subsequently suctioned from the trachea, indicating that the tube and ventilatory pressures do not protect against the passage of fluid from the pharynx to the lower trachea in intubated newborns.[74] They suggest that inadequate control of gastroesophageal reflux may put intubated, tube-fed infants at risk for aspiration.

Table 11-6. Complications of Endotracheal Intubation

Acute	Chronic
Traumatic	Defective primary dentition
Perforation	Palatal grooves
Nasopharynx	Acquired cleft palate
Oropharynx/hypopharynx	Nasal and choanal stenosis
Other injury	Subglotic stenosis
Hemorrhage	Gingival grooves
Laryngeal edema	Granulomas
Phrenic nerve	Tracheal necrosis
Pneumopericardium	Necrotizing tracheobronchitis
Hemopericardium	Tracheomegaly
Mechanical	
Malposition	
In esophagus	
In one mainstem bronchus causing obstruction	
Too high or low	
Obstruction	
Mucus plugs	
Accidental extubation	
Kinking	
Swallowed endotracheal tube	
Physiologic	
Apnea	
Hypoxia	
Rise in blood pressure	
Aspiration	

(Data compiled from refs. 1, 2, 76 and other sources.)

Bhutani and co-workers[75] have reported a 91 percent increase in tracheal volume in ventilated infants, causing what they called tracheomegaly in neonates $<$ 1,000 g birthweight. This change was demonstrated by x-ray. The duration of ventilation was 25.4 $\pm$ 4.9 days.

Prevention of Complications of Endotracheal Intubation

The four major components of preventing complications of endotracheal intubation are (1) proper technique, 2) careful selection of equipment, 3) adequate preparation of the neonate for the procedure, and 4) monitoring of the infant's general condition during the procedure.[76] Adherence to these measures will reduce complications from all tubes and lines. Endotracheal tube complications can be reduced substantially by attention to tube size,[21] limiting the number and duration of intubations, reducing tube malposition by careful tube fixation, notation of tube length at the patient's nose or lip, and stabilization of the head when handling the baby.[76] Complications of suction can be decreased when guidelines are followed for "appropriate suction pressure, length of catheter, and frequency and duration of suctioning."[76] Unnecessary suction raises the risk of complications, while inadequate suctioning increases the risk of airway obstruction. Different polyvinyl chloride (PVC) endotracheal tubes did not alter the incidence or severity of palatal grooves in one study.[77] Heller and Cotton[78] have used illuminated endotracheal tubes for placement, thereby eliminating the need for irradiation. Unfortunately, esophageal

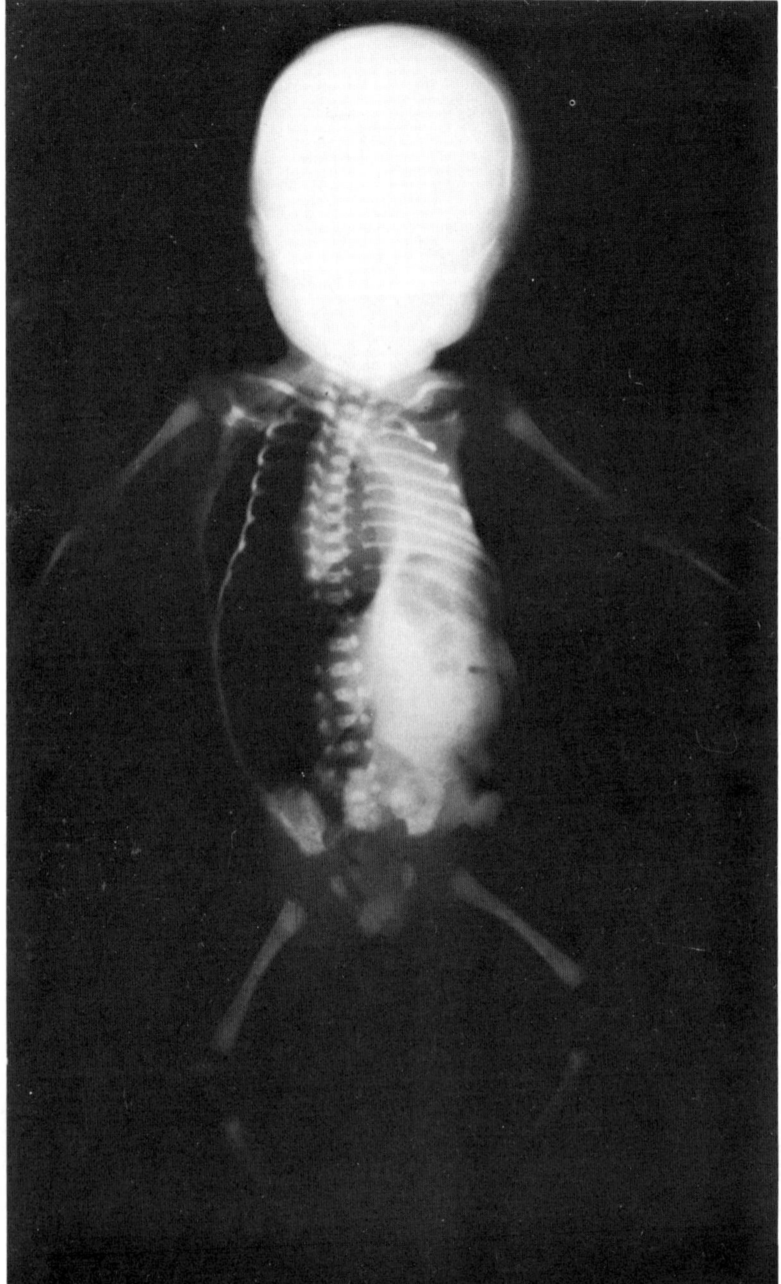

Fig. 11.7. x-Ray showing pneumothorax and pneumoperitonium. Whole-body x-ray of a 24-weeks gestation, 600 g infant who lived for 13 minutes. The massive right pneumothorax displaces the heart and mediastinum to the left and extends into the abdomen, displacing the right hemidiaphragm, liver, and abdominal organs.

Table 11-7. Complications of Endotracheal Suction

Lesion
Hemorrhage
Inadvertent extubation
Perforation: Lung or mainstem bronchus
Bronchopulmonary fistula
Hypoxia
Bradycardia
Systemic hypertension
Increased cerebral blood flow, and increased intracranial pressure
Granuloma formation

(Data compiled from ref. 76.)

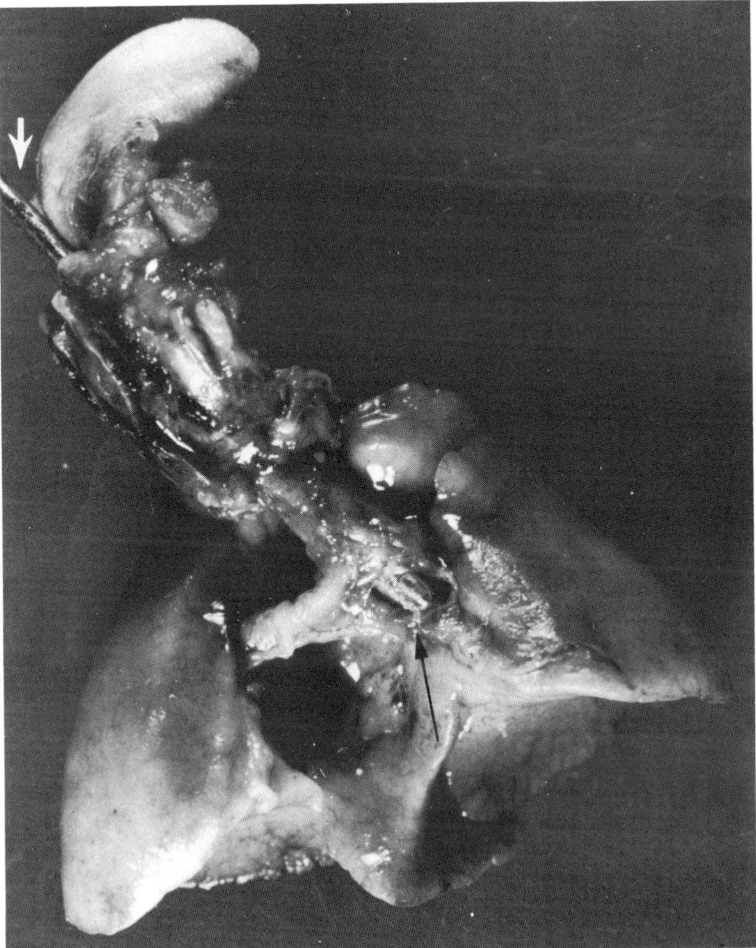

Fig. 11.8. Perforation of bronchus by endotracheal tube. Lungs of the infant whose x-ray is shown in Fig. 11-7. The posterior wall of the right mainstem bronchus was perforated (long arrow) by a probe (white arrow) inserted in the proximal trachea.

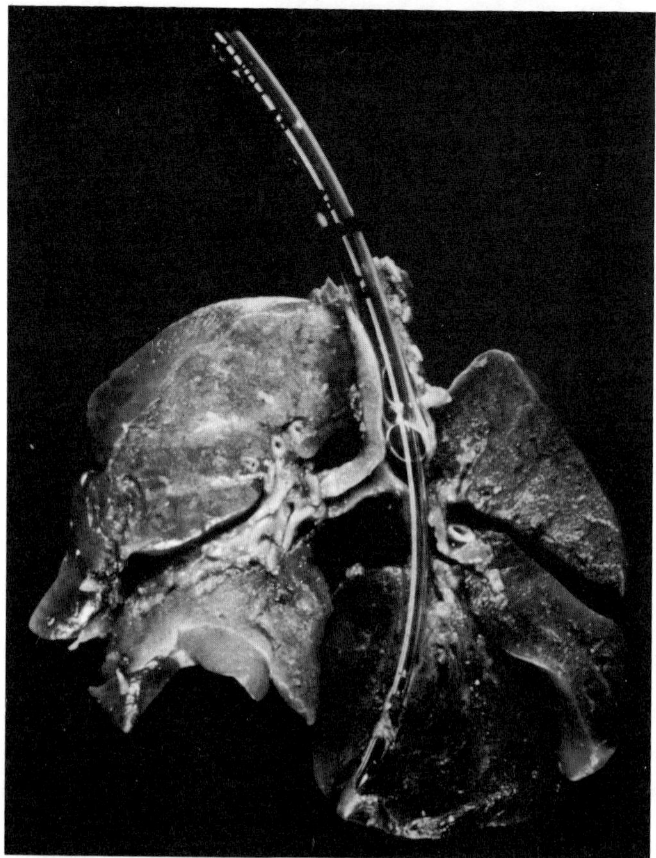

Fig. 11.9. Perforation of lung by endotracheal suction tube. A reconstruction of the process of perforation is made at autopsy. The suction catheter, which is inside an endotracheal tube, enters the right lower lobe bronchus, perforates one segmental bronchus, and ends in a subpleural cyst. A second bronchopleural fistula is present in an adjacent segmental bronchus.

tube malplacement cannot be identified by illumination. Ultrasound localization is likely to become more popular in the future.

COMPLICATIONS OF TUBES AND LINES

This section discusses tubes introduced into the thoracic cavity and gastrointestinal tract, and the various venous and arterial lines used so commonly in the NICU. A list of complications caused by this equipment is presented in Table 11-8.

Tubes in the Thoracic Cavity

A thoracic tube is often employed as an emergency procedure when pneumothorax develops in an infant who probably has "stiff" lungs. The incidence of perforation of the lung has been reported to be as high as 25 percent[79] (Fig. 11-10). Needle aspiration may also lead to lung perforation and, for emergency aspiration, a can-

Table 11-8. Complications of Tubes and Lines

Tubes in thoracic cavity	Tubes in gastrointestinal tract
Infection	Apnea
Scarring	Bradycardia
Visceral perforation	Hypoxia
Lung	Reflux aspiration
Liver	Hemorrhage
Spleen	Perforation
Diaphragm	Misplacement in trachea
Pericardium	
Vessels	
Auxillary	
Pulmonary	
Intercostal	
Obstructions/compression	Peripheral intravenous lines
Aorta	Infiltration
Phrenic nerve	Edema
Hemorrhage	Infection
Visceral perforation	Tissue necrosis
Vessel perforation	Scarring
Fistula	Contracture
Bronchopleural	Loss of function
	Perforation of adjacent artery
Complications common to parenteral lines	Peripheral arterial lines
Infection	Peripheral nerve damage
Hemorrhage	Arterial spasm
Thromboembolism	Ischemia/ischemic necrosis
Infiltration	Central venous lines
Trauma to vessel wall/perforation	Malposition
Improper position	Lymphatic obstruction
Hypernatremia	Cardiac arrhythmia
Heparin overload	Extravasation of fluid
Occlusion of lumen	Pericardial effusion
Breakage of line	Cardiac tamponade
Thrombocytopenia	Hydrothorax
	Hemothorax
	Ascites
Umbilical arterial lines	Umbilical venous lines
Insufficiency of major vessels	Hepatic necrosis
Loss of extremity	Hepatic abscess
Visceral infarcts	Bowel injury from exchange transfusion
Renal artery thrombosis	Cardiac injury
Intestinal ischemia	Pulmonary injury
Total aortic thrombosis	
Hemoperitoneum	
Retroperitoneal hemorrhage	
Hypertension (renal emboli/thrombosis)	
Congestive heart failure	
Hemiparesis and paraplegia	
Mycotic aneurysms	
Thrombocytopenia	
False and aortic aneurysm	
Aortic thromboatheroma	
Urinary ascites from bladder injury	

(Data from refs. 1 and 72 and other sources.)

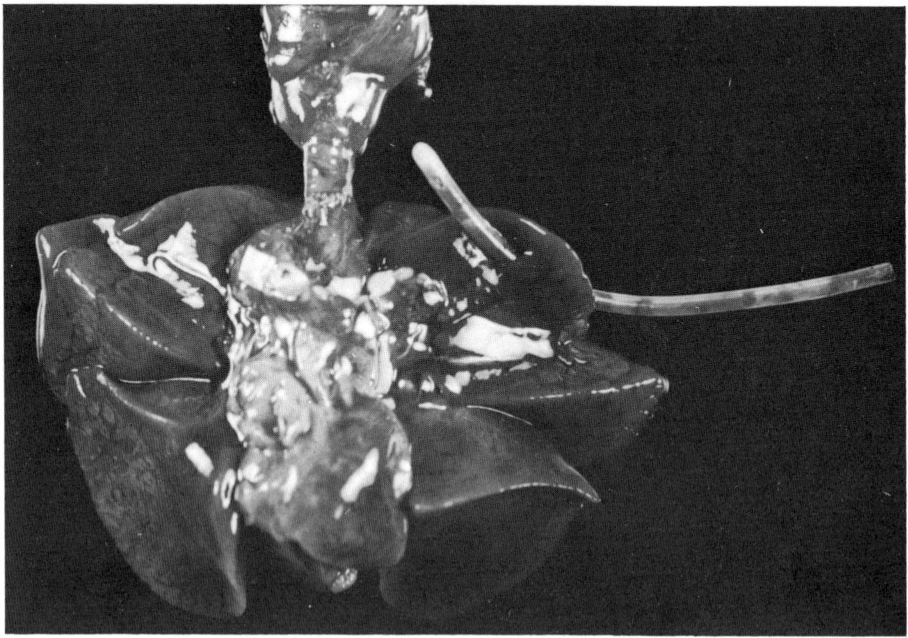

Fig. 11.10. Perforation of lung by chest tube. A chest tube penetrated the upper lobe of the left lung in this infant with severe hyaline membrane disease.

nula/stylet assembly may be safer than a needle.[76] Rapid re-expansion of a lung against a sharp trocar predisposes to lung perforation, a complication that can be reduced by using a curved hemostat rather than a sharp trocar.[76] Persistence of pneumothorax after tube placement should raise the possibility of lung perforation or bronchopleural fistula. Other complications can be reduced by appropriate technique and management.[80]

Tubes in the Gastrointestinal Tract

Tubes in the gastrointestinal tract are generally used for feeding or bowel decompression. Complications are due to trauma or the stress of the procedure, and are listed in Table 11-8. Most of the complications can be reduced by good technique, including careful fixation of the tube.[81] Perforation has been reported with both PVC and silicone tubes.[27,82] The risk with PVC tubes may be higher because they become hardened after insertion. Infants of less than 1500 g weight are considered to be at increased risk.[76] Prolonged tube placement increases the risk of facial scarring from the strapping required to hold the tube in place. Perforation by a tube should be considered when pneumoperitoneum occurs, especially in the absence of other air-leak syndromes.

Complications of Arterial and Venous Lines

Intervention in the form of placement of a vascular line is one of the most common procedures performed on the sick newborn. As recently as 1980, 85 percent of neonates admitted to one NICU had at least one umbilical vessel catheterized, and

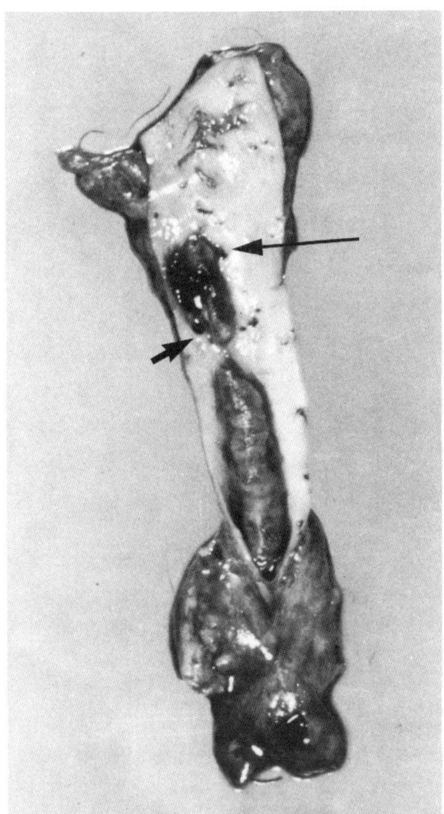

Fig. 11.11. Thombus in abdominal aorta. An umbilical artery catheter was inserted at birth because of severe asphyxia in this full-term infant who lived for 21 days. The thrombus partially occludes the abdominal aorta, and extends into the celiac (long arrow) and renal (short arrow) arteries.

it is estimated that house staff spend 10 percent of their time inserting vascular lines.[83] The major complications are trauma, infection, and thromboemboli (Figs. 11-11 and 11-12). In Table 11-8, a list of complications is presented. It is divided into those common to all lines and those more specific to particular lines. Thromobosis is a significant and frequent complication of any foreign object in the vessel lumen, damage to the endothelium being the major thrombogenic factor.[84] Silastic catheters were considered to cause thrombosis less often than those made with PVC,[85] but recent evidence suggests that added radiopaque material may be a major thrombogenic factor.[86] Ultrasound localization of catheters may replace radiographic methods and thus eliminate the need for radiopaque material.[87] The risk of thrombosis is increased with end-hole catheters.[88]

Peripheral Intravenous Lines

The major complications of peripheral intravenous lines are infection, infiltration, inadvertent perforation of an artery, and those that result from poor placement or improper restraint. The latter can cause circulatory, tissue, and nerve injuries. Complications can be reduced by the elective rotation of infusion sites, but there have been conflicting reports on the role of line material. Batton et al.[89] found that Teflon catheters did not increase complications and could be kept in place longer, but two earlier studies showed a higher incidence of infection with Teflon

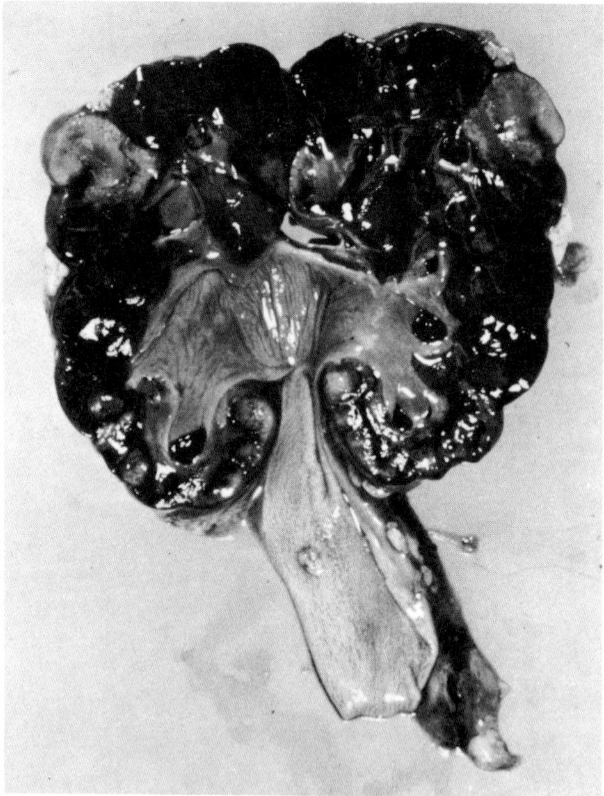

Fig. 11.12. Infarct of kidney. Multiple recent and old infarcts in this small and shrunken kidney resulted from the thrombus shown in Fig. 11.11. The renal artery was occluded by a thrombus. The patient had a history of hematuria and hypertension.

catheters as compared to traditional scalp vein needles.[90,91] Infiltration is an important complication and can be reduced by providing good visibility at the catheter placement site, frequent inspection for infiltration, and removing the line as soon as any infiltration is detected.[76] Damage is directly related to the toxicity of the infusate, the amount of infusate, and the time lag between injury and intervention. Upton and co-workers[92] have described the possible mechanisms of tissue injury. These include direct cytotoxicity, mechanical compression with or without compromise of local circulation, and secondary infection. Dextrose, calcium, and vasopressors cause skin sloughs and full thickness tissue necrosis.[76] Any disruption of skin integrity will predispose to infection.

Chandavasu et al.[93] have suggested multiple skin punctures as a means of reducing the incidence of post-infiltration skin sloughs and tissue necrosis. In an NICU with a yearly census of 1,411 patients, they reduced the incidence of these complications from 3 per week to zero by introducing this technique. They defend their technique by pointing out that hyaluronidase does not eliminate the damaging fluid that has infiltrated, and permits only limited dispersement, while steroids may cause atrophy of subcutaneous fat. Multiple skin punctures increase the pain inflicted on the neonate and carry the risk of infection, since the skin integrity is repeatedly broken. However, sloughing due to necrosis from the infusate is more likely to result in infection and the need for skin grafting.

Peripheral Arterial Lines

The arteries most often used when the umbilical route is not possible include the radial, posterior tibial, and dorsalis pedis. The major risk of catheters in such vessels is ischemia secondary to vasospasm, embolus, or thrombosis. Preventive measures include determining the adequacy of collateral circulation before catheter placement and testing distal perfusion of the limb after catheter insertion.[76] Immediate removal is indicated if ischemia is not relieved. Thrombosis occurs later and its incidence may be reduced by using heparinized catheters (in the wall).[94,95] Heparin infusion may prolong lumen patency,[96,97] but the impact of this technique on thrombosis has not been established,[97,98] and there is some danger of overdosage and the development of a bleeding disorder.[96,99] Hemorrhage is a particular danger with arterial lines, either from perforation of the vessel wall or human error in managing the line or stopcock. Peripheral nerve injury has also been reported.[100]

Central Venous Lines

The frequent need to provide parenteral nutrition for the sick neonate necessitates the insertion of catheters into major veins such as the subclavian and internal jugular. Complications of such central venous lines include insertion failure in 2 to 41 percent of cases, insertion complication in 0 to 41 percent (trauma), and complications after insertion in 0 to 11 percent.[101] Infection is the major problem[102,103]; the risk is increased when pressure transducers are added to the line.[104] Particular attention should be paid to asepsis at insertion and whenever the line is handled,[105] and to infection surveillance. MacDonald and Chou suggest removal of the catheter in culture-proven blood infection,[76] although others have attempted to treat bacteremia with the infusion of antibiotics.[106,107] This latter approach is as yet of unproven value in [neonates who] are particularly susceptible to overwhelming sepsis. MacDonald and Chou have found that treatment of Gram-positive infections, particularly those caused by "Staphylococcus epidermidis" and fungal infections, is unsuccessful with a line in place.[76] We have seen an infant at autopsy at Magee-Womens Hospital with *Candida albicans* sepsis who had a *Candida* thrombus at the catheter tip and migration of this infection along the superior vena cava; the infection destroyed the sinoatrial node in the right atrium, causing cardiac arrythmia (Macpherson, TA: unpublished observations) (Fig. 11-13). Hemorrhage, malposition, and infiltration of infusates are of particular concern with central venous lines. Malposition can cause cardiac arrythmias,[108] while internal bleeding and extravasation of fluid are not easily recognized; diagnosis requires a high index of suspicion. Complications of these lines are more common (72 percent versus 22 percent) and more serious when the line is not optimally situated in the distal superior vena cava (SVC).[109] Thrombosis and emboli are more likely when the catheter tip is in a vein smaller than the SVC. Other, rare complications include perforation of the SVC[110] or heart, causing cardiac tamponade, and perforation into the pleural cavity, causing pleural effusion.[109] Complications of central venous lines can be reduced if their use is restricted to parenteral feeding, thereby reducing the number of times the line is invaded.[76]

Central venous catheter placement via peripheral vessels has been used with some success.[111,112] Its complications have ranged from a frequency of 18 to 26 percent and include occlusion, thrombosis, dislodgement, and failure to insert the

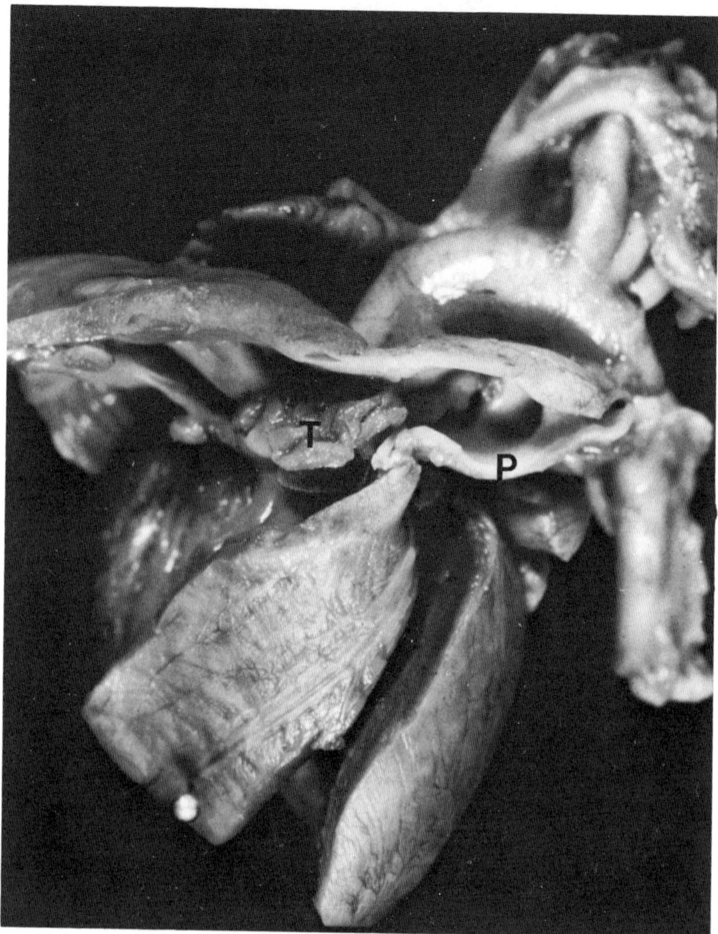

Fig. 11.13. Thromboemboli in right ventricle and main pulmonary artery. This 2-month-old infant was born at 23 weeks gestation and received parenteral nutrition through a jugular-superior vena cava catheter. At autopsy, as shown in the figure, an organized thromboembolus (T), which originated from a superior vena cava thrombus, is adherent to the right ventricular outflow tract and pulmonary artery (P). *Candida albicans* was found in the thrombus in the superior vena cava. Multiple thromboemboli were present in the pulmonary arteries and lungs.

line. The percutaeous route is claimed to be a safe and effective means of providing prolonged parenteral nutrition, particularly for the low-birthweight infant.[111,112] Complications of percutaneous central line insertion in the femoral vein include arterial perforation (14 percent incidence), swelling of the leg or thrombosis (11 percent), and an insertion failure rate of 14 percent.[101]

Umbilical Venous Lines

The value of accurate data on complications of umbilical vein catheterization (UVC) in newborns is well demonstrated by studies done several years ago, when endothelial damage, phlebitis, thrombosis, hepatic necrosis, hepatic abscess, hemorrhage, and sepsis were documented as such complications.[113–117] Publication of the data led to reduction in the use of such lines; their current use is now restricted to exchange transfusion, central venous pressure monitoring, and emergency vascular access when umbilical artery or peripheral vessel access are not possible.[76] Schmidt and Zipursky maintain that no accurate conclusions can be drawn about the incidence of thrombosis from previous reports, since variables such as catheter placement and infusates have not always been taken into account.[118] The complication rates are higher when catheter placement is not beyond the ductus venosus.[119,120]

There is some disagreement over the reasons for thrombosis from umbilical vein catheters. Larroche concluded that neither the caliber of the catheter nor the type of infusate were significant, but rather that duration of catheterization was the critical factor.[114] Campbell considered the size of the infant, the size of the catheter, the type of catheter, the person performing the catheterization, the infusate, the catheter location, and the duration of catheterization to be important.[121] The safest location is thought to be the thoracic portion of the inferior vena cava.[2] Complications are higher when the portal, mesenteric, splenic, or intrahepatic veins are inadvertently catheterized. Accidental transcardiac catheterization of pulmonary vessels has also occurred.[2,76] Krauss and co-workers found positive catheter cultures in over 50 percent of umbilical vein catheters.[122] Liver damage can be reduced if catheter position is confirmed prior to infusion, except in emergencies, when vital infusates can be given slowly via the umbilical vein.[123]

Complications of UVC can be reduced by limiting the indications for and duration of its use, and by close attention to placement and management techniques.[123] The line should be removed promptly when strict indications for its use no longer remain.[76]

Umbilical Artery Lines

Although umbilical artery catheterization (UAC) has fewer complications than UVC, the complications of UAC are important and potentially fatal. Umbilical artery catheter lines are used most frequently for monitoring blood gases and mean arterial pressure in the newborn, but peripheral lines are sometimes necessary when there are contraindicators to the use of UAC, such as necrotizing enterocolitis, omphalocele, omphalitis, peritonitis, and vascular insufficiency of the lower limbs or buttock.[76] Many of the complications of UAC follow thrombus formation.[119] Vascular complications include renal artery thrombosis, visceral infarction, intestinal ischemia, limb ischemia, and total aortic thrombosis. Consequences of these complications include organ failure, hypertension secondary to renal artery occlusion,[124,125] loss of an extremity,[126] neurologic deficits,[127] and even death due to congestive cardiac failure when the aorta is occluded.[128]

As with a UVC, the exact causes for thrombosis with UAC are not known. Placement of umbilical artery catheters is more difficult than that of umbilical vein catheters, thus increasing the likelihood of damage to the intima. Once in place, a large catheter may cause changes in blood flow dynamics, predisposing the vessel to intimal injury.[119] There does not appear to be any consensus on whether high (thoracic aorta at T6 to T10) and low (just above the aortic bifurcation) catheter tip positions carry different risks of thrombosis. Positioning the catheter between these two locations puts the catheter tip near the visceral branches of the GIT and kidney, and does increase the risk of infarction of these organs.

The incidence of thrombosis in UAC depends on the criteria used for diagnosis. Schmidt and Zipursky indicate that aortography will demonstrate UAC-associated thrombosis in 20 to 95 percent of cases; autopsy studies show it in 3 to 56 percent of cases.[118] In another review, the incidence is 1.5 to 38 percent, based on clinical signs of ischemia; 12.5 to 62.5 percent at autopsy; and 24 to 92 percent by contrast studies.[129] Ultrasound techniques will provide more accurate and less invasive means of determining the incidence of UAC-associated thrombosis in the future.

Thrombosis is common in newborns and is not caused by catheters alone; there is a high incidence of spontaneous thrombosis in neonates. Thrombocytopenia has been associated with thrombosis in cases of intravascular catheterization, and may even suggest that in a given patient thrombosis has occurred.[130] In one report, thrombocytopenia was associated with the use of an umbilical artery catheter in 62 percent of cases.[131]

Perforation of an umbilical artery with subsequent perivascular, perivesicular, and intraperitoneal hemorrhage is a potentially life-threatening complication.[132] This complication is more common when difficulty is experienced at the time of insertion. MacDonald and Chou[76] maintain that "many instances of failure to pass a catheter more than a few centimeters are really perivascular dissections with perforation occurring close to the base of the umbilicus." Vessel perforation has also caused bladder injury with the development of uroascites.[133,134] A false abdominal aortic aneurysm was produced by an umbilical artery catheter that was used for an exchange transfusion.[135] As with UVC, infection is a complication of UAC,[122] but the consequences appear to be less serious than those of thrombosis. A few cases of umbilical artery catheter breakage have been reported.[136] We recently had an episode in the nursery in which the catheter was inadvertently cut during manipulation, with migration along the umbilical artery (McPherson TA: unpublished observation).

Vasospasm induced by catheter insertion is an important complication of this procedure. Tolazoline infusion has been used to successfully treat vasospasm due to catheter placement.[137] This drug is employed for the treatment of persistent pulmonary hypertension in the newborn (PPHN); complications of its use include hypotension, altered renal function, gastrointestinal distention, and hemorrhage.[138] However, the complications are dose-related, and are reported as being 30 percent for a 1 to 2 mg/kg/hour dose and 82 percent for a 10 mg/kg/hour dose.[137] Since the dose use for treating vasospasm is much lower than that needed for PPHN, complications in this context are likely to be rare.

Umbilical artery catheter lines often need to be removed because they become occluded. Bosque and Weaver[99] found that umbilical artery catheter occlusion was less frequent with the use of continuous heparin infusion (0 of 18 cases) than with intermittent infusion (8 of 29 cases). Bleeding was not a problem in the continuous infusion group despite the fact that the dosage was 30 times that with the intermittent infusion. Although up to 220 U/kg/day of heparin were given to the continuous infusion group, this was still well below the 576 U/kg/day necessary for heparinization.[99]

It is unlikely that all complications of tubes and lines will be eliminated. However, many may be avoided if those persons inserting them are properly trained, select the best materials, are aware of the potential hazards, prepare the baby adequately, are compulsive in their attention to detail of technique, manage the catheters with care after insertion, and remove them as soon as complications occur or when the tubes are no longer indicated.

Other Complications Involving Vessels

Beyond their use for the insertion of vascular lines, blood vessels are subjected to multiple punctures for blood sampling. Arteriovenous fistulas followed multiple arterial punctures in one neonate who had 90 arterial blood gas determinations over a 13-week period.[139] When a catheter is being placed in a vein, an adjacent artery may be inadvertently damaged. Digital ischemia has resulted when intravenous cannulation inadvertently damaged a neighboring artery.[83] In two cases, amputation of portions of a finger or thumb resulted. This complication can be avoided if the operator knows the vascular anatomy of the area used. It is necessary to instruct the house staff carefully in these techniques, since it is reported that they spend 10 percent of their time inserting lines.[83] This is particularly important because, with prolonged hospitalization, complications arise when more proximal or secondary distal sites are used.[140]

Catheters are often used to inject agents into the circulation. Ultrasound has demonstrated that retrograde blood flow causes a rise in blood pressure at distant sites.[141] Radial artery flush has been shown to cause blood pressure elevations in the aortic arch and common iliac artery that correlate with the volume and velocity of the flush. Butt et al.[141] recommended that small volumes of 0.5 ml be injected over periods of 5 seconds each to reduce the likelihood of microembolization and hypertensive insults that could play a role in the pathogenesis of intraventricular hemorrhage, ischemic cerebral injury, and necrotizing enterocolitis.[141]

RETINOPATHY OF PREMATURITY

According to Biglan and co-workers, "retinopathy of prematurity (ROP) is a condition characterized by abnormalities in development of the capillary network that overlies the nascent retina in premature infants. These abnormalities include vascular congestion, dilatation, tortuosity, arteriovenous shunting, and in advanced stages, incursion of fibrovascular tissue into the vitreous cavity. In the most severe forms, detachment of the neurosensory retina will occur, and this may result in blindness."[142] Perhaps more than any other complication of the newborn, ROP exemplifies the dilemma of the neonatologist: that of a serious complication whose cause is probably related to unavoidable intervention in a sick, premature neonate. In this case the unavoidable treatment is oxygen exposure, and the unknown risk of ROP with the possibility of total blindness. Besides this, ROP is an example of the consequence of a premature assumption about the cause of a particular neonatal complication. The acceptance of oxygen as the sole cause of ROP resulted in harmful changes in clinical practice, and inappropriate litigation.[143] A positive outcome of these and other serious neonatal misadventures is that enthusiasm and resources have been generated to establish collaborative studies to address these issues.

Currrently, ROP refers to the acute vascular abnormalities of the developing

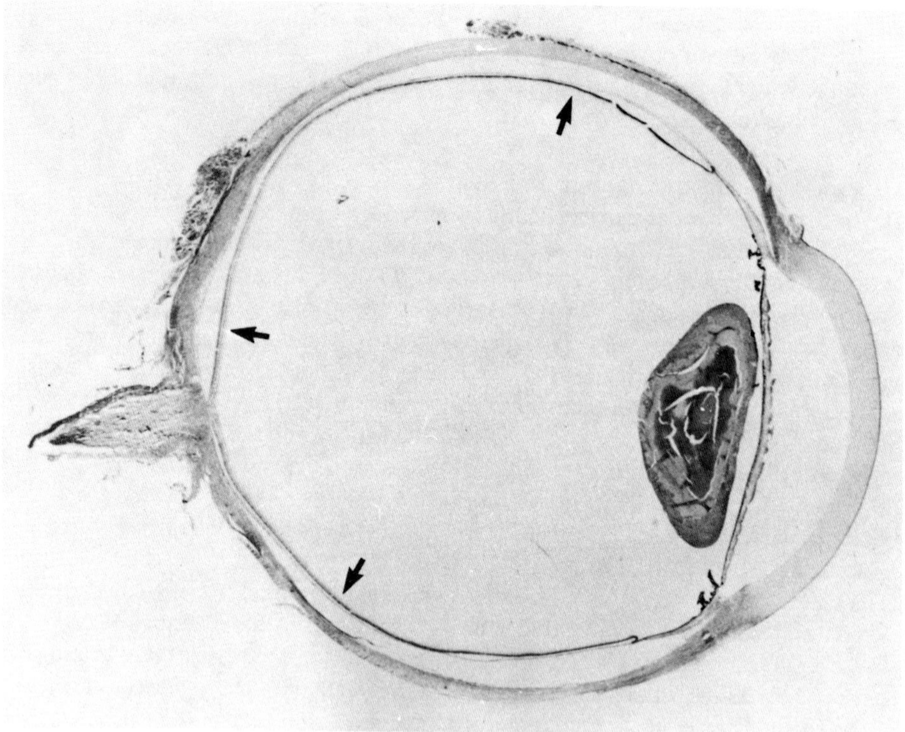

Fig. 11.14. Whole mount of section of an eye with normal retina (arrows).

retinal circulation that are seen during the first 3 or 4 months of age, while retrolental fibroplasia (RFP) refers to a later cicatricial phase observed in the retina and overlying vitreous humor after the more acute phases of ROP subside[142] (Figs. 11-14 & Fig. 11-15). The development of the retinal circulation is completed only at term (nasal aspect) and shortly thereafter (temporal aspect); this late completion is a probable reason why the immature retina is susceptible to ROP and RFP.

Although the precise prevalence of ROP is unknown, Phelps[144] has estimated that its most serious consequence, blindness, develops in at least 500 infants annually in the United States. The prevalence of proliferative disease ranges from 7.5 percent[145] to 1.9 percent at Magee-Womens Hospital.[142] Purohit et al.[146] found RFP in 43 percent of infants of 500 to 749 g birthweight, and 3 percent of those whose birthweight was 1500 to 1750 g. Such comparisons are difficult, since, until recently, there was no uniform system of classification[147] nor any established regimen for patient selection.[148] The ROP collaborative study should provide more accurate information about the prevalence of ROP.

There has been much disagreement about the factors associated with the development of ROP. Biglan and co-workers[142] have tabulated the factors associated with the occurrence of ROP. These factors include low birthweight, oxygen exposure, assisted ventilation, hypercarbia, apnea, sepsis, light exposure, seizures, ACTH, vitamin E, intraventricular hemorrhage, patent ductus arteriosus, indomethacin, blood transfusion, xanthine administration, and maternal bleeding. In

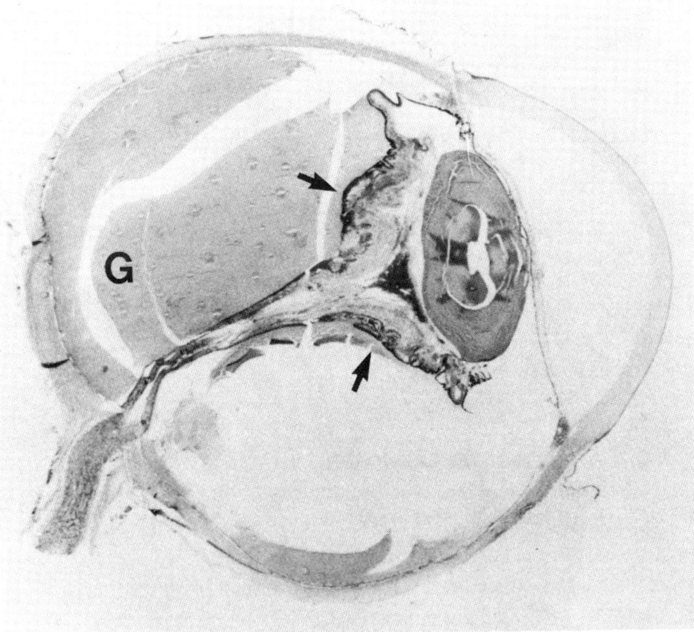

Fig. 11.15. Whole mount of section of eye with RFP. The retina (arrows) is completely detached from the sclera and forms a fibrovascular membrane adherent to the posterior surface of the lens. Gelatinous eosinophilic material (G) occupies the space between the detached retina and sclera.

almost every instance, they list references that both support and refute an association with the various risk factors listed above. Purohit et al.[146] considered maternal diabetes mellitus and antihistamine exposure in the last 2 weeks of pregnancy to be important risk factors for the development of ROP. Although "prematurity and oxygen exposure are the only two factors to have been repeatedly and convincingly demonstrated to be of significance in the pathogenesis of ROP,"[142] ROP has been reported in full-term infants who were not given supplemental oxygen,[149] in the absence of supplemental oxygen,[150] and in anoxic children.[151] In addition, ROP has not always appeared in instances in which infants have been exposed to oxygen for long periods of time.[142] Lucy and Dangman[152] have published an excellent review of the role of oxygen as a risk factor for ROP. The role of light, previously considered to be important, no longer has strong support as a risk factor.[153]

Abundant controversy has also surrounded attempts to prevent the development of ROP. Vitamin E has been the principal actor in this regard, following the claim that vitamin E administration reduced the incidence of RLF.[154] Concerns over study design defects in this and subsequent studies,[142] plus reports of complications of vitamin E treatment,[155–157] leave the role of vitamin E in the prevention of ROP unclear.[142] A list of the adverse effects of vitamin E is given in Table 11-9.[155–159] The American Academy of Pediatrics has not recommended the use of vitamin E for, the prevention of ROP.[160]

The treatment of ROP is also controversial. Since 90 percent of the acute forms of ROP regress,[161] the impact of cryotherapy is difficult to assess. Since large

Table 11-9. Adverse Effects of Vitamin E

Cretinuria
Decreased wound bleeding
Impaired fibrinolysis
Platelet aggregation
Decrease in coagulation factors associated with Vitamin K deficiency
Necrotizing enterocolitis
Intracranial hemorrhage
Hepatomegaly (in kittens)
Mortality (in kittens)
Soft tissue irritation/calcification at injection site
Anti-inflammatory activity
Ascites/hepatomegaly/thrombocytopenia syndrome from dl-Alpha Tocopheryl Acetate (IV)

(Data compiled from refs. 155 to 159.)

numbers of centers are currently evaluating cryotherapy as part of the treatment of ROP in a large collaborative study, the answer about this form of therapy should be forthcoming, including its as yet undetermined risks. Even more uncertain is the treatment of detached retina by surgical reattachment, a procedure now being performed with limited success in the United States.[162–165] The procedure is difficult and associated with complications such as redetachment of the retina, glaucoma, corneal opacification, and phthisis bulbae. Furthermore, the best result may be limited to light perception.[142]

Thus, it is fortunate that most forms of ROP will regress spontaneously, with only 10 percent of patients developing some form of cicatricial RFP.[166] Other complications include strabismus, refractive errors, decreased vision due to optic atrophy,[167] glaucoma, amblyopia, pseudostrabismus, and late retinal detachment.[168–169]

There is still much to be learned about ROP. "If any impact is to be made on reducing ROP as a complication of perinatal care," stated Biglan et al., "the following needs to occur: (1) the risk factors need to be clarified, (2) the angiogenic substance involved in normal and abnormal vascularization of the retina needs to be identified, (3) the incidence of prematurity needs to be reduced, (4) the value of preventive medications such as vitamin E need to be defined, and (5) the value of cryotherapy and surgical reattachment of the retina need to be established."[142]

TOTAL PARENTERAL NUTRITION

The complications of total parenteral nutrition (TPN) are a consequence of the infusate and of the line inserted to deliver the parenteral nutrition. Line complications have already been described in the section on the complications of central venous lines. Total parenteral nutrition was originally instituted to provide nutritional support for infants with surgically treatable gastrointestinal disorders but who were unable to take enteric feedings. It was then extended to use in sick, preterm infants whose nutritional needs could not be met by other means.

Gutcher and Cutz[170] have summarized the major reasons why complications occur with TPN. They cite a variety of reasons, including:

1. Incomplete knowledge about nutritional requirements in premature or ill neonates.

2. The possible inappropriateness of reference standards based on growth patterns in the fetus or healthy term infant for an infant who is premature or critically ill.

3. The possible inability of an infant to process nutrients administered in quantities appropriate for the infant's size.

4. Inadequacy of the monitoring tools for both acute and long-term effects of parenteral nutrition.

Table 11-10. Complications of Parenteral Nutrition

- Liver
  - Cholestasis
  - Fatty liver
  - "Hepatitis"
  - Cirrhosis
  - Hepatocellular carcinoma
- Cholelithiasis
- Choledocholithiasis
- Lung
  - Lipid emboli
  - Endothelial cell lipid
  - Lipid in alveolar macrophages
  - Malassezia furfur vasculitis
- Gallbladder
  - Distention
- Metabolic Deficiency
  - Vitamin D (1–3 months)
    - Rickets
  - Vitamin A
    - (?)Increased incidence of RDS and BPD
  - Copper (late: 6–8 months)
    - Sideroblastic anemia
    - Neutropenia
    - Depigmentation
    - Copper (late: 6–8 months)
    - Functional CNS defects
    - Bone defects
  - Phosphate
    - Bone changes
  - Zinc
    - Dermatitis
  - Taurine
    - Retinal changes
  - Vitamin C
    - Decreased conversion of tyrosine to phenyl
  - Vitamin E (see separate table)
  - Glucose
    - Hypoglycemia
- Metabolic excess
  - Vitamin A
    - Hypervitaminosis A
  - Calcium
    - Hypercalciuria
      - Renal calculi
  - Bone demineralization
    - Rickets
  - Glucose
    - Hyperglycemia
      - Osmotic diuresis
      - Dehydration
      - Azotomia
  - Amino acids
    - Hyperammonemia
    - Hyperosmolar coma
    - Mental retardation
- Tyrosine
  - Intellectual deficit
- Hyperchloremic acidosis
- Liver pathology (early: less than 30 days)
  - Centrilobular cholestasis
  - Pseudoacinar and giant cell transformation of hepatocytes
  - Increased EMH
  - Mild portal inflammation
  - Fibrosis
  - Patchy hepatic necrosis with eosinophilic bodies
  - Kupffer cells with foamy cytoplasm
- Liver pathology (mid: past 30 days)
  - Greater cholestasis
  - Cholangiolar/bile duct proliferation
  - Increased fibrosis
  - Increased periportal inflammation
- Liver pathology (late: past 60 days)
  - Micronodular cirrhosis (biliary type)
  - Severe cholestasis
  - Marked ductular proliferation
  - Excessive bile plugging in ductules and hepatocytes
  - Portal and pericellular fibrosis
  - (?)Hepatocellular carcinoma (1 case reported)

(Data compiled from refs. 170 to 173.)

5. Toxic effects of TPN on multiple organ systems, the causes of many of which remain unknown.

6. A narrow margin between deficiency and toxicity for some nutritional component of TPN.

7. The many steps in ordering, preparing, and administering TPN in which human and technical errors can occur.

There have been several recent reviews of TPN,[170–173] the complications of which have been summarized in part in Table 11-10 and will not be discussed further. In addition, Gutcher and Cutz[170] have listed the indications for parenteral nutrition and the consequences of giving intravenous fat (with supporting references). The complications of intravenous fat that they list include apparent hyperbilirubinemia, apparent hyponatremia, substitution of plant phytosterols in the developing central nervous system, abnormal platelet function, vasculitis secondary to "Malassezia furfur," hyperglycemia, abnormal plasma lipoprotein (lipoprotein X), impaired cellular immune function, and carnitine deficiency.

COMPLICATIONS OF EXCHANGE TRANSFUSION

Rapid removal and replacement of large aliquots of blood in a small infant may cause rapid shifts in blood pressure and cardiac output.[174] Keenan et al.[175] reported serious morbidity in 5.2 percent of exchange transfusions, including seven cases with apnea/bradycardia requiring intervention. There was one exchange transfusion associated with death among 190 infants given 331 exchanges. Hypoglycemia occurs because of hyperinsulinemia resulting from an increase in plasma glucose, which is induced by the rapid infusion of blood with citrate-phosphate-dextrose (CDP).[176] The transfusion of old blood cells may cause hyperkalemia because of leakage of potassium from red cells older than 1 week. Hyperkalemia increases the risk of cardiac arrythmias during the procedure. Old blood (more than 5 days) is deficient in 2,3-DPG and causes increased levels of heme pigments in the plasma, resulting in competition for albumin-binding sites.[174] The many other risks of exchange transfusion are listed in Table 11-11. The incidence of complications is low (1 to 2 percent),[177] and the most common ones are those that are readily recognized and easily treated, being metabolic in nature.[174] Thrombocytopenia can result from multiple exchange transfusions as a result of the dilutional effect[178]; this procedure is the cause of 20 percent of cases of neonatal thrombocytopenia.[179] Normalization of the platelet count may take 7 days.[180] Lang and Valrei[181] have reviewed the additional hazards of blood transfusion.

Post-transfusion viral infection is of more recent concern. Cytomegalovirus (CMV) infection has been reported in 9 to 13 percent of cases with conventional blood and 11 percent with saline-washed red blood cell transfusions.[182] Yeager et al.[183] found that donors with CMV indirect hemagglutination titers above 1:8 transmitted CMV in 13.5 percent of cases, while no transmission occurred when the titer was below 1:8. They also found that the mortality rate associated with CMV was 40 percent, whereas that expected was 6.6 percent. The use of frozen-thawed-washed red blood cells (FTW-RBC)[184] or leukocyte-poor blood[185] can re-

Table 11-11. Complications of Exchange Transfusion

Hypocalcemia
Hypoglycemia
Acidosis
Hyperkalemia
Air embolism
Thromboembolism
Post-transfusion infection
Hepatitis
CMV
AIDS
Septicemia
Hypothermia
Hyperthermia
Thrombocytopenia
Leukopenia
Heparin overload
Deficiency of coagulation factors (V and VIII)
Mortality
Complications related to UVC
Vessel perforation
Portal vein thrombosis
Hyperviscosity
Fluid overload
Graft-versus-host disease
Intraventricular hemorrhage
Necrotizing enterocolitis with bowel perforation
Transfusion reaction

(Data compiled from refs. 174–190.)

duce the risk of CMV transmission. Blood with FTW-RBC contains virtually no plasma, leukocytes, or platelets. The major barrier to transfusing CMV-free blood is that 40 to 100 percent of donors have complement-fixing antibodies against CMV.[186]

There is some concern that immunologic risks such as graft-versus-host disease (GVHD) are associated with exchange transfusions.[187,188] The risk is small, especially if irradiated blood is used.[189] Follow-up of infants who have received granulocyte transfusions has failed to reveal either abnormalities in their immunologic profile or the development of alloantibodies.[190] Other possible complications of granulocyte transfusion include transmission of infectious agents such as hepatitis and CMV, leukocyte aggregation, and pulmonary sequestration of white blood cells[187] (see also Ch. 11).

COMPLICATIONS OF BLOOD SAMPLING

"In practical terms, the removal of 1 ml of blood from a 1 kg infant is equivalent to removing 70 ml of blood from an average adult," observe Blanchette and Zipursky, adding that it is therefore not suprising that "repeated blood sampling, even using capillary samples, can have a profound effect on the hemoglobin concentration of small, premature infants."[191] They further state that blood sampling is the "commonest cause of anemia in premature infants." While most NICUs keep track of blood volumes withdrawn for laboratory testing, Bell et al.[191,192]

have shown that significant blood loss is related to blood on swabs and within non-gradated portions of syringes and tubing. Blanchette and Zipursky calculated that iatrogenic blood loss in their study was 26.9 + 9 ml in "ill" premature infants and 14.6 + 5 ml in "healthy" ones.[191] They indicate that these figures must be interpreted in light of the fact that the premature infant has a total red cell mass of 32.3 to 45.5 mg/kg. Complications such as oozing after venipuncture or arterial puncture, local hematoma, and infection can also occur.

COMPLICATIONS OF DRUG ADMINISTRATION

A full review of drug complications is beyond the scope of this work. Excellent reviews on maternal and fetal drug-related problems have been published elsewhere.[1,5,171] When one considers the frequency with which drugs are administered to the neonate, it is surprising that complications are not more common! Aranda et al.[193] have found that 76.1 percent of neonates receive from 1 to 26 different drugs, with 6.19 + 5.73 drugs per infant and 30 to 63 doses per infant. Among 4,305 administrations, 58.5 percent were given intravenously, 10.1 percent orally, and 9.8 percent intramuscularly. In 15.9 percent of instances, missed medications or errors were made, as judged from the ordered drug regimen. Twenty different drugs accounted for 10 percent of the drugs given, while 8 drugs made up more than 24 percent of the volume.[193] The complexity of drug administration in the newborn has resulted in computation errors in 8 percent of cases, according to Perstein et al.,[194] with many errors being as great as a factor of 10; they recommend that all personnel who make drug computations be tested regularly for computational skills and knowledge of appropriate dosage for age. Koren and coworkers[195] also found tenfold errors when drugs were prepared on the unit. This error rate was reduced by having pharmacists prepare the drugs. The aforementioned drug-related complications can be corrected more easily than the myriad of effects that follow inappropriate drug administration in the neonate.

REDUCING IATROGENIC COMPLICATIONS IN THE NEWBORN

Fletcher and Macpherson[143] have suggested six areas in which attention may reduce the numbers of perinatal complications: (1) recognition, (2) communication, (3) supervision, (4) documentation, (5) long-term follow-up, and (6) research. The first step in reducing iatrogenic complications is the recognition that complications can occur, and awareness of the variety of complications that can result from a given intervention, whether it be diagnostic or therapeutic. This awareness will modify the decision to intervene in the first place, and increase diligence in management when intervention is clearly indicated. This is of particular importance in common tasks that are part of the placement and care of tubes and lines.[76] Vigilance tends to be lower in routine or minor procedures, especially those not requiring specific consent.[143] Recognition must extend beyond NICU personnel to include support personnel, radiology technicians, phlebotomists, monitoring personnel, pharmacists, and engineers responsible for equipment maintenance.

Recognition of new complications is an essential part of progress in neonatal care, and in this regard the autopsy is essential. The role of the anatomic pathologist has been described[196,197] and includes the important function of auditor.[198,199] The fear of litigation should not lessen efforts to get autopsy consent, since medical honesty in identifying new complications is essential to optimal patient care.[143]

Communication can take several forms, ranging from personal discussion among colleagues to publication in referenced journals. Communication beyond one's close colleagues is generally in the form of scientific meetings, abstracts, and publications. These carry a significant delay that could be avoided if other, more rapid means of communication existed, such as a regular newsletter on iatrogenic complications.

Supervision is necessary, and this must be provided not only in the care of the living neonate for interventions such as drug administration and the insertion of vascular lines, but also in the recognition of complications at autopsy.[196] The opportunity for recognition should extend beyond the nursery to the discharged infant. This is particularly so in the compromised neonate who will be attended by several different physicians. The neonatologist has a responsibility for long term follow-up.[200]

It is in the area of research that much still needs to be done. Klebanoff and Rhoads[201] have indicated that the perinatal period is most suited from an epidemiologic perspective for collaborative studies. They suggest that such studies could take several forms, such as: (1) a central clearing house for communications—an effective extension of the "letter to the editor," without the inevitable delays that accompany these letters, (2) surveys of suspected complications initiated by member institutions, and (3) ecological studies generated in part from responses to the surveys named in point 2. They maintain that if items 1 or 2 in this list were in operation in the form of a collaborative group, the recognition of complications such as benzyl alcohol toxicity might have been expedited.

In 1984, the Study Group for Complications of Perinatal Care (SGCPC) was formed in Pittsburgh, with funding support raised by Magee-Womens Hospital. The SGCPC is an international, multicenter, multidisciplinary study group committed to prevention of the complications of perinatal care by individual and collective effort. Its activities to date have included the development of a standardized perinatal autopsy protocol and initiating the development of a uniform system for the categorization of perinatal deaths. Both of these projects are scheduled for completion by December 1987. In early 1987, the SGCPC will conduct several surveys as a first step toward collaborative ecological studies. An annual scientific meeting has already been initiated. Membership is open to all disciplines, and further information on institutional and individual membership can be obtained by writing to:

SGCPC
c/o Trevor Macpherson, M.D.
Magee-Womens Hospital
Department of Pathology
Forbes Avenue and Halket Streets
Pittsburgh, PA 15213
(412) 647-4654

CONCLUSION

According to Klebanoff and Rhoads,[201] "perinatology is a fertile field for collaborative epidemiologic research; all major types of epidemiologic studies can be carried out with less difficulty than in some other subject areas. The relatively short duration of pregnancy, the fact that the large majority of women report for prenatal care and deliver in a hospital, and the acute nature and duration of many perinatal and neonatal conditions can all contribute to the success of prospective studies and clinical trials. There is a need for a variety of cooperative research efforts. The National Institute of Child Health and Human Development has recently funded two cooperative interuniversity networks, one of seven maternal fetal medicine units and one of seven neonatal intensive care units. It is anticipated that each network will collaborate on a modest number of detailed protocols, most of which are likely to be randomized trials. It is clear from the initial steering committee meetings of these groups that they can address only a few of the many issues that need investigation. Other collaborative effects could be productively initiated to contribute to the knowledge base in this rapidly changing field."

REFERENCES

1. Valdes-Dapena M: Iatrogenic disease in the perinatal period as seen by the pathologist. p. 382. In Naeye RL, Kissane JM, Kaufman N (eds): Perinatal Diseases. Wiliams & Wilkins, Baltimore, 1981
2. Ablow RC: Complications of neonatal intensive care. p. 191. In Kassner EG (ed): Iatrogenic Disorders of the Fetus, Infant, and Child. Springer-Verlag, New York, 1985
3. Meyers MA: p vii. In Kassner EG (ed): Iatrogenic Disorders of the Fetus, Infant, and Child. Springer-Verlag, New York, 1985
4. Pepper OHP: Medical Etymology. W.B. Saunders, Philadelphia, 1954
5. Kassner EG, Haller JO: Iatrogenic disorders of the fetus. p. 81. In Kassner EG (ed): Iatrogenic Disorders of the Fetus, Infant, and Child. Springer-Verlag, New York, 1985
6. Kassner EG, Haller JO: Birth trauma, perinatal asphyxia, and iatrogenic respiratory distress. p. 125. In Kassner ED (ed): Iatrogenic Disorders of the Fetus, Infant, and Child. Springer-Verlag, New York, 1985
7. Kassner EG: p. ix. In Kassner EG (ed): Iatrogenic Disorders of the Fetus, Infant, and Child. Springer-Verlag, New York, 1985
8. Fox WW: Mechanical ventilation in the management of persistent pulmonary hypertension of the neonate (PPHN). p. 102. Proceedings of the 83rd Ross Conference on Cardiovascular Sequelae of Asphyxia in the Newborn, 1982
9. Perelman R: Reducing iatrogenic lung disease in the premature newborn. Semin Perinatol 10:217, 1986
10. Reid L, Rubino L: The connective tissue septa in the fetal human being. Thorax 14:3, 1959
11. Macklin MT, Macklin CC: Malignant interstitial emphysema of the lungs and mediastinum as an important occult complication in many respiratory diseases and other conditions: An interpretation of the clinical literature in the light of laboratory experiment. Medicine, 23:281, 1944
12. Caldwell EJ, Powell RD, Mullooly JP: Interstitial emphysema: A study of physiologic factors involved in the experimental induction of the lesion. Am Rev Respir Dis 102:516, 1970
13. Thibeault DW: Pulmonary barotrauma: interstitial emphysema, pneumomediastinum and pneumothorax. p. 307. In Thibeault DW, Gregory GA (eds): Neonatal Pulmonary Care. Addison-Wesley, Menlo Park, CA, 1979
14. Thibeault DW, Lachman RS, Laul VR, Kwong MS: Pulmonary interstitial emphysema, pneumomediastinum and pneumothorax. Am J Dis Child 126:611, 1973
15. Unal D, Perraud P, Tapounie E, et al: Iatrogenic gas effusions of iatrogenic origin in neonatal reamination. Ann Anesthesiol Fr 16:163, 1975
16. Plenat F, Vert P, Didier F, et al: Pulmonary interstitial emphysema. Clin Perinatol 5:351, 1978
17. Brewer LL, Moskowitz PS, Carrington CB, Bensch K: Pneumatosis pulmonalis. Am J Pathol 95:171, 1979

18. Wood BP, Anderson VM, Mauk JE, Merritt TA: Pulmonary lymphatic air: Locating "pulmonary interstitial emphysema" of the premature infant. Am J Roentgenol 138:809, 1982
19. Moskowitz PS, Bensch KG, Carrington CB: Pneumatosis pulmonalis. Pediatrics 68:612, 1981
20. Macklin CC: Transport of air along sheaths of pulmonic blood vessels from alveoli to mediastinum. Arch Intern Med 64:913, 1939
21. Anderson KD, Chandra R: Pneumothorax secondary to perforation of segmental bronchi by suction catheters. J Pediatr Surg 11:687, 1976
22. Pomerance JJ, Weller MH, Richardson CJ, et al: Pneumopericardium complicating respiratory distress syndrome: Role of conservative management. J Pediatr 84:883, 1974
23. Cimmino CV: Editorial. Some radio-diagnostic notes on pneumomediastinum, pneumothorax, and pneumopericardium. VA Med Monthly 94:205, 1973
24. Higgins CB, Broderick TW, Edwards DK, et al: The hemodynamic significance of massive pneumopericardium in preterm infants with respiratory distress syndrome. Clinical and experimental observations. Radiology 133:363, 1979
25. Grosfeld JL, Boger D, Clatworthy HW: Hemodynamic and manometric observations in experimental air-block syndrome. J Pediatr Surg 6:339, 1971
26. Siegel RL, Rabinowitz JG, Sarasohn C: Intestinal perforation secondary to nasojejunal feeding tubes. AJR 126:1229, 1976
27. McAlister WH, Siegel MJ, Shakelford GD, et al: Intestinal perforations by tube feedings in small infants. AJR 145:687, 1985
28. Stocker JT, Madewell JE: Persistent interstitial pulmonary emphysema: Another complication of the respiratory distress syndrome. Pediatrics 59:847, 1977
29. Stocker JT, Drake RM, Madewell JE: Cystic and congenital lung disease in the newborn. p. 93. In Rosenberg HS, Bolande RP (eds): Perspectives in Pediatric Pathology, Vol 4. Year Book Medical Publishers, Chicago, 1978
30. Glenski JA, Thibeault DW, Hall FK, Hall RT, et al: Selective bronchial intubation in infants with lobar emphysema. Am J Perinatol 3:199, 1986
31. Kogutt MS: Systemic air embolism secondary to respiratory therapy in the neonate: Six cases including one survivor. Am J Roentgenol 131:425, 1978
32. Vinstein AL, Gresham EL, Lim MO, et al: Pulmonary venous air embolism in hyaline membrane disease. Radiology 105:627, 1972
33. Northway WH, Rosan RC, Porter DB: Pulmonary disease following respiratory therapy. N Engl J Med 276:357, 1967
34. Philip AGS: Oxygen plus pressure plus time: The etiology of bronchopulmonary dysplasia. Pediatrics 55:44, 1975
35. Joshi VV, Mandavia SG, Stern L, et al: Acute lesions induced by endotracheal intubation: occurrence in the respiratory tract of newborn infants with respiratory distress syndrome. Am J Dis Child 124:646, 1972
36. Larson E: Pathology of chronic complications of neonatal ventilator therapy. p. 410. In Thibeault DW, Gregory GA (eds): Neonatal Pulmonary Care. Addison-Wesley, Menlo Park, CA, 1979
37. Wigglesworth JS: The respiratory system. p. 168. In Wigglesworth (ed): Perinatal Pathology. W.B. Saunders, Philadelphia, 1984
38. Banerjee CK, Girling DJ, Wigglesworth JS: Pulmonary fibroplasia in newborn babies treated with oxygen and artificial ventilation. Arch Dis Child 47:509, 1972
39. Boat TF, Lleinerman JI, Fanaroff AA, et al: Toxic effects of oxygen on cultured human neonatal respiratory epithelium. Pediatr Res 7:607, 1973
40. Taghizadeh A, Reynolds EOR: Pathogenesis of bronchopulmonary dysplasia following hyaline membrane disease. Am J Pathol 82:241, 1976
41. Mayes L, Perkett E, Stahlman MT: Severe bronchopulmonary dysplasia: A retrospective review. Acta Pediatr Scand 72:225, 1983
42. Ehrenkranz RA, Ablow RC, Warshaw JB: Oxygen toxicity. The complication of oxygen use in the newborn infant. Clin Perinatol 5:437, 1978
43. Hansen TN, Gest AL: Oxygen toxicity and other ventilatory complications of treatment of infants with persistent pulmonary hypertension. Clin Perinatol 11:653, 1984
44. Weibel ER: Oxygen effect on lung cells. Arch Intern Med 128:54, 1971
45. Anderson, WR, Strickland MB, Tsai SH, et al: Light microscope and ultrastructural study of the adverse effects of oxygen therapy on the neonate lung. Am J Pathol 73:327, 1973
46. Clark JM, Lambertsen CJ: Pulmonary oxygen toxicity: A review. Pharmacol Rev 23:37, 1971
47. McCord JM: Oxygen radicals and lung injury. The state of the art. Chest 83:35S, 1983
48. Merritt TA, Puccia JM, Stuard ID: Cytologic evaluation of pulmonary effluent in neonates with respiratory distress syndrome and bronchopulmonary dysplasia. Acta Cytol 26:15, 1982

49. Doshi N, Kanbour A, Fujikura T, et al: Tracheal aspiration cytology in neonates with respiratory distress: Histopathological correlation. Acta Cytol 26:15, 1982
50. Metlay LA, Macpherson TA, Doshi N, Milley JR: A new iatrogenic lesion in newborns requiring assisted ventilation. N Engl J Med 309:111, 1983
51. Mimouni F, Ballard JL, Ballard ET, Cotton RT: Necrotizing tracheobronchitis: Case report. Pediatrics 77:366, 1986
52. Boros SJ, Mammel MC, Lewallen PK, et al: Necrotizing tracheobronchitis: A complication of high-frequency ventilation. J Pediatr 100:95, 1986
53. Ophoven JP, Mammel MC, Gorden MJ, et al: Tracheobronchial histopathology associated with high-frequency jet ventilation. Crit Care Med 12:829, 1984
54. Kirpalani H, Higa T, Terlman M, et al: Diagnosis and therapy of necrotizing tracheobronchitis in ventilated neonates. Crit Care Med 13:777, 1985
55. Doshi N, Klionsky B, Kanbour A: Yellow hyaline membrane disease in neonates: Clinical diagnosis by tracheal aspiration cytology. Pediatr Pathol 1:193, 1983
56. Garland JS, Nelson DB, Rice T, Neu J: Increased risk of gastrointestinal perforation in neonates mechanically ventilated with either face mask or nasal prongs. Pediatrics 76:406, 1985
57. Tsao FHC, Zachman RD: Prenatal assessment of fetal lung maturation: A critical review of amniotic fluid phospholipid tests. p. 167. In Farrell PM (ed): Lung Development: Biological and Clinical Perspectives, Vol. 2. Neonatal Respiratory Distress. Academic Press, Orlando, FL, 1982
58. Liggins GC: Premature delivery of fetal lungs infused with glucocorticoids. J Endocrinol 45:515, 1969
59. Kotas RV, Avery ME: The influence of sex on fetal rabbit lung maturation and on response to glucocorticoids. Am J Respir Dis 121:377, 1980
60. Papageorgiu AN: The prevention of respiratory distress syndrome: studies in enhancement of lung maturation. p. 233. In Stern L (ed): Hyaline Membrane Disease. Grune & Stratton, Orlando, FL, 1984
61. Rhodes PG, Graves GR, Patel DM, et al: Minimizing pneumothorax and bronchopulmonary dysplasia in ventilated infants with hyaline membrane disease. J Pediatr 103:634, 1983
62. Morley J: Replacement of pulmonary surfactant. p. 241. In Raivio KO, Hallman N, Kouvalainen K (eds): Respiratory Distress Syndrome. Academic Press, Orlando, FL, 1984
63. Notter RH, Shapiro, DL: Liver surfactant in an era of replacement therapy. Pediatrics 68:781, 1981
64. Mannino FL, Merritt TA: The management of respiratory distress syndrome. p. 427. In Thibeault DW, Gregory GA (eds): Neonatal Pulmonary Care, 2nd, Ed. Appleton-Century-Crofts, Norwalk, CT, 1986
65. Merritt TA, Hallman M, Holcomb K, et al: Human surfactant treatment of severe respiratory distress syndrome: pulmonary effluent indicators of lung inflammation. J Pediatr 108:741, 1986
66. Cilley RE, Zwischenberger JB, Andrews AF, et al: Intracranial hemorrhage during extracorporeal membrane oxygenation in neonates. Pediatrics 78:699, 1986
67. Bartlett RN, Roloff DW, Cornell RG, et al: Extracorporeal circulation in neonatal respiratory failure; a prospective randomized study. Pediatrics 76:479, 1985
68. Bell EF: Prevention of bronchopulmonary dysplasia: Vitamin E and other antioxidents. p. 77. In Report of the Nineteenth Ross Conference on Perinatal Research (March, 1986): Bronchopulmonary Dysplasia and Related Chronic Respiratory Disorders, Columbus, OH
69. Carlo WA, Pacificol L, Chatburn R, et al: Efficacy of computer-assisted management of respiratory failure in neonates. Pediatrics 78:139, 1986
70. Giacoia GP, Chopra R: The use of a computer in parenteral alimination of low birth weight infants. JPEN 5:328, 1981
71. Hermansen MC, Kahler R, Kahler B: Data entry errors in computerized nutritional calculations. J Pediatr 109:91, 1986
72. Ninan A, O'Donnell M, Hamilton K, et al: Physiologic changes induced by endotracheal instillation and suctioning in critically ill preterm infants with and without sedation. Am J Perinatol 3:94, 1986
73. Long JG, Philip AGS, Lucey JF: Excessive handling as cause of hypoxia. Pediatrics 65:203, 1980
74. Goodwin, SR, Graves SA, Haberkern CM: Aspiration in intubated premature infants. Pediatrics 75:85, 1985
75. Bhutani VK, Ritchie WG, Shaffer TH: Acquired tracheomegaly in very preterm infants. Am J Dis Child 140:449, 1986
76. MacDonald MG, Chou MM: Preventing complications from the tubes and lines. Semin Perinatol 10:224, 1986
77. Molteni RA, Bumstead DH: Development and severity of palatal grooves in orally intubated newborns. Am J Dis Child 140:357, 1986

78. Heller RM, Cotton RB: Early experience with illuminated endotracheal tubes in premature and term infants. Pediatrics 75:664, 1985
79. Moessinger AC, Driscoll JM, Wigger JH: High incidence of lung perforation by test tube in neonatal pneumothorax. J Pediat 92:635, 1978
80. Fletcher MA, Eichelberger MR: Thoracostomy tubes. p. 259. In Fletcher MA, MacDonald MG, Avery GB (eds): Atlas of Procedures in Neonatology. J.B. Lippincott, Philadelphia, 1983
81. Fletcher MA: Gastric and transpyloric tubes. p. 283. In Fletcher MA, MacDonald MG, Avery GB (eds): Atlas of Procedures in Neonatology. J.B. Lippincott, Philadelphia, 1983
82. Johnson DE, Foker J, Munson DP, et al: Management of esophageal and pharyngeal perforation in the newborn infant. Pediatrics 70:592, 1982
83. Wehbe MA, Moore JH Jr: Digital ischemia in the neonate following intravenous therapy. Pediatrics 76:99, 1985
84. Chidi CC, King DR, Boles JR: An ultrastructural study of intimal injury by an indwelling umbilical catheter. J Pediatr Surg 18:109, 1983
85. Boros SJ, Thompson TR, Reynolds JW, et al: Reduced thrombus formation with silicone elastomere (silastic) umbilical artery catheters. Pediatrics 56:981, 1975
86. Clawson CC, Boros SJ: Surface morphology of polyvinyl chloride and silicone elastomer umbilical artery catheters by scanning electron microscopy. Pediatrics 62:702, 1978
87. George L, Waldman JD, Cohen ML, et al: Umbilical vascular catheters: localization by two-dimensional echocardio/aortography. Pediatr Cardiol 2:237, 1982
88. Tyson JE, deSa DJ, Moore S: Thromboatheromatous complications of umbilical artery catheterization in the newborn period. Arch Dis Child 51:744, 1976
89. Batton DG, Maisles JM, Applebaum JM: Use of intravenous cannulas in premature infants: A controlled study. Pediatrics 70:487, 1982
90. Corso JA, Agostinalla R, Brandiss MW: Maintenance of polyethylene catheters to reduce risk of infection. JAMA 210:2075, 1969
91. Druskin MS, Siegal PD: Bacterial contamination of indwelling intravenous polyethylene catheters. JAMA 185:966, 1963
92. Upton J, Mulliken JB, Murray JE: Major intravenous extravasation injuries. Am J Surg 137:497, 1979
93. Chandavasu O, Garrow E, Valda V, Alsheikh S, et al: A new method for the prevention of skin sloughs and necrosis secondary to intravenous infiltration. Am J Perinatol 3:4, 1986
94. Hoar PF, Wilson RM, Mangano DT, et al: Heparin bonding reduces thrombogenicity of pulmonary-artery catheters. N Engl J Med 305:933, 1981
95. Kido DK, Pawlin S, Alenghat JA, et al: Thrombogenicity of heparin and non-heparin coated catheters. AJNR 3:535, 1981
96. Rajani K, Goetzman BW, Wennberg RP, et al: Effect of heparinization of fluids infused through an umbilical artery catheter on catheter patency and frequency of complications. Pediatrics 63:552, 1979
97. David RJ, Merten DF, Anderson JC, et al: Prevention of umbilical artery catheter clots with heparinized infusates. Dev Pharmacol Ther 2:117, 1981
98. O'Neill JA, Neblett WW III, Born ML: Management of major thromboembolic complications of umbilical artery catheters. J Pediatr Surg 16:972, 1981
99. Bosque E, Weaver L: Continuous versus intermittent heparin infusion of umbilical artery catheters in the newborn infant. J Pediatr 108:141, 1986
100. Koenigsberger MR, Moessinger AC: Iatrogenic carpal tunnel syndrome in the newborn infant. J Pediatrics 91:443, 1977
101. Kanter RK, Zimmerman JJ, Strauss RH, Stoeckel KA: Central venous catheter insertion by femoral vein: Safety and effectiveness for the pediatric patient. Pediatrics 77:842, 1986
102. Boeckman CR, Krill CE Jr: Bacterial and fungal infections complicating parenteral alimentation in infants and children. J Pediatr 85:117, 1970
103. Eichelberger MR, Rouse PG, Hoelzer DJ, et al: Percutaneous subclavian venous catheters in neonates and children. J Pediatr Surg 16:547, 1981
104. Simmons BP: Guidelines for prevention of intravascular infections. In intravascular infections: Intravenous Therapy Related. US Department of Health and Human Services, Public Health Service, Centers for Disease Control, Atlanta, 1981
105. Eichelberger MR, MacDonald MG, Warg J: General principles of central venous catheters. p. 173. In Fletcher MA, MacDonald MG, Avery GB (eds): Atlas of Procedures in Neonatology. J.B. Lippincott, Philadelphia, 1983
106. Heimanz J, Skelto J, Pizzo PA: Perspective on the management of catheter related infections in cancer patients. Pediatr Infect Dis 5:6, 1986

107. Prince A, Heller B, Levy J, et al: Management of fever in patients with central venous catheters. Pediatr Infect 5:20, 1985
108. Daniels SR, Hannon DW, Meyer RA, et al: Paroxysmal supraventricular tachycardia: A complication of jugular central venous catheters in neonates. Am J Dis Child 138:474, 1984
109. Effmann EL, Ablow RC, Touloukian RJ, et al: Radiographic aspects of total parenteral nutrition during infancy. Radiology 127:195, 1978
110. Kulkarni PB, Dorand RD, Simmonds EM Jr: Pericardial tamponade: complication of total parenteral nutrition. J Pediatr Surg 16:735, 1981
111. Gilhooly J, Lindenberg J, Reynolds JW: Central venous silicone elastomer catheter placement by basilar vein cutdown in neonates. Pediatrics 78:636, 1986
112. Durand M, Ramanathan R, Martinelli B, Tolentino M: Prospective evaluation of percutaneous central venous silastic catheters in newborn infants with birth weights of 510 to 3920 grams. Pediatrics 78:245, 1986
113. Scott JM: Iatrogenic lesions in babies following umbilical vein catheterizations. Arch Dis Child 40:426, 1965
114. Larroche JCL: Umbilical catheterization: Its complications. Biol Neonate 16:101, 1970
115. Brans YW, Ceballos R, Cassady G: Umbilical catheters and hepatic abscess. Pediatrics 53:264, 1974
116. Fraga JR, Javate BA, Venkatessan S: Liver abscess and sepsis due to *Klebsiella pneumoniae* in a newborn. A complication of umbilical vein catheterization. Clin Pediatr 13:1081, 1974
117. Williams JW, Rittenberry A, Dillard R, Allen RG: Liver abscess in newborns. Am J Dis Child 125:111, 1973
118. Schmidt B, Zipursky A: Thrombotic disease in newborn infants. Clin Perinatol 11:461, 1984
119. Wigger HJ, Bransilver BR, Blanc WA: Thrombosis due to catheterization in infants and children. J Pediatr 76:1, 1970
120. Wiedersberg H, Pawlowski P: Anemic necrosis of the liver after umbilical vein catheterization. Helv Paediatr Acta 345:53, 1979
121. Campbell RE: Roentgenologic features of umbilical vascular catheterization in the newborn. Am J Roentgenol 112:68, 1971
122. Krauss A, Albert R, Kannan M: Contamination of umbilical catheters in the newborn. J Pediatr 77:965, 1970
123. MacDonald MG: Umbilical vein catheterization. p. 149. In Fletcher MA, MacDonald MG, Avery GB (eds): Atlas of Procedures in Neonatology. J.B. Lippincott, Philadelphia, 1983
124. Plumer LB, Kaplan GW, Mendoza SA: Hypertension in infants—A complication of umbilical artery catheterization. J Pediatr 89:802, 1976
125. Merten DF, Vogel JM, Adelman RD, et al: Renovascular hypertension as a complication of umbilical artery catheters. J Pediatr Surg 16:972, 1981
126. Gupta JM, Robertson NRC, Wigglesworth JS: Umbilical artery catheterization in the newborn. Arch Dis Child 43:382, 1968
127. Krisnamoorthy KS, Fernandez RJ, Todres ID, et al: Paraplegia associated with umbilical artery catheterization in the newborn. Pediatrics 58:443, 1976
128. Henry CG, Gutierrez F, Lee JT, et al: Aortic thrombosis presenting as congestive heart failure: An umbilical artery catheter complication. Am J Roentgenol 116:475, 1972
129. McDonald MM, Hathaway WE: Neonatal hemorrhage and thrombosis. Semin Perinatol 7:213, 1983
130. Nachman RL, Thomas M, Patel D, et al: Thrombocytopenia as evidence of local thrombus: the umbilical arterial catheter. Pediatrics 50:825, 1972
131. Mehta P, Vasa R, Neumann L, et al: Thrombocytopenia in the high-risk infant. J Pediatr 97:791, 1980
132. Marsh JL, King W, Barrett C, Fonkalsrud EW: Serious complications after umbilical artery catheterization for neonatal monitoring. Arch Surg 110:1203, 1975
133. Dmochowski RR, Crandell SS, Carrier JN: Bladder injury and uroascites from umbilical artery catheterization. Pediatrics 77:421, 1986
134. Vordermark JS II, Buck AS, Dresner ML: Urinary ascites resulting from umbilical artery catheterization. J Urol 124:751, 1980
135. Malloy MH, Nichols MM: False abdominal aortic aneurysm: An usual complication of umbilical arterial catheterization for exchange transfusion. J Pediatr 90:285, 1977
136. Choi SJ, Raziuddin K, Haller JO: Broken umbilical catheter: A report of two cases. Am J Dis Child 131:595, 1977
137. Heath RE: Vasospasm in the neonate: Response to tolazoline infusion. Pediatrics 77:405, 1986
138. Ward RM: Pharmacology of tolazoline. Clin Perinatol 11:703, 1984

139. Ontell SJ, Gauderer MWL: Iatrogenic arteriovenous fistula after multiple arterial punctures. Pediatrics 76:97, 1985
140. Clarke TA, Reddy PG: Intravenous infusion technique in the newborn. Clin Pediatr 18:550, 1979
141. Butt, WW, Gow R, Whyte H, et al: Complications resulting from use of arterial catheters: Retrograde flow and rapid elevation of blood pressure. Pediatrics 76:250, 1985
142. Biglan AW, Brown DR, Macpherson TA: Update on retinopathy of prematurity. Semin Perinatol 10:187, 1986
143. Fletcher MA, Macpherson TA: Reducing complications of perinatal care. Semin Perinatol 10:163, 1986
144. Phelps DL: Vision loss due to retinopathy of prematurity. Lancet 1:606, 1981
145. Kalina RE, Karr DJ: Retrolental fibroplasia: Experience over two decades in one institution. Ophthalmology 89:91, 1982
146. Purohit DM, Ellison RC, Zierler S, et al: Risk factors for retrolental fibroplasia. Experience with 3025 premature infants. Pediatrics 76:339, 1985
147. The Committee for the Classification of Retinopathy of Prematurity: An international classification of retinopathy of prematurity. Arch Ophthalmol 102:1130, 1984
148. James LS, Lanman JT: History of oxygen therapy and retrolental fibroplasia. Pediatrics 57, suppl. 1:591–642, 1976
149. Brockhurst RJ, Chishti MI: Cicatricial retrolental fibroplasia: Its occurrence without oxygen administration in full term infants. Albrecht Von Graefes Arch Klin Exp Ophthalmol 195:113, 1975
150. Adamkin DH, Shott RJ, Cook LN, et al: Non-hyperoxic retrolental fibroplasia. Pediatrics 60:828, 1977
151. Kalina RE, Hodson WA, Morgan BC: Retrolental fibroplasia in a cyanotic infant. Pediatrics 50:765, 1972
152. Lucy JF, Dangman B: A reexamination of the role of oxygen in retrolental fibroplasia. Pediatrics 73:82, 1984
153. Glass P, Avery GB, Siva Subramanian KN, et al: Light and retinopathy of prematurity: What is prudent for 1986. N Engl J Med 313:401, 1985
154. Owens WC, Owens EU: Retrolental fibroplasia in premature infants: II studies on the prophylaxis of the disease. The use of alpha tocopheryl acetate. Am J Ophthalmol 32:1631, 1949
155. Phelps DL: Vitamin E and retinopathy of prematurity. p. 181. In Silverman WA, Flynn JT (eds): Retinopathy of prematurity. Blackwell Scientific, Boston, 1986
156. Finer NN, Peters, KL, Hayek Z, et al: Vitamin E and necrotizing enterocolitis. Pediatrics 73:387, 1984
157. Johnson L. Bowen FW, Abbasi S, et al: Relationship of prolonged pharmacological serum levels of Vitamin E to incidence of sepsis and necrotizing enterocolitis in infants with birth weight 1500 grams or less. Pediatrics 75:619, 1985
158. Zipursky A: Vitamin E deficiency anemia in newborn infants. Clin Perinatol 11:393, 1984
159. Centers for Disease Control: Unusual syndrome with fatalities among premature infants: association with a new intravenous Vitamin E product. MMWR 33:198, 1984
160. American Academy of Pediatrics, Committee on Fetus and Newborn: Vitamin E and prevention of retinopathy of prematurity. Pediatrics 76:315, 1985
161. Cassady J, Schiffman J, Flynn J, et al: Natural history of retinopathy of prematurity (ROP). Second NEI Symposium on Eye Disease Epidemiology. Washington, DC, 1985
162. Charles S: Vitreous surgery for retinopathy of prematurity (ROP) in Syllabus: Retinopathy of Prematurity Conference, Washington DC, 2:858, 1981
163. McPherson AR, Hittner H, Lemos R: Retinal detachment in young premature infants with acute retrolental fibroplasia. Thirty-two cases. Ophthalmology 89:1160, 1982
164. Machemer R: Closed vitrectomy for severe retrolental fibroplasia in the infant. Ophthalmology 90:436, 1983
165. Trese M: Surgical results of stage V retrolental fibroplasia and timing of surgical repair. Ophthalmology 91:461, 1984
166. Schaffer DB, Johnson L, Quinn G, et al: Vitamin E and retinopathy of prematurity. Ophthalmology 92:1005, 1985
167. Keith CG: Visual outcome and effect of treatment in Stage III developing retrolental fibroplasia. Br J Ophthalmol 66:446, 1982
168. Kushner BJ: Strabismus and amblyopia associated with regressed retinopathy of prematurity. Arch Ophthalmol 100:2456, 1982
169. Foster RS, Metz HS, Jampolsky A: Strabismus and pseudostrabismus with retrolental fibroplasia. Am J Ophthalmol 79:985, 1975
170. Gutcher G, Cutz E: Complications of parenteral nutrition. Semin Perinatol 10:196, 1986
171. Pathak A, Bernstein RM, Kassner EG: Complications of drugs, nutritional therapy, and im-

munization. p. 275. In Kassner EG (ed): Iatrogenic Disorders of the Fetus, Infant, and Child. Springer-Verlag, New York, 1985
172. American Academy of Pediatrics. Committee on Nutrition: Commentary on parenteral nutrition. Pediatrics 71:547, 1983
173. Pereira GR: Perinatal nutrition. Clin Perinatol 13:1, 1986
174. Cashore WJ, Stern L: The management of hyperbilirubinemia. Clin Perinatol 11:339, 1984
175. Keenan WJ, Novak KK, Sutherland JM, et al: Morbidity and mortality associated with exchange transfusion. Pediatrics 75, suppl.:417–421, 1985
176. Schiff D, Aranda JV, Chan G, et al: Metabolic effects of exchange transfusion. I. Effect of citrated and of heparinized blood on glucose, nonesterified fatty acids, 2-(4 hydroxybenzeneazo) acid binding and insulin. J Pediatr 78:603, 1971
177. Stern L: Hazards and dangers of exchange transfusion. Can Med Assoc J 100:1009, 1969
178. Podolsak B: Thrombopoiesis in newborn infants after exchange blood transfusion. Z Kinderheilkd 114:13, 1973
179. Castle V, Andrew M, Kelton J, et al: Frequency and mechanism of neonatal thrombocytopenia. J Pediatr 108:749, 1986
180. Heys RF: Steroid therapy for idiopathic thrombocytopenic purpura during pregnancy. Obstet Gynecol 28:532, 1966
181. Lang DJ, Valeri CR: Hazards of blood transfusion. Adv Pediatr 24:338, 1977
182. Demmler GJ, Brady MT, Bijou H, et al: Posttransfusion cytomegalovirus infection in neonates: Role of saline-washed red blood cells. J Pediatr 108:762, 1986
183. Yeager AS, Grumet FC, Hofleigh EB, et al: Prevention of transfusion-acquired cytomegalovirus infections in newborn infants. J Pediatr 98:281, 1981
184. Brady MT, Anderson DC, Milam JD, et al: Prevention of post-transfusion cytomegalovirus infection (PTCMV) in neonates by use of frozen-washed (FS-RBC) red blood cells. Pediatr Res 17:266A, 1983
185. Lang DL, Ebert PA, Rodgers BM, et al: Reduction of posttransfusion cytomegalovirus infections following the use of leukocyte-depleted blood. Transfusion 17:391, 1977
186. Krech U: Complement-fixing antibodies against cytomegalovirus in different parts of the world. Bull WHO 49:103, 1973
187. Naiman JL, Punnett HA, Lischner HW, et al: Possible graft-versus-host reaction after intrauterine transfusion for Rh erythroblastosis fetalis. N Engl J Med 281:697, 1969
188. Parkman R, Mosier D, Umanksy I, et al: Graft-versus-host disease after intrauterine and exchange transfusion for hemolytic disease of the newborn. N Engl J Med 290:359, 1974
189. Kim HC: Red blood cell transfusion in the neonate. Semin Perinatol 7:159, 1983
190. Stegagno M, Pascone R, Colarize P, Laurenti F, et al: Immunologic follow-up of infants treated with granulocyte transfusion for neonatal sepsis. Pediatrics 76:508, 1985
191. Blanchette VS, Zipursky A: Assessment of anemia in newborn infants. Clin Perinatol 11:489, 1984
192. Bell EF, Nahmias C, Sinclair JC, et al: The assessment of anemia in small premature infants. Pediatr Res 11:467, 1977
193. Aranda JV, Collinge JM, Clarkson S: Epidemiological aspects of drug utilization in a newborn intensive care unit. Semin Perinatol 6:148, 1982
194. Perlstein PH, Callison C, White M, et al: Errors in drug computations during newborn intensive care. Am J Dis Child 133:376, 1979
195. Koren G, Barzilay Z, Greenwald M: Tenfold errors in administration of drug doses: A neglected iatrogenic disease in pediatrics. Pediatrics 77:848, 1986
196. Macpherson TA: The role of the anatomical pathologist in perinatology. Semin Perinatol 9:257, 1985
197. Macpherson TA, Valdes-Dapena M, Kanbour A: Perinatal mortality and morbidity: The role of the anatomical pathologist. Semin Perinatol 10:179, 1986
198. Dudley HA: Audit and the pathologist. Proc R Soc Med 68:634, 1975
199. Gambino SR: The autopsy: The ultimate audit. Arch Pathol Lab Med 108:444, 1984
200. Fletcher MA: After discharge from the intensive care nursery: What then for the neonatologist. Semin Perinatol 10:234, 1986
201. Klebanoff MA, Rhoads GG: Collaborative epidemiologic research in perinatology. Semin Perinatol 10:169, 1986

Index

Page numbers followed by *f* denote figures; those followed by *t* denote tables.

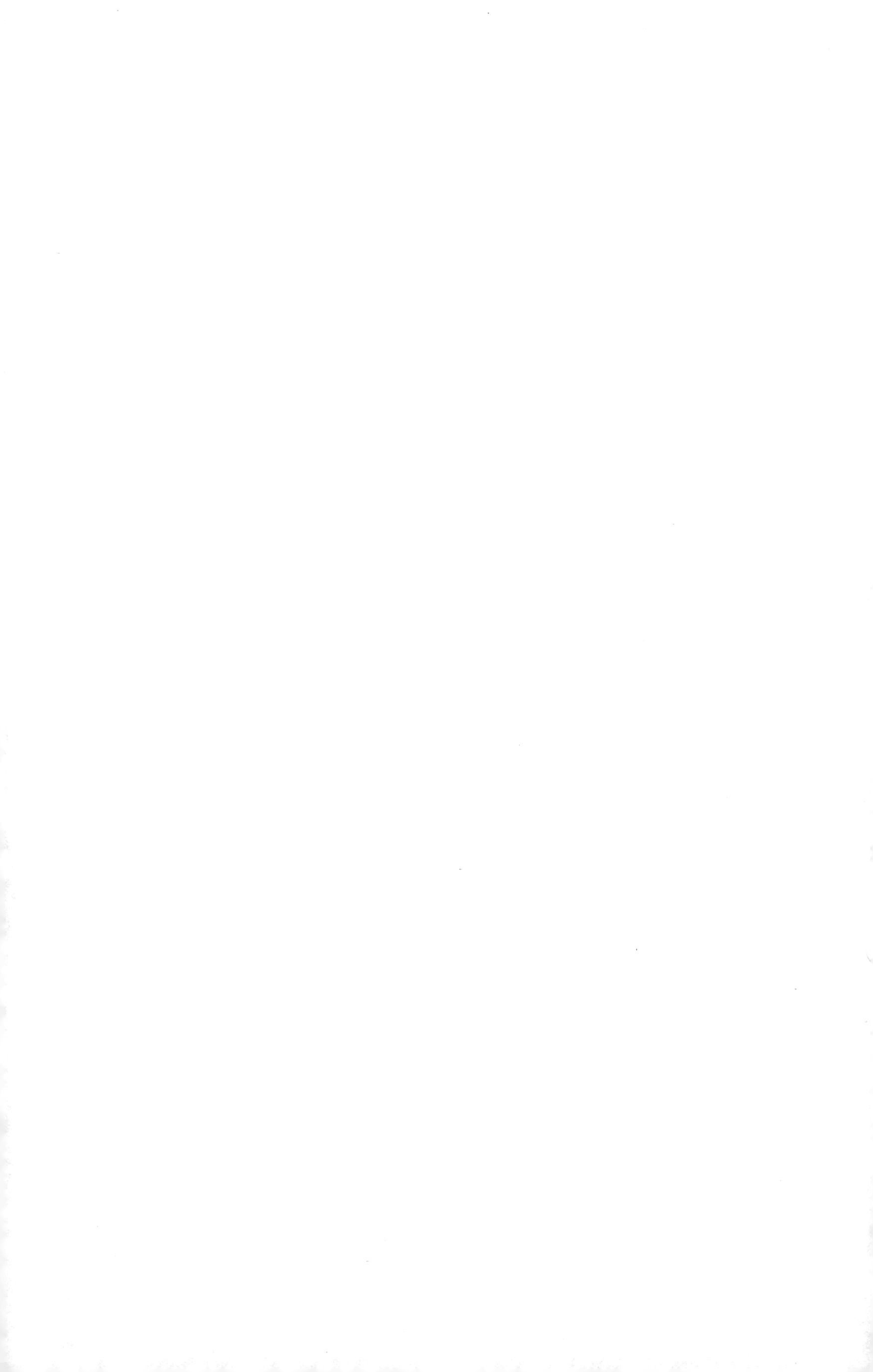